PEDIATRIC COLLECTIONS

Child Abuse: Overview and Evaluation

About AAP Pediatric Collections

Pediatric Collections is a series of selected pediatric articles that highlight different facets of information across various AAP publications, including AAP Journals, AAP News, Blog Articles, and eBooks. Each series of collections focuses on specific topics in the field of pediatrics so that you can keep up with best practices, and make an informed response to public health matters, trending news, and current events. Each collection includes previously published content focusing on specific topics and articles selected by AAP editors.

Visit http://collections.aap.org to view a list of upcoming collections.

TABLE OF CONTENTS

go.aap.org/connect

D1376782

TABLE OF CONTENTS

TABLE OF CONTENTS

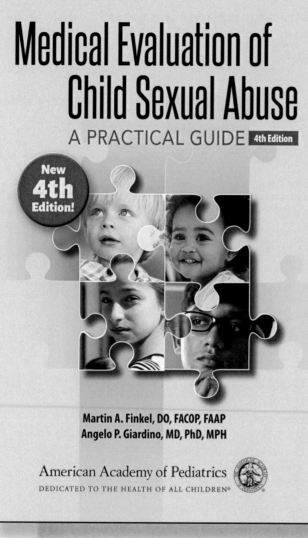
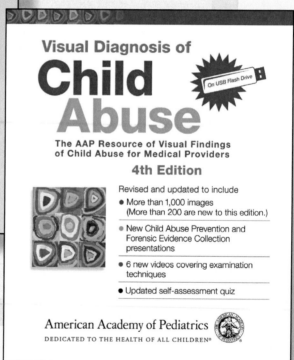
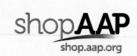

Foreword | Protect the Child

Over 40 years ago, I watched a rudimentary axial image of an infant's head slowly appear on the screen. The technology was state of the art, my medical school hospital proud to have installed a newly minted, first-generation computed tomography (CT) scanner. As the infant lay in the scanner tunnel, the pediatric neurosurgeon and the 3 of us shadowing second-year medical students discussed the history of the infant, how he was under the care of a babysitter when he slipped out of the babysitter's arms, falling headfirst onto the hardwood floor and immediately becoming limp and unresponsive. As the image of a pixelated, vague gray circular area encapsulated by white "crescent moons" emerged on the CT monitor screen, the neurosurgeon shook his head stating that the infant had bilateral subdural bleeds due to the fall, and the poor babysitter will probably feel guilty for what was obviously an accident. When asked how these bleeds occur, the neurosurgeon answered, "A simple fall over a short distance onto a hard surface can cause significant intracranial bleeding in an infant. Why it happens to some but not others is unknown." Later, the infant was found to have a broken right arm, also attributed to the fall. That was in 1978. Yet, while in 1946 Dr. John Caffey described infants with subdural bleeds and long bone fractures probably due to accidents, in 1972 Dr. Caffey, reconsidering what he had been observing over the years, introduced the concept of the shaken baby syndrome. Violent shaking of an infant could lead to subdural hemorrhages, retinal hemorrhages, and long bone fractures. The pattern of injuries in the infant I had encountered was not the result of a simple accidental fall.

During residency 3 years later, I was involved in the care of an infant who had bilateral subdural hemorrhages, bilateral retinal hemorrhages, metaphyseal fractures, and bruises on the face and trunk. The district attorney asked me to testify in court as to the cause of the infant's condition but also asked if I could have the attending physician testify. Now the attending physician, a national expert in his field of pediatrics, had a reputation for being gruff with residents, not wishing to be disturbed from his own academic pursuits. To ask him to testify begged retribution. I very timidly approached the attending physician and asked if he would testify. The attending gave me a very piercing stare, and I prepared myself for the expected rebuke. After a very long pause, the attending said, "Dr. Zenel, there is a point in one's career as a pediatrician you need to take a stand and protect the child." Needless to say, he testified. He also became a treasured mentor.

Since 1962, when Dr. Henry Kempe published his observations on the "Battered Child Syndrome," the definition of "child abuse and neglect" has expanded to include many forms of non-accidental trauma and neglect to the infant, child, and adolescent. There are physical abuse, sexual abuse, psychological abuse, and medical child abuse and neglect (formerly known as Munchausen by proxy). The 2 lessons I learned as a medical student and as a resident hold true today. While medicine advances in technology and knowledge, we need to stay up to date. More importantly, we need to protect the child.

Joseph A. Zenel, MD, FAAP
Editor-in-Chief, *Pediatrics in Review*

Introduction | When Child Abuse Enters the Medical Home

When child abuse or neglect concerns present to the provider and "enters the medical home," the initial responses might very well be a complex combination of fear, denial, and decision paralysis. Even the most experienced pediatrician might feel, "Never. Not this parent"; or maybe judge, "Of course, this family…"; or question, "What do I do now?" This small and important collection of American Academy of Pediatrics (AAP) publications and reports provides guidance and support to the medical home providers.

Be Aware. The scope of the problem of child maltreatment has essentially remained unchanged for the past decade. The National Child Abuse and Neglect Data System, a voluntary data collection system that gathers information from all 50 states, the District of Columbia, and Puerto Rico about reports of child abuse and neglect, examines trends in child abuse and neglect across the country. While sexual abuse reports have declined, reports for other forms of maltreatment have not consistently declined across our country. Our attention to child maltreatment is now framed in a broader view with a solid evidence base on identification and growing knowledge as pediatricians on the effects of child abuse on health and development. Adverse childhood experiences, toxic stress in all forms, but especially interpersonal violence, can alter brain structure, physiology, and over-functioning of the child or teen victim. Awareness that the problem exists and how to address the concern is now more than ever a call to action for the pediatrician. Keeping the diagnosis of child maltreatment on the differential for both physical examination findings and for behavioral changes is the starting point for correct identification and action.

Be Prepared. Our role in identification, evaluation, and treatment for children with a diagnosis of suspected or confirmed child maltreatment can be guided—as with any diagnosis or condition—by evidenced-based guidelines. Listed here are important AAP references that are practical and essential guides when evaluating and treating sentinel injuries, physical abuse, and sexual abuse. The more complex the clinical scenario or patient, the greater the risk for the child is balanced with the need to be thorough in approach, hence the additional resources listed under high-risk populations. Practical things take an impractical amount of time and effort when child maltreatment is a concern. Consultation with other subspecialties, including child abuse pediatricians who can be found by region via the AAP Council on Child Abuse & Neglect website, should be considered depending on the physical or behavior presentations.

Stay Connected. Once a report is made to child protective services, the inherent reaction or next step may be to let the system do its job and to disconnect from the process. A key part of the ongoing evaluation of and then help for the child and family is the connected partnership of the pediatrician and child welfare system. Beyond the mandated report, we play a role in educating caseworkers about everything pediatric so they are best informed about injury, behavior, disease or condition, and of course, child development. Advocating for the parent to establish a safer and more effective parenting style is in our medical home toolbox. Establishing trusted relationships with community partners in child welfare, behavioral health, and home visitation programs is crucial in the ongoing care of these children and families.

Finally, just as we are champions for safety in injury prevention (car seats, helmets, and socket plugs), infection control (immunizations and handwashing), and child development (preschool for all kids, in-office screenings, child find services), we are all inherent child maltreatment prevention champions. As we promote positive parenting in all our early childhood interactions, we have safe and healthy children as our north star. With that in mind and heart, we can be prepared to respond when child abuse enters the medical home and a child needs our advocacy and help.

Andrew Sirotnak MD, FAAP
Editorial Board, *Pediatrics in Review*
Cochair, AAP Council on Child Abuse & Neglect
Director, Child Protection Team & Children's Hospital Colorado & The Kempe Center

Physical Abuse of Children

Jill C. Glick, MD,* Michele A. Lorand, MD,† Kristen R. Bilka, MMS, PA-C‡

*Department of Pediatrics, University of Chicago; Medical Director, Child Advocacy and Protective Services, University of Chicago Comer Children's Hospital, Chicago, IL.

†Division of Child Protective Services, Department of Pediatrics; Medical Director, Chicago Children's Advocacy Center, John H. Stroger, Jr. Hospital of Cook County, Chicago, IL.

‡Department of Pediatrics, University of Chicago; Physician Assistant, Child Advocacy and Protective Services, University of Chicago Comer Children's Hospital, Chicago, IL.

EDITOR'S NOTE

This article stresses the importance of the "sentinel injury," a physical injury that is unusual for the age of the child and may herald more serious injuries, thereby necessitating further evaluation.

Joseph A. Zenel, MD
Editor-in-Chief

Practice Gap

Before receiving a diagnosis of child abuse, 25% to 30% of abused infants have "sentinel" injuries, such as facial bruising, noted by clinicians or caregivers. (1)(2)(3)(4)(5)(6) Although easily overlooked and often considered minor, such injuries are harbingers warning clinicians that pediatric patients require further assessment. Appropriate intervention is critical, and the clinician plays a major role in identifying children who present with signs or symptoms concerning for child physical abuse by ensuring appropriate and expeditious medical evaluations and reports to child protective services.

Objectives   After completing this article, the reader should be able to:

1. Identify which injured children require a child abuse evaluation.

2. Recognize subtle signs and nonspecific symptoms of major trauma in infants.

3. Understand sentinel injuries and their significance.

4. Know which laboratory and imaging studies to obtain when child physical abuse is suspected.

5. Understand the legal obligation to report children with injuries that are suspicious for physical abuse and develop a thoughtful approach to informing parents of this legal obligation.

CASE PRESENTATION

A private practice pediatrician receives a phone call from a community emergency department (ED) physician regarding one of her patients, a 4-month-old infant being treated for bronchiolitis. The ED physician informs her that the baby's chest

AUTHOR DISCLOSURE Drs Glick and Lorand and Ms Bilka have disclosed no financial relationships relevant to this article. This commentary does not contain a discussion of an unapproved/investigative use of a commercial product/device.

radiograph has revealed multiple posterior rib fractures in different stages of healing, and physical examination shows a cluster of small bruises on her cheek. The mother denies a history of trauma and has no explanation for the findings. The ED physician is concerned that the baby has been abused and his plan includes admitting the patient to the hospital to obtain a head computed tomography (CT) scan, skeletal survey, complete blood cell count, coagulation studies, electrolytes, and liver function tests. He also plans to consult with the child abuse pediatrician and arrange for an evaluation of the patient's siblings. Lastly, he tells the primary pediatrician that he will explain the clinical findings to the family and file a report with the child welfare system. The primary pediatrician thanks him for contacting her and, recalling no significant medical history, pulls the patient's chart.

The baby's most recent visit was slightly more than 1 week ago for her routine 4-month health supervision visit. She is a term infant who has no prior medical complaints other than colic at 1 month of age that has resolved. On recent physical examination, the baby appeared well, with normal growth and development, and the mother did not raise any concerns during the visit. The primary pediatrician now notes that she documented a small circular bruise on the baby's chest that the mother stated occurred when a 3-year-old sibling hit the baby with a toy. Having had a longstanding relationship with this mother and family, she accepted this explanation for the bruise.

After reviewing the chart, she explores the current literature and management of suspected child physical abuse, including the American Academy of Pediatrics clinical report on evaluation of suspected child physical abuse. (7) She now understands that the bruise she noted on examination was a sentinel injury that should have prompted further evaluation. As a result of the case, her practice group plans to review and implement guidelines for the identification and evaluation of children presenting with signs or symptoms concerning for physical abuse.

INTRODUCTION

Child physical abuse is a difficult diagnosis to entertain primarily because clinicians are hesitant to accept that caretakers can injure children. The diagnosis is further complicated by the reality that caretakers rarely disclose maltreatment, preverbal or obtunded children cannot provide a history, and signs and symptoms of physical abuse may be subtle and confused with other common pediatric diagnoses.

Clinicians must appreciate that with few exceptions, almost any injury can be either abusive or accidental.

Once considered a strictly social problem, child abuse is now also recognized as a medical problem. A recent survey by the Children's Hospital Association revealed that more than 90% of responding hospitals have child protection teams, and more than 50% have at least 1 of the 324 board-certified child abuse pediatricians in the United States on staff. (8)

Recognition of the profound impact of childhood experiences on adult health and well-being, beginning with Feleitti's landmark adverse childhood experiences study, further solidifies the need for clinicians to recognize possible maltreatment and intervene. (9) Adverse childhood experiences have wide-ranging, cumulative, and direct impacts on adult health, increasing the incidence of chronic diseases and early death. (9)(10) The role of the clinician is therefore not only limited to promoting wellness but also to decreasing or eliminating long-term health consequences resulting from childhood exposure to trauma and violence.

EPIDEMIOLOGY

In 2014, over 3.5 million children were subjects of child maltreatment reports. Of those, 702,000 children (20%) were found to have evidence of maltreatment. (11) This translates to an annual victimization rate of 9.4 children per 1,000 in the United States and a prevalence rate of 1 in 8 children by age 18 years. (12) Neglect is the most common form of child maltreatment, constituting 75% of indicated reports; 17% are attributable to physical abuse. In 80% of child physical abuse cases, a biological parent is the perpetrator. Children in their first postnatal year have the highest victimization rate (24.4 per 1,000), and children younger than age 3 years have the highest fatality rate, comprising over 70% of the nationally estimated 1,580 child maltreatment deaths in 2014. Child welfare data and trends, however, are dubious because of a lack of standardized terminology and differences in report and response types across states.

RISK FACTORS FOR CHILD PHYSICAL ABUSE

Risk factors for abuse are commonly categorized into parental, child, and social characteristics. Identification of risk factors aids in the assessment of abuse but more importantly aids in the ability to counsel parents and develop preventive strategies. Risk factors are not, in and of themselves, diagnostic. Many families have risk factors and never abuse their children, while others have no apparent risk factors and do abuse their children. Child abuse does not discriminate; it affects children of all ages, socioeconomic classes, and ethnic groups.

Parental/household risk factors include substance abuse, mental illness, interpersonal violence (IPV), single and/or teen parent, and a nonrelated adult in the home. Among the social risk factors are social isolation, poverty, lower levels of education, and large family size. Child-related risk factors include prematurity, low birthweight, intrauterine drug exposure, and developmental and physical disabilities. The most significant risk factor for abuse is the age of the child, with infants and toddlers being at greatest risk for serious and fatal child physical abuse.

A clear association exists between particular developmental stages and physically abusive injuries, such as excessive crying and abusive head trauma or toilet training and inflicted scald burns. Awareness of these developmental triggers should guide anticipatory guidance, with the potential for preventing an abusive injury.

IPV is a substantial risk factor for child abuse, and each health supervision visit should include IPV screening. Exposure to violence itself, even if the child is not physically harmed, has significant and long-lasting effects.

WHEN TO CONSIDER THE DIAGNOSIS OF CHILD PHYSICAL ABUSE

Injuries are common in childhood. Although most childhood injuries are accidental, the clinician must appreciate that almost any injury can be abusive. With the exception of patterned marks, very few injuries are pathognomonic for abuse. In the nonverbal child, injuries may be apparent or covert; many children present with nonspecific symptoms and a lack of history. Child physical abuse should be entertained in any infant displaying signs or symptoms potentially explained by trauma, such as irritability, lethargy, vomiting, apnea, seizures, or coma.

Several studies of abused children have demonstrated that antecedent sentinel injuries, such as bruises, intraoral lesions, and skeletal trauma, were noted by medical professionals or caregivers before a subsequent abusive act, while children presenting with accidental injuries were not found to have sentinel injuries. (1)(2)(3)(4)(5)(6) Because infants are essentially nonmobile and nonweight-bearing, they should never have bruising. Therefore, any injury in an infant must be viewed as significant and descriptive language such as "minor" should not be used. Identifying a sentinel injury with appropriate evaluation of the child may be lifesaving.

As children become mobile, the incidence of expected accidental trauma increases, and common childhood injuries such as bruises over bony prominences and toddler's, clavicular, and skull fractures are seen. In contrast to children with abusive injury, witnesses often corroborate accidental injuries in ambulatory children, caregivers seek timely care, they provide a consistent history, and the mechanism described explains the injury observed. Because the incidence of child physical abuse is highest in children younger than age 4 years, the clinician must have a high index of suspicion and add abusive trauma to the differential diagnosis of the ill-appearing young child.

Determining which injured children require an evaluation for child physical abuse should account for the age and developmental ability of the child, the injury sustained, the adequacy of the historical explanation provided, and

TABLE 1. Criteria for Consideration to Initiate a Child Physical Abuse Assessment

Age and Development

- Nonmobile infant with *any* injury
- Injury in nonverbal child
- Injury inconsistent with child's ability
- Statement of harm from a verbal child

Injury

- Any injury in a nonmobile infant
- Uncommon in age group
- Occult finding
- Mechanism not plausible
- Multiple injuries, including involvement of multiple organs
- Injuries of differing ages
- Pattern of increasing frequency or severity of injury over time
- Patterned cutaneous lesions
- Bruises to torso, ear, or neck in child younger than age 4 years
- Burns to genitalia, stocking or glove distribution, branding, or pattern

History

- Chief complaint does not contain caregiver concern for an injury *and* plausible history
- Caretaker response not commensurate to injury
- Unexplained delay in seeking care
- Lack of, inconsistent, or changing history
- Inconsistencies or discrepancies in histories provided by involved caretakers

clinical findings (Table 1). Fundamentally, when injuries are not explained or historical data provided contain inconsistencies or insufficiencies, a child abuse evaluation is warranted. Any child younger than age 2 years who presents with a suspicious injury should have a skeletal survey. Other studies should be obtained based upon clinical concern and findings. Negative studies do not rule out child abuse.

HISTORY OF THE PRESENT ILLNESS AND CHILD PHYSICAL ABUSE

A thorough history of present illness is the single most useful piece of information to aid the clinician in making a correct diagnosis. The detailed history should be obtained in separate interviews with each caregiver, the child (if possible), verbal siblings, and any other persons in the household. Interviews should be conducted such that each parent or caregiver can give a history in his or her own words. He or she should be allowed to provide the entire history without interruption, decreasing the chance that the interviewer unintentionally redirects or suggests a mechanism. Details about the mechanism of injury, the events leading up to the injury, and whether the injury was witnessed or unwitnessed should be elicited. For example, in injuries related to falls, having parents recreate the scene, describing the height of furniture, flooring, and the position of the child before and after the fall, is essential.

A history of the onset and progression of symptoms since the child last appeared well should be obtained. Determining who was caring for the child and asking each of the caretakers how the child appeared by focusing on descriptions of activity and movement (particularly during feeding, bathing, and diaper changing) can aid in determining when a child may have been injured. For infants with intracranial injury, it may be difficult to develop a timeline of when the child was last well because the infant may be thought of as "well-appearing" while asleep when the child actually may be seriously injured. Important features of the history that should raise concern for an abusive injury include: no history of trauma; a history of trauma inconsistent with the severity, pattern, or timing of the injury; injury inconsistent with the developmental capabilities of the child; multiple or evolving histories; discrepant histories from the same caregiver or between caregivers; injury attributed to a sibling or pet; and a delay in seeking medical care.

In addition to a detailed history of the incident, the patient's birth, past medical, developmental, and dietary histories should be obtained. A complete social history identifies risk factors for maltreatment, and a family medical history focusing on illnesses such as bone disease or bleeding tendencies allows for screening and identification of possible underlying medical problems in the patient.

PHYSICAL EXAMINATION AND DIAGNOSTIC EVALUATION

A thorough and well-documented physical examination of any child with concerns for possible child abuse is imperative. The clinician should be aware that children may suffer more than one type of abuse; the physically abused child may also be neglected or sexually abused. The child's mental status, affect, and level of activity should be noted. The child must be undressed and all skin surfaces examined with good lighting. The entire body must be evaluated, including areas that may be overlooked, such as the pinnae, behind the ears, the oral cavity including the teeth and frenula, the soles and palms, the genitals, and the anus. Every cutaneous injury should be described according to color, shape, size, and location. Photographic documentation or drawings should be completed and placed in the medical record. The presence or absence of swelling and the ability to move limbs should be noted. Paradoxical comfort (a baby who is more comfortable when not being held but cries when picked up) may be observed in infants with occult injuries such as rib fractures. An assessment of the child's nutritional status, including completion of a growth chart, is crucial because neglect, malnutrition, and failure to thrive may be comorbidities with physical abuse.

The diagnostic evaluation of suspected physical abuse should always be driven by the history, physical examination, and differential diagnosis. Clinicians must consider the possibility that multiple types of trauma may coexist and recognize that injuries may be occult. Any nonverbal and nonambulatory child with an injury should have a standard child abuse evaluation (Table 2) no matter how "minor" the injury. The most prudent approach is to rule out skeletal trauma in all children younger than 2 years of age with a standard skeletal survey and assess for occult central and/or internal injuries by choosing appropriate imaging and laboratory studies (Table 3).

ABUSIVE HEAD TRAUMA

Abusive head trauma (AHT) has the highest mortality of all forms of child physical abuse, with an estimated fatality rate greater than 20%. Survivors have irreversible sequelae of brain injury, ranging from minor behavioral

TABLE 2. Protocol for the Evaluation of Suspected Child Physical Abuse

History of Present Illness

- Interview primary caretakers separately; note historian's ability to provide history

- Ask caretakers about age-appropriate developmental abilities of child. Observe child if possible

- Develop a timeline from when the child was last agreed upon to be in his or her usual state of good health and note the following:

  o Onset of symptoms and progression

  o The patient's observed mental status and activity level. Ask specifically about how the child appeared at time of hand off between caretakers

- Note if there were any witnesses, photos taken of child, or other corroborating information

Social History

- List all adults having access to the child, including age, relationship, and contact information

- List all children, including age and relationship; identify in which home they reside

- Note history of drug or alcohol abuse, intimate partner violence, mental illness, prior history of involvement with child protective services

Relevant Past Medical History

- Skeletal trauma: child or family history of bone disease, diet history

- Abusive head trauma (AHT) and cutaneous injuries: child or family history of bleeding diathesis, eg, prolonged bleeding after circumcision, umbilical cord removal, or surgery or as a result of past injuries

Physical Examination

- Examine closely for possible intraoral injuries such as frenulum tears; explore all unexposed surfaces: behind ears, genital region, and bottoms of feet

- Growth chart: obtain prior growth data, and with regard to AHT, note trajectory of head circumferences

Photodocumentation

- If photos are obtained, document in the medical record details of the photos taken, including location of injuries, number of photos taken, date, and photographer

- If photodocumentation is unavailable, use a body diagram noting all cutaneous lesions by size, location, and color

Evaluation

- Indicated laboratory and imaging studies for current illness or injury

- Studies to assess occult injuries, such as skeletal survey

- Communication with appropriate subspecialists regarding findings and treatment, including child abuse pediatricians when appropriate for referral and consultation

Mandated Reporting and Safety

- Develop dialogue to inform parents about mandated reporting, safety, and reason for report

- Ensure that forms and phone numbers for reporting are accessible

- Establish office process for specific scenarios with regard to obtaining imaging and laboratory studies and process for transfer to appropriate facility for evaluation and treatment, including protocol for accessing expertise of child abuse pediatrician

- Facilitate thorough sibling assessment, including appropriate imaging, laboratory studies, and interpretation; establish protocol to ensure results of sibling assessments are communicated to others in the investigation, including primary care clinician

- Ensure medical record and photodocumentation accessibility for investigators (consent not required after report to child welfare)

- Discuss disposition of, medical follow-up, and supportive services for patient with child welfare case worker

---

issues and neurodevelopmental delays to significant neurodevelopmental delays, seizures, blindness, and paralysis. (13) The incidence of AHT is 15 to 30 cases per 100,000 infants annually in the United States. AHT occurs most often in children younger than age 2 years and crying is the most commonly identified trigger. Recognizing that the phrase "shaken baby syndrome" implies a specific mechanism, in 2009 the American

Academy of Pediatrics (AAP) recommended that AHT replace this terminology to acknowledge that multiple mechanisms, either separately or together, can cause calvarial, brain, and cervical injuries. (14)

Infants and young children who have AHT can present with signs and symptoms ranging from mild to life-threatening, with a clinical spectrum that includes irritability, vomiting, lethargy, seizures, apnea, coma, and death. Often there are no external findings suggestive of trauma and the history is lacking or misleading. Thus, depending on the extent and severity of the injuries, traumatic brain injury is often misdiagnosed as colic, viral syndrome, otitis media, gastroenteritis, gastroesophageal reflux, or pyloric stenosis. Clinicians must keep AHT in their differential diagnoses and have a high index of suspicion to obtain a thorough history and perform the appropriate diagnostic tests.

Brain injuries seen in 80% of AHT cases include subdural hemorrhage that is interhemispheric, posterior, often layering over the tentorium, and/or a thin subdural layer over either or both of the convexities. Mass effect results not from the subdural trauma itself but rather from significant cerebral edema. The parenchymal damage evolves into a clinical picture consistent with hypoxic-ischemic encephalopathy. Although additional injuries need not be present to diagnose AHT, these neurologic injuries are frequently associated with other traumatic findings, such as retinal hemorrhages, posterior rib fractures, and classic metaphyseal lesions (CMLs). Bruising to the scalp or other parts of the body may or may not be present. The clinician must be mindful to ensure a thorough evaluation for other occult injuries, including neck, internal, and other skeletal trauma.

A short fall leading to fatal head trauma is exceptionally rare, with a calculated risk of less than 1 per 1,000,000 children annually. (15) A unique situation is the development of an epidural hematoma after minor blunt trauma in which a temporal linear skull fracture may sever the middle meningeal vessels and lead to an accumulation of blood that results in mass effect. This is one circumstance in which a child may be neurologically intact after minor or trivial trauma but experience deteriorating mental status and acute symptoms as a result of mass effect.

Head and neck imaging must be obtained for any child for whom there are concerns for AHT. A CT scan is the initial imaging modality of choice because it can be performed quickly in the critically ill child. However, CT scan does not reveal parenchymal injuries, cannot reliably differentiate between subdural and subarachnoid collections, and involves substantial radiation exposure. Magnetic resonance imaging (MRI) should be performed once the patient is stable, ideally a few days after admission, to optimize visualization of the parenchyma and evaluate for edema, stroke, and thromboses. MRI can also elucidate the location of extra-axial fluid collections and aid in the aging of intracranial hemorrhages. MRI imaging of the spine is also indicated because studies have now demonstrated injury to the cervical spine, such as ligamentous injury and spinal subdural hemorrhage, in children with AHT. (16)(17) MRI is also preferred over CT scan when clinical findings such as rapidly increasing head circumference or focal neurologic issues suggest remote injury. MRI does not entail radiation exposure, but it is a longer study that most often requires sedation.

Retinal injuries such as hemorrhages, schisis or tearing, and folds are associated with AHT and may be seen in up to 80% of cases. Hemorrhagic retinopathy from AHT is classically described as multilayered, with hemorrhages that are too numerous to count and extend to the ora serrata. This very specific finding is unique to AHT and is not due to increased intracranial pressure, blunt head trauma, or cardiopulmonary resuscitation. Retinoschisis and macular folds are reported almost exclusively in children who have sustained violent craniorotational injury and are specific to this mechanism. Any infant or child who has intracranial injuries suspicious for abuse should be evaluated by an ophthalmologist who can meticulously and precisely document the ocular findings, preferably with use of photo imaging. The rate of healing varies from days to weeks and aging of retinal hemorrhages is imprecise. Of note, an ophthalmologic examination is not a screening tool for AHT but is indicated when there is evidence of intracranial injury.

CUTANEOUS INJURIES

The skin is the most frequently injured organ in child abuse, with bruises, bites, and burns accounting for many child maltreatment injuries. Although cutaneous injuries are very common in childhood, they are rare in the preambulatory child: "those who don't cruise don't bruise." (18)(19) Considerable data support that bruising is not only extremely uncommon in infants but highly correlated with child abuse. (20)(21) Thirty percent or more of seriously injured or fatally abused children have been noted to have bruises, which are sentinel signs (Figure 1), reported on physical examination before subsequent severe or fatal abuse. These data support the directive that any nonmobile infant who has a bruise must receive a full child abuse evaluation (Table 2) and a report to child welfare for investigation. (3)(4)(5)(6)

TABLE 3. Child Physical Abuse Medical Evaluation: Imaging and Laboratory Studies

STANDARD CHILD PHYSICAL ABUSE MEDICAL EVALUATIONS

Skeletal Injuries

- Skeletal survey (with views according to the collaborative practice parameter issued by the American College of Radiology and the Society for Pediatric Radiology)
- Follow-up skeletal survey is indicated in 2 weeks when abuse is suspected on clinical grounds and/or initial findings are abnormal or equivocal
- Core laboratory studies for bone health: calcium, magnesium, phosphate, and alkaline phosphatase
- If concerns for vitamin D deficiency (elevated alkaline phosphate, abnormal bone density, or dietary concerns), consider 25-hydroxyvitamin D and parathyroid hormone level

Central Imaging

- Head computed tomography (CT) scan (useful for screening, and/or monitoring an ill child)
- Magnetic resonance imaging (MRI) of head and spine (useful for elucidating extra-axial spaces, parenchymal disease, and spinal injury)

Routine Trauma Laboratory Tests

- Hematologic: complete blood cell count and platelets
- Coagulation: international normalized ratio, prothrombin time, and activated partial thromboplastin time
- Metabolic: glucose, blood urea nitrogen, creatinine, calcium, magnesium, phosphate, albumin, and protein
- Urinalysis: urine toxicology screen, order myoglobin if urinalysis positive for blood and red cells are not seen on smear
- Liver function tests: aspartate aminotransferase and alanine aminotransferase (>80 U/L [1.34 μkat/L] is concerning for occult injury)
- Pancreatic enzymes: amylase and lipase

ADDITIONAL POTENTIAL TESTS

Ophthalmologic Examination

- Indicated if evidence of either acute or remote central nervous system trauma
- Not a screening tool for abusive head trauma

Abdominal (Thoracoabdominal) Imaging: CT Scan With Intravenous Contrast

- Elevated liver or pancreatic enzyme values
- Comatose patient
- Evidence of trauma with delay in care (liver function tests may have decreased to normal levels)

Concerns for Bleeding Diathesis (Family History or Clinical Concerns)

- von Willebrand antigen, von Willebrand activity (ristocetin co-factor), Factor VIII, Factor IX, platelet function assay
- Hematology consultation

Metabolic Diseases

- Genetics consultation

As children start to ambulate, the incidence of bruising increases. Bruise location and morphology are important factors to consider when assessing for child physical abuse in ambulatory children. Accidental injuries tend to occur over bony prominences (shins and elbows) in contrast to bruises due to abuse, which are located on the face, head, neck, torso, flanks, buttocks, and thighs. The mnemonic "TEN 4" is useful to recall which bruise locations are concerning for abuse: Torso, Ear, Neck, and 4 signifying children younger than age 4 years and any bruising noted in infants younger than 4 months. (20) Bruising and abrasions that occur on more than one body surface, are in multiple stages of healing, and are patterned or well demarcated are more likely to be the result of abuse. Patterned injuries reflect the shape of the instrument, such as loop marks from a cord or cable, linear bruises from belts, or multiple parallel linear bruises equally distributed from a slap with a hand. Contrary to some common beliefs, children do not bruise more easily than adults and bruises cannot be aged precisely. The appearance of a bruise is related to many factors, including the state of hemoglobin degradation, the color of skin pigment, the depth of the bruise, the location on the body, the lighting in the room, and the patient's metabolism and circulation. Bruises of differing colors do not signify different times or incidents. Finally, because bruises or soft-tissue injury may be painful for days, the presence of tenderness does not necessarily mean the injury is acute.

Determining whether marks or bruising from corporal punishment constitutes abuse is a difficult task. Legally, some states condone corporal punishment as an acceptable form of behavioral modification while others define it as a form of child maltreatment and require reporting to child welfare. The AAP and the American Academy of Child and Adolescent Psychiatry do not condone corporal punishment due to its limited effectiveness and potential deleterious effects. Although known to be immediately effective, spanking and corporal punishments have significant adverse outcomes, such as increased aggression and decreased development of appropriate behavior. (22)(23)(24) Both groups advise against the use of corporal punishment and encourage alternative methods of behavioral modification – such as time out, loss of privileges, positive reinforcement, and opportunities for positive touch like hand holding and hugging – that have healthier, long-lasting effects. From a practical standpoint, each clinician must be versed in his or her state laws. More importantly, the clinician must develop a thoughtful and culturally sensitive

dialogue with parents that promotes alternative methods of discipline.

Bite marks are another patterned skin injury noted in abused children. Clinicians can discern between animal and human bites by assessing the shape: animal bite marks are puncture wounds with a sharply angulated arch, while human bite marks are crush injuries consisting of an ovoid pattern of tooth marks that may surround an area of central bruising. In general, adult bite marks measure greater than 2 cm between the maxillary canines. Consultation with a forensic odontologist may assist in the evaluation of well-demarcated bite marks. Multiple bites on different body planes, bites on soft-tissue areas, and bites on areas generally covered by clothing should raise a suspicion of abuse. Bites to the genitalia, buttocks, and/or breasts should raise a concern of possible sexual abuse. Acute bites to the genitalia, buttocks, and/or breasts may warrant collection of forensic evidence for DNA by swabbing the area with a cotton swab moistened with distilled water.

Hot liquid, grease, steam, hot objects, chemicals, electricity, or microwave ovens may cause abusive burns. Compared to accidental burns, abusive burns are more severe, more likely to be full-thickness, and require more extensive treatment, including grafting. Children who are abusively burned are most often younger than 4 years and inflicted immersion burns to the buttocks and genitalia are commonly associated with toilet training.

Abusive burns most often take the form of immersion scald burns, characterized by well-demarcated areas of confluent depth with no splash or cascading flow pattern. Immersion burns may involve the buttocks, perineum, extremities, hands, or feet. Circumferential burns affecting the feet and/or hands are sometimes referred to as having a "stocking" or "glove" distribution. In immersion burns, the position in which the child was held may be surmised by the burn pattern and depth. If the child's buttocks come into contact with the tub surface, a "doughnut" type pattern may be noted with relative sparing of the part of the anatomy coming into contact with the tub. Sparing of the flexion creases is often observed. Persons who inflict these burns generally do not suffer burns themselves. A careful scene reconstruction and investigation, including water temperature, may help determine the length of time the child was held in the water. Generally, the hotter the water, the shorter the duration of submersion. Partial-thickness burns develop in minutes at 48.9°C (120°F) but take mere seconds at 65.6°C (150°F). (25)

Children often come into contact with hot objects, such as irons, hair tools, radiators, and stovetops. Resultant burns are related to the heat of the object and period of contact with

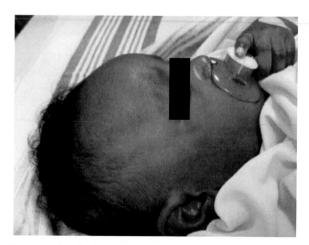

Figure 1. Infant displaying bruising that represents a sentinel sign for physical abuse.

the skin. Both abusive and accidental contact burns can result in a patterned mark, making discernment based on appearance difficult. Suspicious contact burns require a thorough scene investigation and corroboration, particularly if the child is nonverbal. In general, abusive contact burns are deeper and leave a clear imprint while those that result from grazing against a hot object are not as deep or well-demarcated.

The most common differential diagnosis of inflicted cutaneous injury is accidental injury. Dermatologic and other conditions such as congenital dermal melanocytosis (mongolian spots), phytophotodermatitis, Henoch-Schönlein purpura, Ehlers-Danlos syndrome, vasculitis syndromes, bleeding dyscrasias, eczema, malignancy, and cultural practices such as cupping and coining (cao gio or gua sha) may lead to cutaneous lesions that appear initially concerning for abuse. Some conditions that may be confused with or mimic burns are impetigo, staphylococcal scalded skin syndrome, herpes, and contact dermatitis. A careful history, physical examination, and diagnostic tests should clarify whether an accident or one of these conditions is the cause of the findings. As always, clinicians should be mindful that the child who has an underlying medical problem might also be physically abused.

SKELETAL INJURIES

Fractures are the second most common type of child physical abuse. Accidental fractures are common in ambulatory children but not in nonambulatory children. Most abusive fractures occur in nonambulatory children, representing 55% to 70% of fractures in children younger than age 1 year and 80% of all abuse fractures found in children younger than 18 months of age. (26) Age is the single most important risk factor for abusive skeletal injury.

Understanding that different types of fractures result from different forces applied to the bone aids in determining if a given history is plausible. Transverse fractures are due to forces that are perpendicular to the bone or bend the bone, torus or buckle fractures are due to axial loading or compression along the long axis of the bone, spiral fractures are due to twisting, and oblique fractures are due to a combination of transverse and twisting forces.

Abusive skeletal injury may involve any part of the skeleton, but fractures of the extremities are most common. Any fracture can result from abuse, and no fracture is pathognomonic for abuse. Some fractures, however, have a higher specificity for abuse, such as posterior or lateral rib fractures or CMLs, also known as "corner" or "bucket handle" fractures. These fractures occur at the ends of long bones, resulting from twisting that causes a planar fracture through the spongiosum of the metaphysis.

Some uncommon fractures, such as sternal, spinal, and scapular fractures, are also highly suggestive of child abuse in the absence of a credible and corroborated trauma history. Any child who presents with multiple fractures or fractures in differing stages of healing should raise concern for nonaccidental trauma.

The most common differential diagnosis of abusive fracture is accidental fracture. Some fractures, such as clavicular fractures, may be due to birth trauma. Underlying medical conditions and metabolic bone diseases should be considered in the differential diagnosis of skeletal trauma and include osteogenesis imperfecta, Menkes syndrome, hyperparathyroidism, hypophosphatasia, and Fanconi syndrome. Although vitamin D deficiency is prevalent, rickets is not, and research demonstrates that the incidence of fractures in skeletal trauma is not influenced by vitamin D deficiency. (27)(28)

IMAGING OF SKELETAL INJURIES

Skeletal injuries may be clinically silent in children younger than age 2 years and in developmentally delayed or nonverbal children. A skeletal survey to identify acute or healing fractures should be performed when there is concern for any form of child physical abuse. If an abused child has siblings who are younger than 2 years, skeletal surveys should be performed to evaluate these siblings. The current recommendation by the American College of Radiology for skeletal survey consists of 21 dedicated views, including oblique views of the chest to aid in the detection of rib fractures. (29) Although the clinician must be mindful of radiation exposure, the discovery of an occult injury is a major determinant in the diagnosis of child abuse and, thus, outweighs radiation risk. Infants may have positive skeletal surveys in up to 20% of cases. (30)

Some fractures with high specificity for child abuse, such as rib fractures and CMLs, may not be apparent on the initial skeletal survey. With healing and new bone formation, these injuries become more obvious. Thus, a repeat skeletal survey obtained 10 to 14 days after the initial survey is recommended to re-evaluate for fractures. Bone scans are no longer obtained as a complementary test to detect possible injury because of their serious limitations, including problems with motion artifact, inability to estimate age of injury, and lack of specificity. Due to radiation exposure concerns, CT scan is not a preferred imaging modality to detect fractures. If chest or abdominal CT scan is performed for other reasons, it can be useful in detecting nondisplaced rib fractures. Skull fractures in the line of the axial plane are often missed on head CT scan. The addition of 3-dimensional CT scan reconstruction enhances the identification and morphology of skull fractures and helps ensure their detection and diagnosis.

Aging of bone fractures is imprecise and must be based upon history and clinical examination findings as well as radiographic known patterns of healing. In young children with long bone fractures, new bone is visible within 1 to 2 weeks, followed by callous development, disappearance of the fracture line, and finally resolution. Some fractures, such as skull fractures or CMLs, do not follow a predictable healing process and cannot be aged based on radiographs alone.

CHEST AND ABDOMINAL INJURIES

Abdominal trauma is the second leading cause of fatalities due to child physical abuse. This is likely due to delays in seeking medical care, a misleading history of no or only trivial trauma, and the greater severity of injury in abusive as compared to accidental abdominal trauma. Early signs and symptoms, such as loss of appetite, vomiting, and abdominal pain, are nonspecific and may be misdiagnosed. Furthermore, physical examination generally does not reveal bruising to the chest or abdomen. Some children with abdominal trauma may be battered and have "distracting injuries," such as AHT or a fracture, that may delay recognition of the abdominal injury. Because signs and symptoms of chest and abdominal injuries may be subtle or overlooked, meticulous physical examination is imperative. Signs and symptoms of occult abdominal trauma vary, depending on the age of child and presence of associated injuries such as intra-abdominal hemorrhage or peritonitis. The clinician should palpate the chest wall to examine for rib deformities. Chest wall tenderness and/or palpable callus may suggest the presence of healing rib fractures. Auscultation for equal breath sounds as well as clear heart tones and bowel sounds and palpation of the abdomen must be performed. Because the physical examination results can be misleading, with a lower sensitivity for trauma in younger children, laboratory screening should be considered, particularly in any nonverbal or nonambulatory child.

Relative to accidental abdominal trauma, abusive abdominal trauma occurs more often in infants and toddlers, is more severe, and requires a higher rate of surgical intervention. The peak age for abusive abdominal injury is between ages 2 and 3 years. This may be due to child-related behavioral risk factors, such as increased activity level, normal exploration, normal negativism, and toilet training.

Abusive injuries to almost every visceral structure have been reported. The most commonly injured organs are the liver and spleen, followed by duodenal and proximal jejunal ruptures or hematomas and pancreatic, vascular, and/or renal trauma. Other injuries may involve the bladder, large intestine, stomach, mesentery, and adrenals. The most common mechanism for abdominal injury is focused blunt force trauma to the abdomen that compresses, crushes, or tears the viscera. Because the forces are focused internally, abdominal bruising is rare, and clinicians should not be lulled into a false sense of security by the absence of abdominal bruising. The major diagnostic differential diagnosis for abusive abdominal injury is accidental abdominal injury, which is readily elucidated by history (or lack thereof).

Any child in whom abdominal trauma is suspected should undergo screening, including liver function tests, pancreatic enzymes, hemoglobin to assess for blood loss, and urinalysis to check for hematuria. Plain radiographs are rarely diagnostic but may reveal indirect evidence of visceral injury, such as dilated loops of bowel, air fluid levels, free air, bowel wall air, periportal tracking, or mass effect on the bowel. Abdominal CT scan with contrast is the preferred imaging modality to assess for intra-abdominal injury and is indicated when hepatic enzymes aspartate aminotransferase and alanine aminotransferase measure more than 80 U/L (1.34 μkat/L). (31) Liver enzyme values acutely rise but then rapidly fall after blunt trauma; liver enzymes due to infection or liver disease do not resolve in this pattern. In children who have subacute abdominal trauma, liver enzymes may have normalized by the time of evaluation. (32)

Thoracic injuries are mostly related to crush or major blunt trauma and may involve the heart, lungs, rib cage, and mediastinum. Pulmonary hemorrhage and edema due to airway obstruction, shearing injury to the thoracic duct resulting in a chylothorax, pneumomediastinum, pneumopericardium, and commotio cordis have all been described as a result of abusive trauma.

REPORTING TO CHILD WELFARE AND THE ROLE OF THE CLINICIAN

As mandated reporters, clinicians are required to make a report to child welfare when there is reasonable cause to believe that an injury is the result of abuse or neglect. The clinician need only suspect that maltreatment has occurred to initiate a report. The clinician's role is to initiate evaluation and ensure appropriate treatment and safety of the patient. The final determination of child abuse requires a coordinated interdisciplinary investigation. Access to the expertise of a child abuse specialist is ideal because he or she is accustomed to collaborating with law enforcement, child welfare, and the legal system.

Primary care clinicians may be challenged by their responsibility to inform the caregiver or parent(s) of a report suspicious for child maltreatment. They are understandably concerned about the safety and disposition of their young patients as well as the potential stress and reaction of the family to an investigation. Anticipating a negative family reaction may cause hesitation in reporting. However, the clinician must keep in mind his or her role as the child's advocate and recognize that the report is a medical intervention that may be lifesaving. Developing a thoughtful dialogue to inform a parent of the need to make a report can ease the stress on the reporter as well as the parent.

Clinicians often wonder what happens after a report is made. In every state, a child welfare organization is responsible for investigation of the child maltreatment allegation. The investigative agency may substantiate (indicate) or not substantiate (unfound) a particular allegation. Unsubstantiated findings do not necessarily mean that child maltreatment did not occur. Most investigations do not result in removal of a child from a home and may, in fact, provide opportunities for augmenting the family by offering support to caregivers, such as home visits, parenting classes, access to transportation for follow-up care, and individual or group therapy.

Some cases may progress in the legal system. When there is urgent and immediate concern for a child's safety, the case may be heard in juvenile/family court and result in the temporary removal of a child to ensure his or her safety, health, and well-being. These children are assigned their own attorney, known as a guardian ad litem.

Criminal court testimony is requested when a specific person has been charged with an act leading to an abusive injury. Unlike juvenile court, in which evidence is based upon preponderance (more likely than not), criminal court requires evidence beyond a reasonable doubt. "Managing Child Abuse: General Principles" is an excellent reference (33) that provides a very thoughtful stepwise approach to reporting and navigating the subsequent legal process.

No matter which direction a report may take, the clinician must advocate for his or her patient to have necessary resources and an appropriate medical home.

PREVENTION AND FUTURE HORIZONS

The monetary cost to society of child abuse has been estimated to be $80.3 billion per year. (34) However, this does not adequately reflect the true loss of a child due to untimely and preventable death. Child maltreatment is now recognized as a major public health problem and a significant contemporary source of morbidity and mortality. Appreciation of the adverse impacts of early stressors on adult health has been transformational in validating the role of the pediatric clinician in promoting wellness not only in childhood but also into adulthood. Knowledge of child physical abuse continues to evolve, providing more clarity, as demonstrated by the recent understanding of the significance of sentinel injuries. Increased awareness of child maltreatment by primary care clinicians along with timely intervention ideally can lead to effective prevention of the adverse outcomes of child maltreatment and, along with more dedicated research, to effective primary prevention.

Summary

- On the basis of research and consensus, the diagnosis of child physical abuse must be entertained whenever an infant or nonverbal child presents with any injury. Substantial evidence supports that any form of trauma in a baby is significant and deserves complete evaluation. (1)(2)(3)(4)(5)(6)

- Clinicians must consider child abuse in the differential diagnosis of any young child with injuries or symptoms where there are discrepancies between the sustained injuries and the history and/or patient's developmental capabilities. On the basis of strong research and consensus, child abuse is recognized not only as a major source of mortality and morbidity in childhood but also as a direct cause of increased adult morbidity and early death. (9)(10)

- On the basis of consensus, primary care clinicians are in a position to identify children with injuries concerning for child abuse, initiate an appropriate and thoughtful medical evaluation, report to child welfare, and appropriately seek child abuse pediatric consultation.

CME quiz and references for this article are at http://pedsinreview.aappublications.org/content/37/4/146.

To view PowerPoint slides that accompany this article, visit http://pedsinreview.aappublications.org and click on the Supplemental tab for this article.

Physical Abuse of Children

Jill C. Glick MD
Michele A. Lorand MD
Kristen R. Bilka MMS, PA-C

Pediatrics in Review

American Academy of Pediatrics
DEDICATED TO THE HEALTH OF ALL CHILDREN®

Child Sexual Abuse

Antonia Chiesa, MD,* Edward Goldson, MD*

*Pediatrics, University of Colorado School of Medicine, Children's Hospital Colorado, Aurora, CO

Education Gaps

1. Clinicians should be aware that, in most cases, sexual abuse of a child is distinctly different from adult sexual assault. Usually there is no physical evidence of the abuse and delayed disclosure is common.

2. Developmental and behavioral histories are important components of a medical history for a sexual abuse diagnosis. Clinicians must be aware of normal sexual behaviors in children. The child's developmental level also informs the approach to evaluation, including how much information can be obtained directly from the child.

Objectives   After completing this article, readers should be able to:

1. Review the epidemiology of child sexual abuse.

2. Recognize the history, signs, and symptoms of sexual abuse.

3. Recognize which patients require emergent evaluation and physical examination for sexual abuse or assault.

4. Describe the behavioral and emotional consequences of child sexual abuse.

5. Describe the normal process of disclosure.

6. Employ effective strategies for interviewing suspected victims of sexual abuse or assault.

7. Recognize that most children examined for sexual abuse have normal examination findings.

8. Discuss common abnormal anogenital findings associated with sexual abuse and differentiate them from those associated with accidental trauma and other medical conditions.

9. Plan appropriate collection of forensic evidence and laboratory evaluation during a sexual abuse concern.

10. Follow mandated reporting laws when there are suspicions of child sexual abuse.

AUTHOR DISCLOSURE Drs Chiesa and Goldson have disclosed no financial relationships relevant to this article. This commentary does not contain a discussion of an unapproved/investigative use of a commercial product/device.

ABBREVIATIONS

CDC	Centers for Disease Control and Prevention
HIV	human immunodeficiency virus
SANE	Sexual Assault Nurse Examiner
STI	sexually transmitted infection

INTRODUCTION

Child sexual abuse is one of the most challenging forms of child maltreatment encountered by pediatric clinicians. It is a highly emotional topic in our society, and although the legal and medical definitions appear to be relatively straightforward, it is very difficult to operationalize them in real-life circumstances. Social contexts affect awareness and cultural norms. High-profile cases with sports figures and clergy as well as the spread of the Internet, social media, and access to sexualized imagery have raised awareness of this phenomenon but also added to its complexity. (1) Parents look to pediatric clinicians for support and prevention messaging. Societal factors can also influence the interpretation of sexual behaviors, making it difficult to determine what is normal or may be an indicator of abuse. In addition, the gathering of information concerning the event(s) can be difficult, and the physical evidence for sexual abuse can be absent or unclear, making a definitive statement that abuse has occurred difficult to accomplish. One key concept is vital: child sexual abuse is distinctly different in most circumstances from the acute sexual assault of an adolescent or adult patient. Knowledge of the unique features of this type of maltreatment informs the approach to evaluation and management. A 2013 American Academy of Pediatrics Clinical Report "The Evaluation of Children in the Primary Care Setting When Sexual Abuse Is Suspected" is a valuable resource. (2)

DEFINITIONS

Sexual abuse occurs when a child or youth is engaged in sexual activities that are developmentally inappropriate and for which the child is emotionally or physically unprepared. (3) It involves the sexual gratification of an adult with little regard to cultural taboos or the needs and the developmental level of the child. Moreover, it can combine a variety of forms of abuse, including physical and psychological abuse, both of which can have profoundly disturbing effects on the developing child or youth. Sexual abuse can be divided broadly into 2 forms: contact and noncontact abuse. Noncontact abuse involves exposing the child to sexual acts that he or she cannot comprehend. It includes exposure to or inclusion in pornography. It also includes exhibitionism by which the child is exposed to inappropriate sexualized content. (4) Contact abuse can be divided into acts involving nonpenetration, such as touching and fondling or masturbation. The other forms of contact abuse involve penetration of the vagina, mouth, or anus.

EPIDEMIOLOGY

Although sexual abuse may appear to many to be a new phenomenon, it has a long, dark history. The abuse of children has been a part of the history of all cultures for millennia. Reports from England and France in the 18th and 19th centuries leave a clear record that children were experiencing sexual abuse with some frequency. It was not until the 1970s that child welfare agencies and other professionals increasingly recognized the breadth and consequences of sexual abuse in all of its forms. (4)(5)

In 2014, there were an estimated 702,000 substantiated victims of child maltreatment, of whom 8.2% were victims of sexual abuse. (6) Prevalence data vary, depending on the population, abuse definitions, and survey design. Recent estimates note a rate of non-peer-related childhood sexual abuse at 11% for females and 2% for males. (7) When peer and stranger assaults are included in questionnaires, the rates increase, especially during the period of adolescence. (7) Children are more likely to be abused by a person they know than by a stranger. (6)

PSYCHOLOGICAL ENVIRONMENT

The psychological environment in which child sexual abuse occurs is influenced by the victim's age, developmental level, and relationship with the perpetrator. Preschool children have limited communication skills, which makes it hard for the child to articulate his or her distress. Adolescent girls are at higher risk than boys. (7) Adolescents seek independence, but at the same time want to be accepted by others and experiment with new relationships and ways of interacting with others. As a result, they may place themselves at risk of being sexually exploited, often without taking into consideration the consequences of their behavior. Developmentally disabled individuals are at particularly high risk for sexual abuse due to their physical or cognitive limitations. (8)

Children of single parents and those living in homes with other psychosocial stressors appear to be at greater risk. (9) Children living in families where there is parental conflict or a poor relationship between the child and parent are also considered at risk. (10) Nonoffending caretakers may be complicit or deny that abuse is taking place. (11) Conversely, families may fear the social ramifications if abuse is revealed. Importantly, clinicians must remember that there is no association between sexual abuse and ethnicity or socioeconomic status. (12)

Children are curious, seek attention and affection, and trust authority. There is a disparity in power between a child and an adult that is associated with the child's dependence on the adult for support, nurturance, and guidance. Most children have a basic trust of adults, particularly those in their immediate environment, such as family members and close friends. Accompanying this trust is the child's belief that the adult is all-knowing and all-powerful. All of these factors can set the stage for the child to not trust or to question his or her intuition. The power and trust can be misused, resulting in the sexual exploitation of a naïve child. This is referred to as "accommodation" (13) and can be psychologically confusing to the child. (14) Perpetrators may use fear tactics against the child or threats to the victim's family as a means of continuing the abuse and maintaining secrecy. (15) As such, children can be seen as natural victims. With the component of secrecy that is invariably a part of sexual abuse, the child remains vulnerable to abuse, often without knowing that he or she has been abused.

"Grooming" is somewhat unique to child sexual abuse. (16) The perpetrator initially pays the child special attention, thus gaining his or her confidence. Over a period of time, the relationship becomes sexualized, with the perpetrator violating the child's privacy and initiating sexual conversations or contact. The perpetrator may seek to justify this behavior under the guise that these experiences are normal or instructive. (16)

Interpreting behaviors and situations in the context of a custody dispute can be difficult. On the one hand, children in this situation may be at greater risk for abuse, but there is also a perception that false allegations are more common. (17) Parental separation is often accompanied by strong emotions, unmet needs, conflict, and differences in supervision practices by either parent. (18) In addition, many of the factors that precipitate separation may also lead to abuse. These could include personality disorder, substance abuse, violence, and perversion. It is unclear if the number of substantiated reports of sexual abuse in custody disputes is markedly greater than in the general population. (19)(20) Some cautious skepticism may be helpful in dealing with these cases, but it should not be the guiding rule. (21) Applying an objective and evidence-based approach is warranted. Because the medical evaluation is unlikely to yield "proof" of abuse, the pediatric clinician's role may be to remain neutral but supportive.

OFFENDER CHARACTERISTICS

Although sexual offenders have some associated risk factors, there is no standard offender profile. They come from all socioeconomic and ethnic groups as well as diverse marital and educational backgrounds. They may have no personal history of sexual abuse or psychopathology. They may not have a prior criminal record, although there appears to be some association with other antisocial behaviors. Conversely, they may be depressed, hostile individuals with pre-existing mental health or criminal problems. Many, but not all, may have a history of being abused themselves as children and a tendency toward substance abuse. (22)

INDICATORS

Child sexual abuse may have a variety of presentations to the medical setting. Parents may seek guidance from the clinician due to less specific worries about inappropriate caregivers or seemingly unrelated behaviors such as sleep disturbance, academic problems, or other mental health symptoms. (Although such behaviors are not specific indicators, it is prudent to consider all forms of abuse when evaluating a child for behavioral issues.) Alternatively, they may present after a child makes a specific disclosure or if an event was witnessed. Some patients, usually adolescents, present after an acute sexual assault.

A comprehensive medical history is critical. In the absence of clear physical examination findings, information that may support a diagnosis of abuse comes from the history, including a thorough review of systems and behavioral history. (23)(24) Clinicians should have a baseline understanding of what is considered normal sexual development to assess appropriately for abnormal behaviors that may be associated with sexual abuse.

Sexuality is defined as the way individuals define themselves in relation to gender and includes sexual knowledge, attitudes, and behaviors. It is influenced by family, culture, experience, and education. Sexuality is shaped by biology and psychology. Sexual development can be considered to have 2 distinct components: physical development and psychosocial development. Physical development is the result of biochemical changes as the child matures; psychosexual development involves the emotional and attitudinal changes associated with developing physical sexual maturity.

Sexual behaviors appear during infancy and progress through childhood (Table 1). They follow a relatively typical trajectory based upon development. Normal sexual activity during childhood involves "consenting, developmentally appropriate activities that are mutually motivated by curiosity and pleasure involving peers in terms of cognitive level."(25) An awareness of normal sexual behavior is important for clinicians working with children and youth to differentiate typical sexual play from behaviors that may be considered problematic or that can emerge following sexual abuse. (26)

TABLE 1. Behaviors Associated with Normal Sexual Development

AGE	NORMAL BEHAVIOR
Infancy	Oral gratification, penile erections with bladder and bowel distention, genital self-stimulation in both genders by 18 months.
2-3 years	Gender identification, enjoy displaying nude body.
3-6 years	Display sexual behavior and understand gender differences; masturbation is common. Like to touch bodies, may include genitals and breasts of parents. Child identifies with parent of same sex.
6-7 years	Still interested in sexuality, but overt behaviors are diminished. Remain curious about sex; use "dirty" words but are more modest than younger children. Learn from peers.
Puberty/adolescence	Display fewer family-related sexual behaviors and more interest in peers.

No single behavior is associated absolutely with sexual abuse, but there is a strong suggestion of association between certain sexual behaviors and sexual abuse (Table 2). Children with a history of abuse or exposure to inappropriately sexualized material tend to display behaviors that are imitative of adult sexual behavior. (27) Sexual behavior is also related to a child's family context. Family nudity is related to greater sexual behavior across all ages. (28) In general, sexually abused children exhibit a greater frequency of age-inappropriate sexual behaviors than either normative or psychiatric outpatient samples. (28) More sexual behavior is seen in children with medical evidence of sexual abuse or a history of penetrative abuse, abuse by an immediate family member, abuse by more than 1 perpetrator, or abuse over a long period of time.

Of note, abnormal sexual behaviors may not always be attributed to the experience of sexual abuse. (29) However, when present, they warrant an evaluation. The evaluator should consider psychological stressors (emotional abuse, physical abuse, parental separation) and family dysfunction as alternative causes of the behavior. Children who are inappropriately exposed to sexualized material may also act out the behaviors or in response to what that they have observed (eg, television, Internet, printed images, social media, sexual violence). If, after such an evaluation, concerns about abuse persist, a report to authorities should be considered and medical and behavioral health evaluations should be obtained. (2)

TAKING A HISTORY

The medical history guides evaluation and treatment as well as the subsequent report to authorities. In cases for which some information has already been gathered by other investigators, the clinician may not need to obtain additional information, unless there are missing details relevant to

the child's medical needs. The medical history should include all standard components, including any seemingly unrelated past history, because children may have other unidentified medical issues. The basis for concerns of sexual abuse likely are provided by the caregiver but could be supplemented by information from law enforcement or social services. The type, timing, and chronicity of abuse inform testing and treatment recommendations. Review of systems should identify any genitourinary or gastrointestinal symptoms that may be relevant, such as dysuria, discharge, enuresis, encopresis, genital pain, or bleeding, or any somatic complaints that could be associated with abuse. Numerous medical signs and symptoms have been associated with sexual abuse. In several series, symptoms mimicking urinary tract infections were commonly seen in children with substantiated reports of abuse. (30) However, as with behaviors, many signs and symptoms are not specific for abuse and can be seen in children who have not been abused. (29)(31) A detailed family and social history can help to identify other risk factors.

The physical examination should be explained in advance to the child and caregiver, describing the genital

TABLE 2. Abnormal Sexual Behavior

• Puts mouth on sex parts.	• Makes sexual sounds.
• Asks to engage in sex acts.	• Engages in kissing with the tongue.
• Masturbates with object.	• Undresses other people.
• Inserts objects in vagina/anus.	• Asks to watch explicit television.
• Imitates sexual intercourse.	• Imitates sexual behavior with dolls.

examination in the context of a full-body evaluation. When possible, it is best to use the terms preferred by the child and family when referring to the genitalia. Giving the child a sense of power and control over the examination can minimize retraumatization.

In general, if the child is young, information should be obtained from the caregiver without the child present. Taking a history from the child directly may be appropriate for older, verbal children. (32) Asking the child if he or she has any specific questions about his or her health or body may elicit general concerns or more specific worries related to abuse. (32) In older children, asking about their understanding regarding the reason for the visit can be a natural step for starting the history. If a child begins to disclose the abuse, the best approach is to follow-up with nonleading, general questions such as "What happened?" or "Tell me more." (32) Avoid directed questions that assume a specific response. The history should focus on medically pertinent information, recognizing that information for purely forensic purposes maybe obtained and recorded at another time by specially qualified interviewers.

Knowledge of child development is vital to understanding the challenges and limits to an objective interviewing approach that employs open-ended and developmentally appropriate questions. Repeating back statements and asking for confirmation or clarification are additional techniques that may be helpful. Younger children are vulnerable to suggestion and tend to be more concrete in their verbal skills and responses. (32) For example, a young child may describe genital or anal contact as "inside," but this does not necessarily indicate penetration beyond the labia or buttocks. (33)(34) It can be linguistically and perceptually difficult for a child to describe his or her experience. A lack of findings associated with penetration should neither discredit statements nor prompt a more invasive evaluation (such as a pelvic examination or anoscopy) if not otherwise indicated. Even early school-age children may not be able to answer questions regarding timing or duration of events, especially if the abuse occurred on multiple occasions or in the more distant past. Older children and adolescents are more likely to give a linear, chronologic history. (32)

Before beginning the genital examination of more verbal children, review body safety with the child about who is allowed to look at or touch the genital and anal areas. (For younger children, this includes caregivers who have toileting and hygiene responsibilities.) Starting the conversation in this manner is helpful both as an entrée into a discussion about abuse concerns and to model healthy communication

for the child and caregiver. Clinicians should explore with the child if anyone else has attempted to look at or touch in an inappropriate manner. Speaking with a child in the presence of a caregiver is reasonable for younger children; providing the opportunity for a private conversation is acceptable for older children and adolescents.

If the child discloses sexual abuse in the medical setting, proper documentation is necessary. When possible, an examiner should use direct quotations, including the questions that were asked of the patient. Documentation should be objective and detailed. If the child does not disclose, clinicians should not insist on more information or continue to ask questions. It is important to avoid repeated interviews of children. Ideally, the investigation of child abuse should include a forensic interview of the victim by specially trained professionals. Most clinicians do not have this forensic training; some communities have dedicated child abuse experts who conduct more extensive interviews or whose examination and medical history are recorded as part of the investigative process. Many communities have Child Advocacy Centers that facilitate a multidisciplinary approach to forensic interviews in child sexual abuse cases and involve social service; law enforcement; and mental health, medical, and legal resources. (35)

DISCLOSURE

Because relationship dynamics often include elements of secrecy or a child's sense of helplessness and entrapment, disclosures of sexual abuse may be delayed and confusing. Disclosures are often received with disbelief. Accusations may be retracted if the child is unable to cope with pressure from the perpetrator and the effects that disclosure might have on the perpetrator, the family, and the child. (36) The disclosure process is complicated and poses a unique challenge to child sexual abuse evaluation.

Children often do not disclose sexual abuse, either because of coercion or a lack of understanding that the abuse is wrong. (37) When children finally do disclose, the disclosure may be delayed months to years after the initial incident and may be neither spontaneous nor complete. (38) Children are more likely to disclose when the offender is no longer in their lives. Disclosures often follow questioning by a parent, teacher, or physician about inappropriate touching. (39) The questions are usually prompted by a concern regarding a medical or behavioral symptom noted in a child. Children tend to disclose a single piece of their story at a time to assess the parent's or interviewer's reaction to what has been disclosed. If the reaction is considered negative, the disclosure may be squelched or recanted. (37) Consequently, partial disclosures, with more information revealed over time, are common. (39)

MEDICAL EVALUATION AND PHYSICAL EXAMINATION

An emergent medical evaluation is indicated when there is concern about:
1. Any acute injury
2. Significant abnormal physical or psychiatric symptoms
3. The need for prophylactic treatment of infection or pregnancy
4. Safety of child or family
5. Parental anxiety/worry
6. The need for forensic evidence collection

In general, forensic evidence collection can be reasonably considered in any female pubertal patient up to 120 hours after the assault. For prepubertal children, 72 hours is generally accepted as the cutoff for determining whether forensic evidence collection is indicated. (40) If the reported sexual abuse occurred beyond these timelines and there are no other acute medical problems or safety issues, the patient can be seen on a nonurgent basis by either the primary clinician or a pediatric sexual abuse expert. (40)

Not all clinicians have the same training and comfort level with sexual abuse evaluations, including those within the emergency department setting. All clinicians should know community resources. Photographic documentation of the genital and anal areas, with either specialized camera equipment or a colposcope, is common in sexual abuse evaluations. Many clinicians working in this field routinely use a peer review process to discuss cases and review documentation. When photographs are part of the examination, evaluators should follow a clear process for secure storage to ensure confidentiality. Some additional sensitivity may be needed if the child's victimization involved photographing the child.

For the younger child who has a history that is not suggestive of injury, the examination is usually noninvasive and the need for forensic evidence collection often is limited. Therefore, an evaluation similar to a health supervision visit that includes the genital and anal area may be all that is indicated. A family may feel more comfortable having the examination conducted in the primary care setting by a clinician with whom they have an established relationship. Ideally, the setting should be a child-friendly environment where the examination is explained in advance, there is no coercion, and the child can ask questions about his or her health. Even in the absence of a diagnostic finding for abuse or forensic evidence, completing a medical evaluation for any child who may have been sexually abused can be useful. The examination may be particularly therapeutic for the child and family when they hear from a trusted clinician that the child's body is healthy and normal in appearance.

Some families have worries about a girl's virginity. Although this term has little medical relevance, the cultural context may be very significant, and the child and family may need support around their concerns. Clinicians should abstain from framing a diagnosis around the concept of virginity. A more prudent approach is to understand the cultural context of the family, validate the child's maltreatment regardless of physical findings, reassure the family about the potential for healthy sexual development, and refer the child for evidence-based mental health treatment when needed.

Chaperones should be present for the examination. (41) Besides the medical chaperone, it is appropriate to let the child decide who else is present in the room for support. Suspected perpetrators of the abuse should not be present. The child should be gowned and the examination cover from "head to toe" to identify other medical conditions or signs of abuse. Examining the entire body also helps to build rapport and place the child more at ease.

Older females can be examined in the lithotomy position (supine with thighs separated, knees flexed, and feet supported in stirrups). A speculum examination is reserved for pubertal females only, although such examination is not needed in most cases. Speculum examination is very rarely indicated for the prepubertal girl unless there are concerns for conditions such as intravaginal injury or a foreign body. When necessary, a speculum examination or vaginoscopy should be performed under anesthesia with the guidance of an experienced child abuse expert or pediatric gynecologist.

Younger children can be examined in the supine position, with the feet placed together near the buttocks and the knees abducted, often referred to as the "frog leg position." Very young children may be more comfortable in their parent's lap in a version of the frog leg position. The lateral decubitus position, with the patient's knees tucked in toward the chest, may be helpful in examining the anal area. The knee-chest position requires that the child remain prone, with the head on or near the examination table, and the knees bent under the body so that the child's hips are elevated. With lifting of the buttocks and labial separation, the posterior edge of the hymen can be better visualized. This technique can be reserved for children in whom there is a question of an abnormality of the posterior hymen. The examiner should be sensitive to any information regarding the position of the victim during the assault.

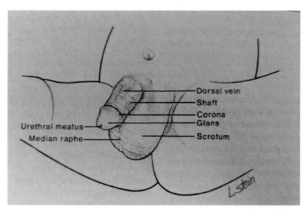

Figure 1. Male anatomy. Finkel M. Physical examination. In: Finkel MA, Giardino AP, eds. *Medical Evaluation of Child Sexual Abuse: A Practical Guide.* 3rd ed. Elk Grove Village, IL: American Academy of Pediatrics; 2009:65. Copyright © 2009 American Academy of Pediatrics. Reproduced with permission.

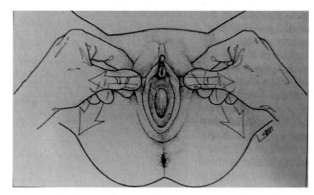

Figure 3. Labial traction. Finkel M. Physical examination. In: Finkel MA, Giardino AP, eds. *Medical Evaluation of Child Sexual Abuse: A Practical Guide.* 3rd ed. Elk Grove Village, IL: American Academy of Pediatrics; 2009:73. Copyright © 2009 American Academy of Pediatrics. Reproduced with permission.

Along with any other injury or signs of abuse, the examiner should document the child's Sexual Maturity Rating stage and provide a full description of the genital and anal anatomy. Working knowledge of basic anatomy (Figs 1 and 2), normal variants, and findings that may be confused with sexual abuse trauma is required. If photographic documentation is not available, a body diagram with genital views may be a helpful addition to the chart. To see the entirety of the external female genital anatomy, gentle labial separation with downward and outward traction is usually needed for the examination (Fig 3). This can generally be accomplished with minimal discomfort to the patient. The examiner should be careful not to apply too

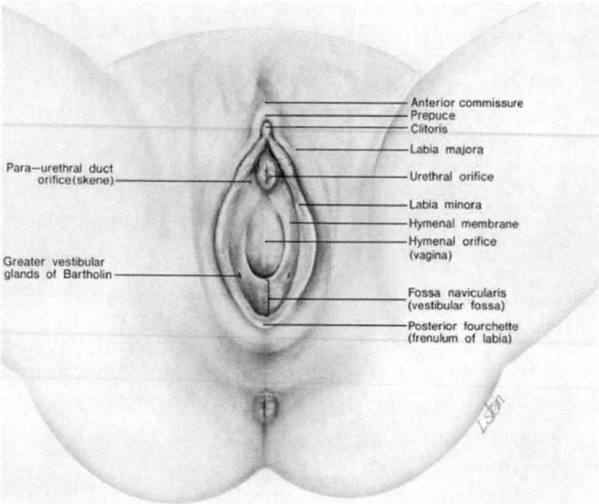

Figure 2. Female anatomy. Finkel M. Physical examination. In: Finkel MA, Giardino AP, eds. *Medical Evaluation of Child Sexual Abuse: A Practical Guide.* 3rd ed. Elk Grove Village, IL: American Academy of Pediatrics; 2009:59. Copyright © 2009 American Academy of Pediatrics. Reproduced with permission.

much labial separation so as to cause an iatrogenic dehiscence in the area of the posterior fourchette.

The hymen, a ring of tissue that surrounds the vaginal opening (Fig 4), is recessed and less readily visible. In the absence of a major pelvic deformity, all females are born with a hymen. The misconception that the hymen tissue completely covers the vaginal opening until it is "broken" with first intercourse is still prevalent and even reinforced in the lay culture. However, complete obstruction of the vaginal canal by a hymen without an opening is an abnormal variant that is known as an imperforate hymen. The condition may require surgical intervention at the onset of menstruation.

There is wide variation in the normal configuration of the hymen (Figs 5 and 6). The tissue can be loose and folded upon itself, resulting in a bunched or redundant appearance. This is the most common configuration among infants and adolescents. Children younger than age 3 years typically have a circular or annular hymen. During the toddler years, hymens may take on a half moon or crescentic appearance. Occasionally, the hymen has a very small opening (microperforate). A band of tissue that stretches across the hymenal opening is a septum, and a hymen with this feature is described as septate.

Before puberty, the hymen is very thin and can be almost transparent. With puberty comes an increase in estrogen and a subsequent increase in the hymen's thickness and ability to stretch, which explains why there is not necessarily injury to the hymen with penetration of the vaginal orifice. (42) A cotton swab may be used to help delineate folded-over edges of an estrogenized hymen. (Such examination should be avoided in a prepubertal child because any contact with the fragile hymen tissue before it is fully estrogenized can be painful.) Alternatively, a drop of clean saline can help "float"

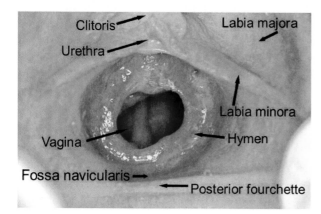

Figure 4. Anatomic terms for structures of the prepubertal female introitus. Kristine Fortin and Carole Jenny. *Pediatrics in Review*. 2012;33:19-32. © 2012 by American Academy of Pediatrics. Reproduced with permission.

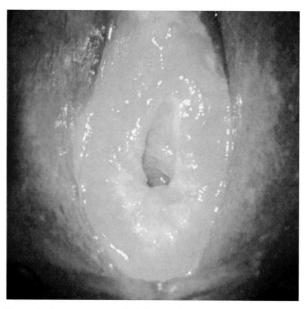

Figure 6. Thick, estrogenized adolescent hymen. Kristine Fortin and Carole Jenny. *Pediatrics in Review*. 2012;33:19-32. © 2012 by American Academy of Pediatrics. Reproduced with permission.

the edges of the hymen and make identification easier. Normal variations in the hymen edge can be confused with healed trauma. (43) The diagnosis of healed injuries, indicative of penetrating trauma, is best left to experienced examiners due to the challenges in differentiating between normal variants. Any question about the significance of findings should prompt referral to a specialist.

Acute injuries can include abrasions, contusions, and commonly lacerations through the hymen. Injuries can heal quickly, within days. (44) In describing any physical finding, it is common to use a "face of the clock" orientation. For example, with the child in the supine position, a finding may be noted at the "3 o'clock position" of the hymen.

A common misconception among families, professionals, and even medical clinicians is that sexual abuse can be diagnosed based on physical examination alone. In

reality, most children with a proven history of sexual abuse (based on perpetrator confession) have normal findings on genital examination for many reasons. (24)(34) In many situations, the type of sexual contact is not injurious, such as rubbing the genitals outside of clothing or exposing the child to pornography. Other contact, such as fondling, may cause minor irritation or a superficial injury that heals quickly. (44) Because delayed disclosures are common, some children do not receive timely medical examinations, allowing more serious injuries the time to heal completely.

ANOGENITAL FINDINGS

Because sexual abuse takes many forms, a variety of medical findings is possible, some of which are more specific for abuse than others. Given the legal ramifications, it is important for the examiner to differentiate conditions that may mimic abuse or could be caused from other conditions. Also, some injuries involving the genitalia are abusive but not sexually motivated, such as bruises and burns from physical abuse. Sexual abuse can cause nonspecific findings, such as erythema or dysuria that results from rubbing or fondling. (30) These nuances can make clinical decision-making a challenge.

The interpretation of physical findings should be based on empiric evidence (regarding specificity for trauma or sexual contact), although any correlating clinical history should be included as part of the rationale for diagnosis. An updated guideline suggests that differentiation of sexual

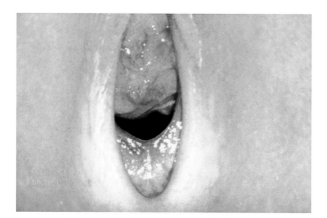

Figure 5. The unestrogenized hymen of a school-age child. Kristine Fortin and Carole Jenny. *Pediatrics in Review*. 2012;33:19-32. © 2012 by American Academy of Pediatrics. Reproduced with permission.

abuse from other conditions based on physical findings (Table 3) must take into account that certain findings can be common in children without a history of abuse (including mimics of abuse), some findings do not have expert consensus for sexual abuse, and some findings are due to trauma or sexual abuse (history dependent). (23)

FORENSIC EVIDENCE AND LABORATORY EVALUATION

Determination of the need for forensic evidence collection is based on both timing and type of sexual contact. Sometimes referred to as a "rape kit," a forensic evidence collection kit is generally supplied by a law enforcement agency. Contents vary but generally include: a detailed set of instructions, consent forms, and the tools necessary to collect specimens (body fluid, hair, nails) from the victim's body to identify DNA and trace evidence or for toxicology in the case of a drug-facilitated assault.

In prepubertal children, the collection is usually limited by the type of contact and the desire to minimize additional emotional trauma. The exchange of body fluid is less common in younger children, who are more likely to experience contact such as fondling or noncontact abuse. In many cases of child sexual abuse, there is no forensic evidence. (45) When it is found, studies have confirmed that for prepubertal victims, evidence (from body fluids) is much more likely to be obtained from the child's clothing or the scene than from the child's body. (45)(46)(47) In general, evidence collection is considered for the prepubertal child within the first 72 hours of contact, although it is unlikely to yield positive results after 24 hours. (45)(47) For pubertal children with a history of penile-vaginal penetration, the ability to collect sperm from inside the vaginal canal is possible for up to 120 hours. (40) Except under very rare circumstances of penetrating trauma, intravaginal or intra-anal swabs of the prepubertal child are not recommended and can actually cause substantial pain or injury.

Upon completion of the collection, it is important to maintain and document the "chain of evidence," which refers to the procedure used by professionals to ensure that any forensic evidence is appropriately secured and handed-off so as to avoid tampering. Many communities have well-established Sexual Assault Nurse Examiner (SANE) programs. (40) SANEs are specially trained in the area of sexual assault assessment and forensic evidence collection. Increasing numbers of these individuals are becoming certified to conduct pediatric examinations.

The decision to test for or treat sexually transmitted infections (STIs) is based on timing and type of sexual contact, clinical history, including other contacts with a STI, perpetrator risk factors, and parental concern for abuse. A minority of prepubertal victims test positive. (48)(49) The prevalence of STIs in the general adolescent population is high enough to recommend testing for all patients. In prepubertal children, a diagnosis of human immunodeficiency virus (HIV) infection, syphilis, gonorrhea, or *Chlamydia* infection are indicative of sexual abuse in the absence of perinatal acquisition, blood transfusion, or rare nonsexual transmission. *Trichomonas vaginalis* is considered highly suspicious. The presence of herpes and anogenital warts is less specific. (50) Although their presence should prompt an inquiry into any concerns of abuse, both can be passed through casual contact. These conditions may be more highly associated with sexual abuse in older children who manage toileting and hygiene independently.

The Centers for Disease Control and Prevention (CDC) publishes treatment guidelines that provide recommendations for laboratory tests and treatment regimens (https://www.cdc.gov/std/tg2015/). (51) Due to potential legal consequences, screening tests that have high specificity are

TABLE 3. Physical Findings

Indicative of trauma	Vaginal, hymenal, perineal, or anal lacerations or contusions; complete, healed transections of the hymen between 4 and 8 o'clock; bite marks; oral palate abrasion; torn oral frenulum
Indicative of sexual contact	Semen, sperm; syphilis (not acquired at birth); gonorrhea; human immunodeficiency virus infection (not acquired at birth or by intravenous route); pregnancy
No consensus regarding specificity for sexual abuse	Herpes, deep notch of the hymen, anal dilation, genital or anal warts
Normal variants	Perianal or hymenal skin tags, superficial notches of the hymen, diastasis ani, intravaginal ridges
Other medical conditions, including those that can be confused with sexual abuse	Vaginitis, labial adhesions, anal fissures, lichen sclerosus et atrophicus, rectal prolapse, urethral prolapse, molluscum contagiosum

recommended. Nucleic acid amplification tests (NAATs) have been studied in prepubertal populations but are only used in limited circumstances. (52) Besides vaginal and urethral samples, throat and rectal samples may be indicated (Table 4).

Follow-up convalescent testing of serum for blood-borne diseases is also required at the intervals noted later in this article (Table 5). (51)

Postexposure prophylaxis should be considered in cases of acute assault where there is a risk of body fluid exchange (Table 6). (51)(53) Single-dose treatments for *Chlamydia*, gonorrhea, and *Trichomonas* infections are recommended. (51) Human papillomavirus vaccination is indicated for females ages 9 through 26 years and males ages 9 through 21 years. Hepatitis B prophylaxis depends on the vaccination status of the victim, type of sexual contact, and disease risk of the offender. Depending on the clinical scenario, hepatitis B treatment can include immunization and/or hepatitis B immunoglobulin. Given the lower risk for STI and higher rates of follow-up, empiric treatment for prepubertal children is not generally required unless sexual contact risk is high or there is concern by the caregiver. For more detail or for information regarding drug allergy, refer to CDC guidelines.

There are multiple options for HIV prophylaxis, and the regimens are complicated. Prophylaxis is less likely to be effective 72 hours after exposure. (54) Therefore, consultation with a specialist, who can also discuss whether prophylaxis is warranted, is advisable. Serious adverse effects from HIV medications are less common, but the course of treatment is 4 weeks. Adolescent patients are less likely to adhere to treatment recommendations, (55)(56) so a detailed process of informed consent should be initiated with the patient and family to ensure compliance.

Acute assault considerations should include a discussion about pregnancy prophylaxis. Pregnancy testing should be completed before the administration of any medication. Levonorgestrel can now be delivered in a one-time dose and is effective up to 5 days after an assault to prevent pregnancy. (57) Other medications have also been studied and are effective.

BEHAVIORAL AND EMOTIONAL CONSEQUENCES

Sexual abuse of children and adolescents, even in the absence of significant physical injury, can have profound adverse psychosocial consequences. (58) Children's behaviors may change over time as they process their experience

TABLE 4. Sexually Transmitted Infection Testing

INFECTION	SPECIMEN	TEST
Neisseria gonorrhoeae	Swabs of the posterior pharynx and anal mucosa in boys and girls, swabs of vulva in prepubertal girls or vaginal canal in postmenarchal girls, swabs of the urethra in boys (if urethral discharge present, a meatal specimen is adequate)	Culture
	Vulvar secretions from prepubertal girls or vaginal secretions from postmenarchal girls or urine sample from girls (no data for use with urine from boys or extragenital sites for girls/boys)	NAATs
Chlamydia trachomatis	Swabs of anus in both boys and girls, swabs of vulva in prepubertal girls or vaginal canal in postmenarchal girls, a meatal specimen only if urethral discharge in boys; pharyngeal specimens not indicated	Culture
	Vaginal specimens or urine from girls/adolescent males (no data for use with urine from boys or extragenital sites for girls/boys)	NAATs
Trichomonas vaginalis	Swabs of vulvar or vaginal mucosa/secretion	Culture wet mount
Bacterial vaginosis	Swabs of vulvar or vaginal mucosa/secretion vaginal specimen	Wet mount
Human immunodeficiency virus	Serum	Antibody PCR
Syphilis	Serum	RPR
Hepatitis (A,B, and C)	Serum	Antibody PCR
Herpes simplex virus	Swab of lesion	Culture PCR

NAAT=nucleic acid amplification test; PCR=polymerase chain reaction; RPR=rapid plasma reagin.

TABLE 5. **Follow-up Sexually Transmitted Infection Testing**

	HEPATITIS B SURFACE ANTIGEN	HEPATITIS B SURFACE ANTIBODY	HEPATITIS C ANTIBODY	HUMAN IMMUNODEFICIENCY VIRUS ANTIBODY	RAPID PLASMA REAGIN
Baseline	X	X	X	X	X
6 Weeks				X	X
3 Months				X	
6 Months	X (if baseline antibody negative and after immunization)	X (if baseline antibody negative and after immunization)	X	X	X

through different developmental stages. (59) Some children respond minimally; others may have more extreme reactions. Very young children, who are more concrete in their understanding of right and wrong, may cope well with little adverse effect, especially if contact is limited and not injurious and their caregiver is protective.

Variable lists of behaviors associated with abuse can be found, many of which are nonspecific and can result from other causes of emotional stress. Some of the more common manifestations include psychiatric disturbances such as depression, anxiety, posttraumatic stress disorder, low self-esteem, and sexual dysfunction. (58) Younger children may act out or have problems in school. They may appear anxious or sad. A range of internalizing and externalizing behaviors can be observed in adolescents. Some respond with social withdrawal, aggression, self-mutilation, substance abuse, school problems, truancy, promiscuity, (60) prostitution, and runaway behavior. Others develop distorted body images leading to eating disorders. Still others may have suicidal ideation or attempts. Many describe a sense of powerlessness, betrayal, and stigmatization. (61)

Studies have shown that belief by the mother (or at least a protective adult caregiver) in a child's disclosure is a positive mediator for a more favorable psychological outcome. (11)(62) Children with abuse involving penetration, violence, a close relationship with the perpetrator, multiple offenders, of longer duration, or with more frequent contact are usually at higher risk for negative impact. (63) Factors associated with greater distress include higher levels of cognitive functioning, children who blame themselves or view their experiences as threatening, a dysfunctional family or lack of social support, other forms of abuse, and close relationship between the mother and the offender. (64)

Evidence-based mental health treatments are available. When children are identified and appropriately referred, good outcomes are possible for those with a history of sexual abuse. Therefore, it is essential to know about community resources available for families. The National Child Traumatic Stress Network is an organization that offers helpful resources for professionals and families (http://www.nctsn.org/). Long-term follow-up and monitoring of these patients

TABLE 6. **Most Common Prophylaxis Regimens**

CONDITION	PROPHYLAXIS	
Hepatitis B	Depends on vaccination status of victim, type of contact, and disease risk of offender	
Gonorrhea	Weight ≥45 kg	Ceftriaxone 250 mg IM once
	Weight <45 kg	25–50 mg/kg IM once, not to exceed 125 mg IM
Chlamydia	Weight ≥45 kg	Azithromycin 1 g PO once
	Weight <45 kg	Erythromycin base or ethylsuccinate 50 mg/kg/day PO divided into 4 doses daily for 14 days
Trichomonas	Weight ≥45 kg	Metronidazole 2 g PO in a single dose OR tinidazole 2 g PO in a single dose
	Weight <45 kg	Metronidazole 15 mg/kg per day PO divided into 3 doses daily for 7 days, not to exceed 2 g/day

IM=intramuscularly; PO=orally.

is important because of their risk for adverse behavioral health issues.

MANDATED REPORTING IN THE UNITED STATES

Mandatory reporting of sexual abuse by medical clinicians is required in all states. Reports should be made in cases of abuse or suspected abuse. Clinicians should be aware of specific statutory requirements and institutional policies where they practice. Good faith immunity clauses exist to protect clinicians from liability should they report in error. Reporting is not a violation of Health Insurance Portability and Accountability Act confidentiality laws. Failure to report a suspected case can result in repercussions for the clinician.

PRIMARY CLINICIAN ROLE IN PREVENTION

Professionals can support parents by emphasizing goals for healthy child sexual development, including privacy, open communication, empathy, and accountability. Clinicians can introduce and model these concepts in the primary care setting. For example, this can be accomplished in the context of anticipatory guidance for toilet training, embedding the concepts of hygiene with personal space and safety. Children and families need a trusted source, such as a primary care clinician, for asking questions, sharing feelings, and learning appropriate information.

Summary

- Based on consistent observational evidence, physical signs and symptoms alone cannot be used to definitively diagnose sexual abuse. Most children with a proven history of sexual abuse have normal findings on genital and anal examinations. (24) The history is a very important factor in the evaluation of child sexual abuse.

- Based on observational data and consensus opinion, some physical examination findings are more specific for sexual abuse than others. (23) Acute vaginal, hymenal, perineal, or anal lacerations or contusions, without an accidental history, are most indicative of sexual abuse.

- Based on observational data, forensic evidence is rarely recovered in cases of prepubertal sexual abuse. When it is found, studies have confirmed that for prepubertal victims, evidence (from body fluids) is much more likely to be obtained from the child's clothing or the scene than from the child's body. (45)(46)(47) In general, evidence collection for the prepubertal child can be considered within the first 72 hours of contact, although it is unlikely to yield positive results after 24 hours.

- Based on strong evidence, effective mental health treatments are available for children who have experienced child sexual abuse.

- Mandatory reporting laws exist in all 50 states for clinicians who have a suspicion of child abuse.

References for this article are at http://pedsinreview.aappublications.org/content/38/3/105.

Parent Resources from the AAP at HealthyChildren.org

- What to Know about Child Abuse: https://www.healthychildren.org/English/safety-prevention/at-home/Pages/What-to-Know-about-Child-Abuse.aspx
- Foster or Adopted Children Who Have Been Sexually Abused: https://www.healthychildren.org/English/family-life/family-dynamics/adoption-and-foster-care/Pages/Foster-or-Adopted-Children-Who-Have-Been-Sexually-Abused.aspx
- What is a Child Abuse Pediatrician?: https://www.healthychildren.org/English/family-life/health-management/pediatric-specialists/Pages/What-is-a-Child-Abuse-Pediatrician.aspx
- Sexual Behaviors in Young Children: What's Normal, What's Not: https://www.healthychildren.org/English/ages-stages/preschool/Pages/Sexual-Behaviors-Young-Children.aspx

For a comprehensive library of AAP parent handouts, please go to the *Pediatric Patient Education* site at http://patiented.aap.org.

Child Psychological Abuse

Melissa Kimber, PhD, MSW, RSW,* Harriet L. MacMillan, CM, MD, MSc, FRCPC*
*McMaster University, Hamilton, Ontario, Canada

AUTHOR DISCLOSURE Dr Kimber has disclosed that she receives funding from the Public Health Agency of Canada to develop curricula on family violence, including child maltreatment. Dr MacMillan has disclosed that her institution receives funding from the Public Health Agency of Canada to develop panCanadian guidance and curricula on responding to family violence, including psychological abuse, and that she is principal investigator on the project. She receives honoraria as a speaker for continuing medical education presentations on topics that include psychological abuse and receives compensation as an expert witness on all aspects of child maltreatment. This commentary does not contain a discussion of an unapproved/investigative use of a commercial product/device.

How to Deal with Emotional Abuse and Neglect: Further Development of a Conceptual Framework (FRAMEA). Glaser D. *Child Abuse Neglect.* 2011;35(10):866–875

Psychological Maltreatment. Hart SN, Brassard MR, Binggeli NJ, Davidson HA. In: *The APSAC Handbook on Child Maltreatment.* Myers JEB, Berliner JN, Briere J, et al, eds. Thousand Oaks, CA: Sage Publications; 2002:79–104

Psychological Maltreatment. Hibbard R, Barlow J, MacMillan H, et al. *Pediatrics.* 2012;130(2):372–378

Interventions to Prevent Child Maltreatment and Associated Impairment. MacMillan HL, Wathen CN, Barlow J, et al. *Lancet.* 2009;373 (9659):250–266

Understanding Emotional Abuse. Rees CA. *Arch Dis Child.* 2010;95(1):59–67.

The Prevalence of Child Maltreatment Across the Globe: Review of a Series of Meta-analyses. Stoltenborgh M, Bakermans-Kranenburg MJ, Alink LRA, van IJzendoorn MH. *Child Abuse Rev.* 2015;24(1):37–50

Distinguishing Between Poor/ Dysfunctional Parenting and Child Emotional Maltreatment. Wolfe DA, McIsaac C. *Child Abuse Neglect.* 2011;35(10):802–813

Considered synonymous, child emotional and psychological abuse (hereafter referred to as *psychological abuse*) is a type of maltreatment that can be difficult for clinicians to detect and assess. Increasingly thought to be the most prevalent form of child maltreatment, psychological abuse involves nonphysical interactions by a caregiver toward a child, including acts of commission that place a child at risk for emotional harm. Pertinent issues for pediatricians include its prevalence, its determinants and risk factors, its negative short- and long-term outcomes, how to assess psychological abuse, and how to collaborate with child protection agencies.

Psychological abuse is arguably the most poorly understood form of child maltreatment; compared with physical and sexual abuse, much less is known about its presentation, causes, consequences, prevention, and treatment. For the pediatrician, a key part of identifying psychological abuse is being attuned to interactions between children and their caregivers. Psychological abuse of a child or adolescent often manifests as a repeated pattern of behavior, but it can also involve a single incident. Examples of psychologically abusive behavior by caregivers include spurning (eg, ridiculing or humiliating), terrorizing (eg, threatening violence against a child or a child's loved ones), isolating (eg, restricting social interactions), corrupting/exploiting (eg, involving in illegal activities), and denying emotional responsiveness (eg, providing no praise).

Although single incidents of these behaviors do not necessarily constitute psychological abuse, 1 severe incident, such as terrorizing a child, could be considered psychologically abusive. A caregiver may use 1 or more of these behaviors briefly or over a longer period. Exposure to psychological abuse has occurred if a caregiver's behavior inflicts harm or places a child at risk for harm. Examples of emotional impairment include a child or adolescent engaging in maladaptive behavior or feeling unloved, unwanted, or only of value to serve the means, desires, and purposes of the caregiver. In addition to physical and sexual abuse, psychological abuse can co-occur with neglect, including physical, medical, and psychological neglect. Notably, the term *psychological maltreatment* includes both psychological abuse and psychological neglect.

Much less is known about the prevalence, antecedents, correlates, and outcomes of psychological abuse compared with other types of maltreatment. In addition, the studies that estimate the prevalence of psychological abuse are disproportionately focused on North American samples. Importantly, psychological abuse is likely the most underreported form of child maltreatment to child welfare authorities. Based on a recent meta-analysis of studies addressing psychological abuse, the prevalence was estimated to be only 0.3% when based on reports by professionals but was as high as 36% when determined by self-reports. Given that psychological abuse often lacks overt indicators of its occurrence, it is not surprising that prevalence rates based on reports by professionals are significantly lower than those based on self-reports of victimization.

No single factor causes psychological abuse. Rather, it can be best understood within what is referred to as the ecological model, which considers the balance of risk and protective factors at the individual, family, community, and societal levels. The experience of multiple and chronic stressors is associated with psychological abuse. For example, caregivers with unstable employment or housing situations report experiencing greater stress and may be more likely to commit psychological abuse. In addition, those who experience changes in family demographics (eg, death of a family member, onset of marital separation, pregnancy) or family conflict (eg, custody disputes, financial strain, disparate co-parenting practices) are at greater risk for committing psychological abuse. Similarly, caregivers with mental health problems, with substance abuse, or who are living in homes where there is intimate partner violence have a greater likelihood of being psychologically abusive toward a child. Importantly, pediatricians should be attuned to the possibility that children and adolescents with intellectual or cognitive disabilities may be especially vulnerable to psychological abuse.

Compared with their nonmaltreated peers, individuals who have been psychologically abused in childhood or adolescence are more likely to have internalizing symptoms, such as depression, anxiety, and posttraumatic stress disorder, as well as externalizing symptoms, including antisocial behavior. Other problems associated with a history of psychological abuse include eating and weight-related disorders, lower educational attainment, and impairment in peer relationships that continue into adulthood.

Detection and assessment of psychological abuse is complicated by the fact that it often co-occurs with other forms of maltreatment. Pediatricians need to be alert to its occurrence. The effects of psychological abuse can vary according to its intensity, duration, and frequency. In addition, the behavioral and emotional effects of psychological abuse can be attenuated by a warm and supportive relationship with a nonoffending caregiver or other adult. Similarly, some children and adolescents demonstrate remarkable resilience in the face of psychological abuse.

It is important for clinicians to ask about relationships in the family from as many members as possible, but this should be done individually to protect anyone disclosing abuse from retaliation. Developmentally and cognitively appropriate, nonjudgmental questions and probing around caregiver discipline practices and how conflict is handled in the home and between family members can yield important information. Similarly,

eliciting when caregivers have been proud and disappointed with their child's or adolescent's behavior can provide insights into caregiver expectations as well as use of praise and discipline. Although interviewing caregivers together to ask general questions about the family and its parenting practices is useful, it is important to meet with each parent and child individually to discuss such issues as feelings of safety and self-worth within the family and to avoid increasing the risk of any intimate partner violence between the caregivers. Similarly, it is crucial to interview a child privately to avoid any undue influence by a caretaker on the child's responses and to avoid any risk of harm to the child who discloses maltreatment by a caregiver accompanying the child.

Guidance on asking for a history from people outside the family who are involved in the child's life, such as child care providers and teachers, is included in the reading list, as is further information about differentiating psychological abuse from questionable caregiving practices. Psychologically abusive caregiving includes making the caregiver's love conditional, deliberately withholding displays of love or affection unless the child meets the caregiver's needs, not responding to the child's psychological or emotional needs, and using discipline that is demeaning by lowering the child's sense of worth or frightening her/him (calling the child crude or rude names, threatening the child's well-being in an attempt to control the child's behavior). But it is not uncommon for parents to face challenges in communicating with their children, and an important consideration is whether the interactions exceed the threshold for psychological abuse. Parents may display rigidity in their emotional expression or use verbal or nonverbal pressure inappropriately to have their children adhere to their expectations. Although these caregivers could benefit from parenting support, their behaviors are not necessarily indicators of psychological maltreatment as would be overt threats or attempts to frighten or intimidate a child.

In most jurisdictions in North America, the threshold for reporting to child protection authorities is having a suspicion of harm to a child, regardless of the type of maltreatment. For the most part, suspicion of psychological abuse is based on history or direct observation of caregiver-child interactions and child/adolescent emotional and behavioral well-being. When there is a history of behaviors that indicate a child is at risk for harm from psychological abuse, it is important to communicate to child protection personnel the child's thoughts, feelings, and behaviors as well as specific statements made by the child about interactions with caregivers. Similarly, documenting statements made by the child's siblings, the offending and nonoffending caregiver(s), teachers, and child care personnel are critical to detailing a repeated pattern of caregiver behavior that is or can be detrimental to the child's well-being. Importantly, clear evidence of harm is *not* a prerequisite for reporting psychological abuse: if a clinician *suspects* that psychological abuse has or may be occurring, a report to the authorities should be made in accordance with state laws. But, as always, prevention is the best intervention, and from a family's first visit, pediatricians have the opportunity to discuss approaches to parenting and to work with parents about being sensitive to their child's needs.

(The reading list provides additional information relating to strategies for reporting and follow-up, which assist the pediatrician to prioritize the safety and well-being of the child.)

COMMENTS: Self-reports of psychological abuse greatly outnumber reports by health professionals. The implication, obviously, is that we pediatricians are missing not only many but in fact the majority of cases. Given the reality that our society underfunds social support services for children and mental health services for everyone, we are faced with a difficult quandary. In most states, suspicion of maltreatment, rather than proof, is the mandated legal trigger for reporting. If, as we should, we assess more vigorously for suspicion of psychological abuse, the new referrals to often overwhelmed child protection agencies pose the risk of doing more harm than good by collapsing the system under the weight of so many reports. In a recent commentary in *Pediatrics* [Parsing Language and Measures Around Child Maltreatment, 2017;139(1):e20163475], Campbell et al argue that addressing the underlying "social determinants of health," such as "household poverty, poor education, and parental mental health" through evidence-supported interventions within the medical setting is a more effective strategy for protecting the well-being of our children than "collapsing the full spectrum of social determinants of health under one umbrella term: child maltreatment." We have some serious thinking, and advocacy, to do.

– Henry M. Adam, MD
Associate Editor, *In Brief*

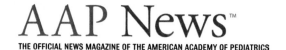

AAP News™

THE OFFICIAL NEWS MAGAZINE OF THE AMERICAN ACADEMY OF PEDIATRICS

:: July-29-2013

'Practical' Guide Helps in Evaluation of Children Who Report Sexual Abuse

Alyson Sulaski Wyckoff, Associate Editor

I s anything bothering you? Tell me why you're here today.

These are open-ended, non-suggestive examples of questions pediatricians can use when evaluating a patient who has disclosed sexual abuse. The importance of the quality of the interview is one point discussed in an updated clinical report that can help pediatricians respond to claims of possible child abuse raised in the clinical setting.

Guidance on interviewing children when sexual abuse is suspected is provided in a revised clinical report that also addresses diagnosis, examination and testing, as well as dealing with parents and tapping resources for referral.

An update to a 2005 document, the report is a resource for pediatricians seeking to learn more about making the diagnosis, doing exams, testing for sexually transmitted infections, dealing with parents and tapping resources for referral. The report's appendix highlights eight conditions that can be mistaken for possible sexual abuse.

The Evaluation of Children in the Primary Care Setting When Sexual Abuse is Suspected is published in the August 2013 issue of *Pediatrics*. (See page 31 of this collection.)

"The major difference in this report and others is this is really very practical advice — like nuts and bolts," said Carole Jenny, M.D., M.B.A., FAAP, lead author of the report from the AAP Committee on Child Abuse and Neglect.

Dr. Jenny said it takes into account pediatricians who have experts in the community as opposed to those in areas where there may not be a single child abuse doctor in the whole state.

Sexual abuse of children occurs commonly, is underdiagnosed and can have lifelong effects. In 2006, 1.8 children per 1,000, or 135,000 children, were victims, according to one national study. Other studies say 5% to 25% of adults reported being sexually abused as children.

Victims often wait years before revealing abuse. One study cited in the report notes that more than half of sexually abused children do not disclose their abuse until they are adults.

A major factor in the child's long-term mental health outcome is whether he or she was believed and supported, according to Dr. Jenny. Yet one of the misperceptions surrounding child sexual abuse — sometimes believed by medical and legal experts — is that kids lie. "I don't think there's any evidence to think that this is an extensive problem," she said. "Kids are much more likely not to talk about it than to make something up."

Still, very young children can be suggestible, Dr. Jenny said, such as in the case where a parent constantly asks a young child coming home from a visitation with the other parent if somebody touched him or her.

Parents should not repeatedly press a child to reveal details of an incident of abuse because this can contaminate the interview. "We want to keep the child's words as clear as possible in their own perceptions," Dr. Jenny noted.

Advice in the clinical report includes the following:

Guidance for pediatricians

- Understand state child abuse reporting laws and how to report.
- Be aware of normal, developmentally appropriate variations in children's sexual behaviors, as well as normal and abnormal genital and anal anatomy.
- Stay up-to-date on community resources for help in evaluation of alleged abuse.
- Seek second expert opinions when a child's physical exam is thought to be abnormal.
- Know when and where to refer cases of acute abuse or assault that require forensic testing, prophylaxis for sexually transmitted infections, HIV and emergency contraception.

Interviewing children about possible sexual abuse

- A child spontaneously disclosing abuse should know it's OK to talk about it.
- During the interview, the child should be separated from the parent, if possible. (The parent will be present for the exam if that is the child's preference.)
- When there is no pre-established relationship with the patient, spend time talking about nonthreatening issues. The child should know it's the doctor's job to keep kids healthy, and it's OK to talk about difficult subjects.
- Don't ask leading or suggestive questions.
- Use developmentally appropriate language, with translators if necessary. The parents can be asked about terms the family uses.
- Record descriptions of abuse given by the child verbatim, using quotation marks. Attribute the remarks to the child. Record impressions but identify them as such.
- Do not coerce the child to talk about abuse, and don't offer rewards for doing so.
- Be supportive and empathic, but don't act shocked, outraged or dismissive.

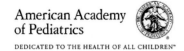

Guidance for the Clinician in
Rendering Pediatric Care

CLINICAL REPORT

The Evaluation of Children in the Primary Care Setting When Sexual Abuse Is Suspected

abstract

This clinical report updates a 2005 report from the American Academy of Pediatrics on the evaluation of sexual abuse in children. The medical assessment of suspected child sexual abuse should include obtaining a history, performing a physical examination, and obtaining appropriate laboratory tests. The role of the physician includes determining the need to report suspected sexual abuse; assessing the physical, emotional, and behavioral consequences of sexual abuse; providing information to parents about how to support their child; and coordinating with other professionals to provide comprehensive treatment and follow-up of children exposed to child sexual abuse. *Pediatrics* 2013;132:e558–e567

Carole Jenny, MD, MBA, James E. Crawford-Jakubiak, MD, and COMMITTEE ON CHILD ABUSE AND NEGLECT

KEY WORD
sexual abuse

ABBREVIATIONS
AAP—American Academy of Pediatrics
HIV—human immunodeficiency virus
NAAT—nucleic acid amplification test
STI—sexually transmitted infection

INTRODUCTION

Sexual abuse of children and adolescents is a common problem that is potentially damaging to their long-term physical and psychological health. The Fourth National Incidence Study on Child Abuse and Neglect[1] estimated that in 2006, 1.8 children per 1000 (or a total of 135 300 children) were victims of sexual abuse. Other national studies have found that 5% to 25% of adults reported being sexually abused as children, depending on the population studied and the methods used to define sexual abuse.[2–7] Pediatricians are likely to care for sexually abused children in their practices, even though many victims wait years before telling anyone about their abuse.[8,9] More than half of sexually abused children do not disclose their abuse until they are adults.[10]

A history of childhood sexual abuse can have lifelong deleterious effects on a child's physical and mental health. Sexual abuse increases the risk of developing posttraumatic stress disorder, anxiety disorder, depression,[11,12] low self-esteem,[13] and social phobias.[14] Children exposed to sexual abuse are more likely to need hospitalization for mental illness.[15] Adult survivors of child sexual abuse are more likely to become victims of intimate partner violence and sexual assault.[16,17] They are at higher risk of developing obesity,[18] sexual problems,[19] irritable bowel syndrome,[20] fibromyalgia,[21] and sexually transmitted infections (STIs), including infection with the human immunodeficiency virus (HIV).[22,23] They use more medical services as adults than those without a history of child sexual abuse[21,24] and are more likely to develop addictions to tobacco, drugs, and alcohol.[25–27]

www.pediatrics.org/cgi/doi/10.1542/peds.2013-1741

doi:10.1542/peds.2013-1741

All clinical reports from the American Academy of Pediatrics automatically expire 5 years after publication unless reaffirmed, revised, or retired at or before that time.

PEDIATRICS (ISSN Numbers: Print, 0031-4005; Online, 1098-4275).

In summary, child sexual abuse occurs commonly and can have lifelong effects on victims' physical and mental health. When the issue of possible sexual abuse is raised in the clinical setting, it is important for pediatricians to know how to respond to and evaluate the child, when to refer the child for evaluation by other professionals, when to report the case to the appropriate investigative agency, and how to counsel parents to decrease the long-term deleterious effects of the abuse. This clinical report updates an American Academy of Pediatrics (AAP) report from 2005 titled "The Evaluation of Sexual Abuse in Children."[28]

RESPONDING TO A PARENT'S CONCERN ABOUT POSSIBLE SEXUAL ABUSE

When a parent brings up the possibility of sexual abuse of his or her child, the pediatrician should immediately exclude the child from the discussion. Children (particularly young children) might be influenced by hearing their parents' concerns about abuse. Sometimes parents are overconcerned about normal childhood sexual behavior.[29] In those cases, reassuring and educating the parents will probably assuage their fears. Parents' overconcern could be related to their own adverse experiences in childhood, and in such cases, a more in-depth assessment to assist the parent is needed. Occasionally, parents might have concerns about possible sexual abuse because of relationship issues that arise between caregivers. Many of these concerns are raised in good faith but ultimately unfounded. Notwithstanding these caveats, every concern about possible sexual abuse should be approached objectively, thoughtfully, and with an open mind.

The pediatrician faces many challenges in evaluating possible sexual abuse to determine which cases warrant an immediate intervention in the office and which cases warrant reporting to investigative agencies or referral for evaluation by other professionals. In all these cases, the pediatrician should carefully document the parent's concerns, take a detailed history of the nature of the child's disclosure from the parents' perspective, ask what questions the parent used in eliciting the disclosure, and document a complete medical history, social history, and review of systems for urogenital and behavioral problems. It is important to note in the record the source of the information documented in the medical record. For example, be sure to say, "Mother tells me that the child said . . .," rather than writing, "The child said. . . ."

Often, a child will present to the pediatrician after direct disclosure to another person regarding sexual abuse. Less commonly, a child presents to the pediatrician with an abnormal genital or anal examination, pregnancy, an STI, or sexual abuse witnessed by a third party or by discovery of sexually graphic images or videos in the possession of a potential perpetrator. The general pediatrician's response depends on what resources are available in the community. Many communities and regions have specialized clinics or child advocacy centers where children can be referred when concerns of sexual abuse arise. In areas without these resources, the general pediatrician is often the most knowledgeable professional in the community regarding the evaluation and interviewing of children. If pediatricians find that their regions do not offer specialized abuse-related services (eg, child advocacy centers or hospital-based child protection programs), it is important for them to educate themselves about childhood genital and anal examinations and about how to interview children to get enough information to make appropriate decisions about reporting to child protective service agencies, referring to counseling facilities, or referring to pediatric clinics specializing in abuse evaluations. The AAP offers a variety of educational materials on child abuse to physicians, including a comprehensive CD-ROM,[30] textbooks on child abuse,[31,32] and educational offerings at the National Conference and Exhibition.

Whenever the issue of possible child sexual abuse arises in the office setting, 5 important issues should be addressed.

1. **The child's safety.** Is the child safe to go home? Is the child at imminent risk of additional harm if sent back to an environment where a possible perpetrator has access to the child? Is the child likely to be harmed or punished for disclosing abuse? Is there concern that the child might be coerced or intimidated to recant the disclosure? If any of these questions are answered "yes" or "maybe," this is a child protection emergency, and the appropriate authorities (child protective services or law enforcement) should be contacted immediately.

2. **Reporting to child protection authorities.** If the child is not at imminent risk, the pediatrician should decide whether child protective services should be contacted about the allegation. It is important to remember that in every state, and in all provinces and territories in Canada, it is mandated that professionals report *suspected* child abuse and neglect to the appropriate government agency (child protective services or police agencies, including tribal agencies). Studies have shown that some pediatricians are hesitant to involve outside agencies,

even if they strongly suspect abuse has occurred.[33] Pediatricians worry about the intrusion of agencies into family life, the risk of the child being separated from the parents, or the possibility that the family will leave the practice if reported to a child protection agency. Some pediatricians have experienced negative interactions with child protection agencies, which could make them distrustful of an agency's response and its effect on the family.[34] Some physicians might overestimate their ability to manage the situation within their practice. Physicians should not let these concerns act as barriers to protecting a child. In the United States, physicians are protected against liability for reporting a reasonable suspicion of child abuse and neglect if the report is made in good faith. This is also the case in many other jurisdictions, but because laws can vary, it is important for physicians to be familiar with the laws that pertain to their practice. Still, the safety of the child should take precedence over the physician's fear of lawsuits.

One problem lies in the definition of *suspected*. If a parent is going through a contentious divorce and the child is having symptoms of anxiety and depression, should abuse be suspected? If a child is sexually acting out with peers, should abuse be suspected? Each pediatrician will need to consider the facts of the individual case when making the decision to report suspected child abuse while bearing in mind the statutory requirements for reporting suspected abuse in his or her state. The threshold for reporting is low. The pediatrician should report when there is a reasonable suspicion that the child was abused. The child protective services agency then has the responsibility to conduct a thorough investigation to determine whether abuse has occurred.

3. **The child's mental health.** In every case, the patient should be assessed for possible mental health problems, and if any are identified, appropriate emergency mental health care should be sought. The initial disclosure of abuse can be extremely stressful for a young person. It is important to consider the possibility that symptoms of depression and posttraumatic stress disorder might already have developed. The family might be angry at the child because the disclosure has introduced stress into the family or because the threatened loss of a family member could result in financial insecurity. A disclosure of sexual abuse is perhaps one of the most explosive events that can occur in a family.

4. **The need for a physical examination.** If sexual abuse is suspected, a thorough examination should be performed to rule out injury, particularly if a child is reporting genital or anal pain or bleeding. If the abuse occurred in the distant past and the asymptomatic child is going to be referred to a specialty center for medical evaluation, examination might be deferred. If the child reports dysuria, a urinalysis is indicated. Rarely, acute sexual assault can cause severe genital or anal injury that can lead to excessive blood loss (a medical emergency).

5. **The need for forensic evidence collection.** Children who have had recent sexual contact involving the exchange of bodily fluids should be immediately referred to a specialized clinic or emergency department capable of collecting evidence using a forensic evidence kit.[35] Many states recommend that forensic evidence be collected if less than 72 hours have passed since the assault. Some states require evidence kits to be performed as late as 96 hours after assault. Some evidence supports limiting collection of forensic evidence in prepubertal children to those who present within 24 hours after assault.[36,37] As more laboratories use DNA testing to analyze forensic specimens, however, the time for collection of useful forensic evidence might be extended beyond the current 72-hour standard.[38,39] Pediatricians should familiarize themselves with the relevant policies of the jurisdiction in which they practice. The referral center also should be capable of evaluating the child for the appropriateness of antiretroviral HIV prophylaxis,[40] postexposure prophylaxis for STIs,[41] and pregnancy prophylaxis. HIV and pregnancy prophylaxis should be given as soon after the sexual contact as possible and are not recommended more than 72 hours after contact.

INTERVIEWING CHILDREN ABOUT POSSIBLE SEXUAL ABUSE

Depending on the community services available, the pediatrician should be prepared to conduct a basic interview with a verbal child about an abuse experience. Often, this is necessary to make the appropriate decision about referral to another facility or to report to child protective services. Several fundamental guidelines inform this process.

1. If the child spontaneously discloses abuse, it is important that the person hearing the disclosure respond by telling the child it is okay to talk about it with adults. If the child begins to make a disclosure and the physician says, "I'm

not the person you should tell this to," the child might be hesitant to disclose at another time.

2. The child should be separated from the parent for the interview if at all possible. Parents can subtly or not-so-subtly influence the child's statements. Separation from the parent is particularly important if the parent is a suspected perpetrator or is supportive of the suspected perpetrator, to prevent the child from feeling intimidated or threatened. The parent will later be present for the examination if that is the child's preference.

3. If the pediatrician has not already established a relationship with the patient, some time should be spent talking about nonthreatening issues, such as school, friends, or pets. It is difficult for a child to be asked painful or embarrassing questions without first feeling safe and supported by the adult asking the questions.

4. Pediatricians should tell children that it is their job as doctors to keep children healthy and that it is okay for children to talk about difficult or uncomfortable subjects with their doctors.

5. The pediatrician should not ask leading or suggestive questions. It is important to begin with open-ended, general questions about the child's likes and dislikes or about the people in the child's family. Then ask about things the child is worried or confused about, or about things that have happened to the child that have been unpleasant or stressful. A question should never suggest an answer. Examples of open-ended questions include the following:

"Is anything bothering you?"

"Tell me why you're here today."

"Do you think he would want you to tell me what happened?"

Examples of incorrect questions are as follows:

"Who touched your privates?"

"I know that Uncle Joe hurt you; tell me about it."

6. Developmentally appropriate language should be used with the child. The terms and concepts understood by a 12-year-old are very different from those understood by a 4-year-old. Be aware of the terms the child uses for the genitalia and anus. The parents should be asked in advance which terms the family uses for private parts and bathroom activities.

7. Any descriptions of abuse given by the child should be recorded word for word (using quotation marks) in the medical record, using the child's own language, and should be attributed to the child. When practical, the response should be recorded together with the question. For example, "When asked why she was not wearing underwear, the patient answered that . . ." or "Without my asking, the child stated that. . . ." Careful notes should be taken during the interview. Video or audio recording of the interview is not needed unless this is part of the pediatrician's regular practice.

8. The child should not be urged or coerced to talk about abuse. The child should be allowed to talk about it if he or she wants to, but there should never be an expectation that the child must disclose to the professional. The child should not be rewarded after a disclosure. (For example, "Tell me what happened with Uncle Joe, and then you can go back to your mom" is not an appropriate statement.) Forcing a child who has been abused to give a disclosure can be experienced by the

child as revictimization and loss of control and can make an already painful experience worse.

9. The pediatrician should remember that this is a *medical* interview and that he or she is obtaining information needed to make the appropriate diagnostic and treatment decisions. If the child makes an initial disclosure to the pediatrician, it is likely that the child will be interviewed again by another adult professional. Parents and children can be told this before the interview begins. Professionals with advanced training in forensic interviewing conduct a very different type of interview than the medical interview conducted in the clinical setting. Although it is important to avoid multiple interviews of the child, in many situations the interview will be a 2-stage process in which the initial evaluator obtains minimal facts to evaluate the need to report to the authorities, and a forensic evaluator conducts a more detailed interview.

10. The pediatrician should be supportive and empathic. Treat the patient with the same respect and caring given to all your patients. If the child tells you about abuse, show appropriate concern; do not act shocked, outraged, or dismissive.

11. Appropriate language should be used to interview children. Translators should be used if necessary, and the child's use of words to describe body parts should be understood.

12. If the pediatrician records his or her impression of the child's emotions during the examination or interview, these subjective impressions should be identified as such (eg, "It was my impression

that the child seemed agitated."). Similarly, if an observation is made that may bear on the truthfulness of the history, it should be clearly identified as separate from fact (eg, "I noted that the child and her mother used identical words when answering this same question. I therefore considered the possibility that the answers may have been rehearsed.").

THE PHYSICAL EXAMINATION WHEN SEXUAL ABUSE IS SUSPECTED

Studies have shown that pediatricians often have not been properly trained to examine the genitals and anuses of children when abuse is suspected.[42] Some of the most basic knowledge, such as the appropriate identification of anatomic structures, has not always been part of pediatric residencies or physicians' continuing education.[43,44] Appropriate techniques for evaluating children's anogenital regions are an important part of pediatric education.

When the question of sexual abuse arises in the medical setting, the pediatrician might want to consider whether the child should be triaged to another facility for evaluation, such as a child advocacy center or a specialized abuse assessment clinic at a children's hospital (after considering the safety questions discussed previously). If the pediatrician does not think that the situation constitutes an emergency, he or she should consider referring the child for evaluation if he or she is not confident that he or she has the necessary examination skills. Unnecessary multiple anogenital examinations should be avoided because they can be upsetting to a sexually abused child. On the other hand, routine examination of the genitals and anus (appropriately chaperoned)[45] during well child examinations can help patients and parents understand that anogenital health is as important as the health of other parts of the body and will familiarize pediatricians with normal anatomic structures.

The anogenital examination should be preceded by a thorough general physical examination. Children who have experienced one type of abuse also are at risk for other types of abuse or neglect. In addition, the general physical examination establishes the physician's role and is likely to be an event the child has previously experienced at a physician's office.

The nature and process of the examination should be explained to the child in age-appropriate language before the examination takes place. An appropriate chaperone must be present. Most children will want a same-gender parent in the room during the examination. If a parent is not available, a second medical professional should be in the room to reassure the child, to assist the examining physician, and to act as a chaperone. A parent or caring professional at the head of the examination table can provide support for the child as well as reasonable assurance and distraction during the examination. Use of appropriate gowns and drapes can protect the child's modesty and make the child feel less vulnerable.

The examination of the genitalia and anus does not require the use of instruments in most cases. For girls, separation of the labia and gentle labial traction while the child is supine with the knees bent and hips abducted (frog-leg position) will adequately expose the genital structures. Speculum examinations are contraindicated in prepubertal children in the office setting. If intravaginal trauma is suspected, vaginoscopy should be performed under anesthesia.

In an adolescent, an examination for sexual abuse should follow the recommendations of the AAP regarding intravaginal examination using a speculum.[46] In many cases, a speculum examination is not needed in the absence of signs or symptoms of genital disease but is usually indicated after acute vaginal sexual assault to document injuries and to collect forensic specimens.[47] Girls should receive their first cervical cytologic examination (Papanicolaou test) at 21 years of age unless there are special circumstances, such as immune suppression or infection with HIV.[46,48]

For boys, the examination of the genitals consists of inspection of the penis and scrotum, documenting any noted trauma or scarring and any other abnormalities.

Examination of the anus is performed in most cases by external inspection with gentle traction of the buttocks to expose the anal sphincter while the child is supine with the knees pulled up to the chest (cannon-ball position). Anoscopy or a digital rectal examination is not routinely indicated.

Documenting the findings of the anogenital examination is important. In specialty centers, the examination is usually documented with photographs or videos. In the pediatric office, a detailed description of the structures will suffice. If photographs are taken, however, they should be treated as a confidential part of the medical record, and care should be taken to label them for proper identification.

An expert committee that has written practice standards for medical examinations in child advocacy centers recommends that all examinations be reviewed by an expert clinician.[49] This usually entails a secondary review of photographs or videos to verify the physical findings. If the examination findings are deemed to be abnormal or consistent with trauma, pediatricians also should have a secondary review of physical findings, either by having a clinician experienced in forensic anogenital examinations review the photographs or by referring the child to a center specializing in child abuse. Studies have shown there to be better agreement on interpretation of examination findings when clinicians have had extensive experience and education in the evaluation of child sexual abuse.[50]

All pediatricians should gain experience in the anogenital examination of children and adolescents. Many conditions can mimic trauma. It is important to recognize these findings and to distinguish them from lesions caused by child abuse.[51] The Supplemental Appendix reviews genital and anal conditions that can be confused with sexual abuse.

Most sexually abused children have normal anogenital examinations.[52,53] Many types of molestation (eg, oral genital contact or fondling) leave no permanent scars or marks. Even children who have been sexually penetrated often have normal examinations.[53,54] Anogenital tissues heal quickly and completely after many types of anal or genital trauma.[55,56] A normal examination of the genitals and anus neither confirms nor rules out sexual abuse. This fact should be mentioned in the assessment portion of the record. After the examination, it is important to reassure the child that he or she is healthy.

TESTING FOR STIs

STIs occur infrequently in prepubertal sexually abused children. A recent multisite prospective study of 536 children evaluated for suspected sexual abuse revealed that 8.2% of the female children younger than 14 years had an STI.[57] *Chlamydia trachomatis*

infections were found in 3.1% of the girls, and *Neisseria gonorrhoeae* infections were found in 3.3%. Only 1 girl tested positive for syphilis (0.3%), and none tested positive for HIV. Five of 12 girls with genital lesions tested positive for herpes simplex virus. Five of 85 symptomatic girls (5.9%) had *Trichomonas vaginalis* identified on a wet mount. Girls with vaginal discharge were more likely to have an STI.

Because STIs are not common in prepubertal children evaluated for abuse, culturing all sites for all organisms is not recommended if the child is asymptomatic. Each case should be evaluated individually for STI risk. Factors that should lead the physician to consider screening for STI include the following[41]:

1. Child has experienced penetration of the genitalia or anus.

2. Child has been abused by a stranger.

3. Child has been abused by a perpetrator known to be infected with an STI or at high risk of STIs (intravenous drug abusers, men who have sex with men, or people with multiple sexual partners).

4. Child has a sibling or other relative in the household with an STI.

5. Child lives in an area with a high rate of STI in the community.

6. Child has signs or symptoms of STIs.

7. Child has already been diagnosed with 1 STI.

Sexually abused adolescents are at higher risk of STIs and should be screened for all STIs, as would any sexually active adolescent presenting for routine care.

Genital and anal infections with *N gonorrhoeae* are rarely acquired perinatally, and outside the newborn period they are considered likely to be caused by sexual abuse.[58] *C trachomatis* infections in children older than

3 years also are likely to be sexually transmitted.[59] *T vaginalis* infection also should raise a concern of possible abuse.[60] Herpes simplex virus and genital warts (human papillomavirus) can be sexually transmitted in children, but these infections are not diagnostic of abuse by themselves.[61] HIV infections in children who have not been exposed to the virus perinatally, through blood products, or by needle sticks are also highly likely to be caused by abuse.[62] In any case of an STI in a child, a careful investigation into risk factors and contacts should be conducted, a thorough medical and social history should be obtained, and the child should be evaluated for possible sexual abuse.

The recommendations for laboratory methods best used to detect infection with *C trachomatis* and *N gonorrhoeae* in abused children are evolving. Current standards require these organisms to be confirmed by culture in cases of suspected sexual abuse that involve the legal system.[41] However, a recent multicenter study found that commercially available nucleic acid amplification tests (NAATs) are highly sensitive and specific for these organisms and that these tests provide "a better alternative than culture as a forensic standard."[63] The study also found that NAATs performed on urine specimens worked as well as vaginal swabs to detect infection in both prepubertal and postpubertal girls, obviating more invasive tests. All positive NAAT results in this study were confirmed by genotypic and sequence analysis tests, leading to a high positive predictive value for *C trachomatis* and *N gonorrhoeae*.

In medicolegal cases, culture-based tests have been preferred because of their high specificity (nearing 100%). This would make the possibility of a false-positive result highly unlikely. Unfortunately, culture-based tests for *C trachomatis* and *N gonorrhoeae* are very insensitive. In addition, many laboratories no longer offer culture-based tests, making it impossible to screen victims for infection using culture methods. If laboratories do maintain limited culture facilities, they would be more likely to provide false results, given limited experience with cultures. Because NAATs provide highly sensitive detection of organisms and their specificity approaches that of culture, the AAP recommends the use of NAATs when evaluating children and adolescents for genital infections with *C trachomatis* and *N gonorrhoeae*.

All positive test results should be considered presumptive evidence of infection and, if used, should be interpreted with caution. Positive results should be confirmed using additional tests in populations with a low prevalence of the infection or when a false-positive test could have an adverse outcome. When establishing a protocol to evaluate positive NAAT results for *N gonorrhoeae* or *C trachomatis*, experts in laboratory medicine and pediatric infectious diseases should be consulted to determine appropriate secondary tests. All positive specimens in suspected abuse cases should be retained by the laboratory for additional testing.

Recently, various rapid antigen tests, DNA hybridization tests, and NAATs have been developed for *Candida* species, *Gardnerella vaginalis,* and *T vaginalis*.[64] These tests have not been extensively studied in children and should not be used at this time. Bacterial vaginosis (the vaginosis associated with *G vaginalis*) and genital candidiasis are not specific indicators of sexual abuse.

By recommending the use of NAATs for *N gonorrhoeae* and *C trachomatis* in cases of suspected sexual abuse of children, the AAP recognizes that pediatricians' first priority should be protecting the health of children. The pediatrician should be considered primarily a provider of health care for children and should prioritize ensuring the health and well-being of their patients rather than focusing on the legal outcome of criminal cases. In practice, rarely have cases of suspected sexual abuse been adjudicated on the basis of a positive test result for an STI alone in the absence of a history, physical finding, or other confirmatory evidence of abuse. Although properly collected, tested, and confirmed laboratory specimens can aid in the prosecution of sex offenders, the pediatrician's main responsibility lies in protecting the child's health.

The Food and Drug Administration has not approved NAATs for the diagnosis of *C trachomatis* or *N gonorrhoeae* infections of the throat or anus. The Food and Drug Administration does allow laboratories to use NAATs for testing nongenital specimens if the individual laboratory undergoes internal validation of the method used in a method verification study. In verification studies, positive and negative specimens are compared with reference standards or with results from a second laboratory.[65] No studies have been published evaluating the use of nongenital-site NAATs in prepubertal children. However, studies in adults have had promising results when using some NAATs to test for rectal or pharyngeal *N gonorrhoeae* and *Chlamydia* infections in high-risk populations.[66–68] At this point, the use of NAATs in children for rectal or pharyngeal specimens is not warranted until more research is available. If used, they should be interpreted with caution.

If diagnosed with an STI, the child should be treated promptly. When there is a possibility that the child has been exposed to HIV, proper follow-up or prophylaxis is needed. When appropriate, consideration should be given to treating the patient with emergency contraception.

WORKING WITH FAMILIES TO MITIGATE THE ADVERSE EFFECTS OF SEXUAL ABUSE

When children disclose sexual abuse, people close to them are usually deeply affected. Parents often have feelings of guilt for not protecting their children[68,69] and might experience intense anger at the abusers. A child's disclosure can exacerbate a parent's own feelings about his or her adverse childhood experiences. Previous family conflict (eg, marital conflict, substance abuse issues) can be aggravated. Some parents want to sweep the disclosure under the rug to avoid dealing with the painful reality. Family members can feel protective of the accused abuser, especially if that person is another family member. Families should be given the following guidance about how to respond to children who disclose abuse.

1. Parents should understand that medical professionals are required to report suspected abuse to the proper authorities for investigation. It is not an option for the pediatrician to keep the disclosure secret.

2. It is important for families to cooperate with agencies investigating the alleged abuse.

3. Studies have shown that the long-term outcomes of children who have experienced sexual abuse are better if they are believed and supported after a disclosure.[11,70] The parents' initial response to the disclosure is important. If the parents show extreme distress and become nonfunctional, the child will feel less secure and less protected. If the parents are openly emotional and weeping, the child might feel that he or she has to recant or minimize the abuse to decrease the parents' distress.

Parents should respond in a calm and protective manner, assuring the child that the abuse was not his or her fault and that they will do all they can to protect the child and keep him or her safe.

4. Parents should not independently try to question the child or accuse the child of lying. If the child wants to talk about the abuse experience, the parent should listen and be supportive, but it is not helpful to repeatedly question the child or force the child to describe the abuse in detail. This type of questioning can be damaging to the legal adjudication of the case.

5. Pediatricians can provide guidance to families by recognizing the importance of mental health assessment after childhood trauma and by familiarizing themselves with mental health treatments that have been shown to be effective in ameliorating the effects of abuse.[71] Children should be treated by therapists with proper training and experience in dealing with child trauma. Options are available to facilitate the delivery of psychological services to abused children through child advocacy centers, community mental health centers, and victims' compensation programs.

GUIDANCE FOR PEDIATRICIANS

1. Pediatricians should understand the mandatory child abuse reporting laws in their states and should know how to make a report to the responsible agency in their jurisdiction that investigates cases of alleged child sexual abuse.

2. Pediatricians should recognize that sexual abuse of children occurs commonly, and they should be prepared to respond appropriately in their clinical practices.

3. Pediatricians should be aware of normal, developmentally appropriate variations in children's sexual behaviors.[29]

4. Pediatricians should be aware of community resources available to assist in the evaluation of alleged child abuse.

5. Pediatricians should be educated about normal and abnormal genital and anal anatomy in children.

6. Pediatricians should seek a second expert opinion in cases of child sexual abuse when the child's anal or genital examination is thought to be abnormal.

7. Pediatricians should know when and where to refer cases of acute alleged sexual abuse or assault that require forensic testing, prophylaxis for STIs and HIV, and emergency contraception.

8. Pediatricians should know the importance of using nonleading, open-ended questions if they are asking questions about possible abuse.

9. Pediatricians should understand how to support children and families when child sexual abuse is suspected.

10. Pediatricians should be aware of the effects of sexual abuse on children's mental health and be able to refer abused children to mental health professionals who have expertise in treating child trauma.

11. Advice on protection of children from sexual abuse should be part of the anticipatory guidance given to parents in the medical home. The AAP Web site provides guidance for pediatricians (http://www.aap.org/en-us/advocacy-and-policy/aap-health-initiatives/Medical-Home-for-Children-and-Adolescents-Exposed-to-Violence/Pages/Sexual-Abuse.aspx) and for parents (http://www.aap.org/en-us/about-the-aap/aap-press-room/news-features-and-safety-tips/Pages/Parent-Tips-for-Preventing-and-Identifying-Child-Sexual-Abuse.aspx) about preventing child sexual abuse. In addition, the AAP developed an educational toolkit for "Preventing Sexual Violence" (https://www2.aap.org/pubserv/PSVpreview/pages/main.html).

LEAD AUTHORS
Carole Jenny, MD, MBA, FAAP Former Committee Member
James E. Crawford-Jakubiak, MD, FAAP

COMMITTEE ON CHILD ABUSE AND NEGLECT, 2011–2012
Cindy W. Christian, MD, Chairperson, FAAP
James E. Crawford-Jakubiak, MD, FAAP
Emalee G. Flaherty, MD, FAAP
John M. Leventhal, MD, FAAP
James L. Lukefahr, MD, FAAP
Robert D. Sege MD, PhD, FAAP

LIAISONS
Harriet MacMillan, MD, American Academy of Child and Adolescent Psychiatry
Catherine M. Nolan, MSW, ACSW, Administration for Children, Youth, and Families
Janet Saul, PhD, Centers for Disease Control and Prevention

STAFF
Tammy Piazza Hurley

REFERENCES

1. Kellogg N; American Academy of Pediatrics Committee on Child Abuse and Neglect. The evaluation of sexual abuse in children. *Pediatrics.* 2005;116(2):506–512

2. Sedlak AJ, Mettenburg J, Basena M, et al. Fourth National Incidence Study of Child Abuse and Neglect (NIS-4): 2004–2009. Washington, DC: US Department of Health and Human Services, Administration for Children and Families; 2010. Available at: www.acf.hhs.gov/programs/opre/abuse_neglect/natl_incid/index.html. Accessed November 4, 2012

3. Saunders BE, Kilpatrick DG, Hanson RF, Resnick HS, Walker ME. Prevalence, case characteristics, and long-term psychological correlates of child rape among women: a national survey. *Child Maltreat.* 1999;4(3): 187–200

4. Tjaden P, Thoennes N. Full Report of the Prevalence, Incidence, and Consequences of Violence Against Women: Findings From the National Violence Against Women Survey. Washington, DC: US Department of Justice, National Institute of Justice; 2000. Available at: https://www.ncjrs.gov/pdffiles1/nij/183781.pdf. Accessed November 4, 2012

5. Finkelhor D. Current information on the scope and nature of child sexual abuse. *Future Child.* 1994;4(2):31–53

6. Finkelhor D, Turner H, Ormrod R, Hamby SL. Violence, abuse, and crime exposure in a national sample of children and youth. *Pediatrics.* 2009;124(5):1411–1423

7. Finkelhor D, Ormrod RK, Turner HA. Lifetime assessment of poly-victimization in a national sample of children and youth. *Child Abuse Negl.* 2009;33(7):403–411

8. Hanson RF, Self-Brown S, Fricker-Elhai AE, Kilpatrick DG, Saunders BE, Resnick HS. The relations between family environment and violence exposure among youth: findings from the national survey of adolescents. *Child Maltreat.* 2006;11(1):3–15

9. Kogan SM. Disclosing unwanted sexual experiences: results from a national sample of adolescent women. *Child Abuse Negl.* 2004;28(2):147–165

10. Smith DW, Letourneau EJ, Saunders BE, Kilpatrick DG, Resnick HS, Best CL. Delay in disclosure of childhood rape: results from a national survey. *Child Abuse Negl.* 2000;24(2):273–287

11. Roesler TA. Reactions to disclosure of childhood sexual abuse. The effect on adult symptoms. *J Nerv Ment Dis.* 1994;182(11): 618–624

12. Jonas S, Bebbington P, McManus S, et al. Sexual abuse and psychiatric disorder in England: results from the 2007 Adult Psychiatric Morbidity Survey. *Psychol Med.* 2011;41(4):709–719

13. Deblinger E, Mannarino AP, Cohen JA, Steer RA. A follow-up study of a multisite, randomized, controlled trial for children with sexual abuse–related PTSD symptoms. *J Am Acad Child Adolesc Psychiatry.* 2006;45(12):1474–1484

14. Swanston HY, Plunkett AM, O'Toole BI, Shrimpton S, Parkinson PN, Oates RK. Nine years after child sexual abuse. *Child Abuse Negl.* 2003;27(8):967–984

15. Simon NM, Herlands NN, Marks EH, et al. Childhood maltreatment linked to greater symptom severity and poorer quality of life and function in social anxiety disorder. *Depress Anxiety.* 2009;26(11):1027–1032

16. Boxer P, Terranova AM. Effects of multiple maltreatment experiences among psychiatrically hospitalized youth. *Child Abuse Negl.* 2008;32(6):637–647

17. DiLillo D, Guiffre D, Tremblay GC, Peterson L. A closer look at the nature of intimate partner violence reported by women with a history of child sexual abuse. *J Interpers Violence.* 2001;16(2):116–132

18. Messman-Moore TL, Walsh KL, DiLillo D. Emotion dysregulation and risky sexual behavior in revictimization. *Child Abuse Negl.* 2010;34(12):967–976

19. Midei AJ, Matthews KA. Interpersonal violence in childhood as a risk factor for obesity: a systematic review of the literature and proposed pathways. *Obes Rev.* 2011;12(5):e159–e172

20. Feiring C, Simon VA, Cleland CM. Childhood sexual abuse, stigmatization, internalizing symptoms, and the development of sexual difficulties and dating aggression. *J Consult Clin Psychol.* 2009;77(1):127–137

21. Walker EA, Gelfand AN, Gelfand MD, Katon WJ. Psychiatric diagnoses, sexual and physical victimization, and disability in patients with irritable bowel syndrome or inflammatory bowel disease. *Psychol Med.* 1995;25(6):1259–1267

22. Finestone HM, Stenn P, Davies F, Stalker C, Fry R, Koumanis J. Chronic pain and health care utilization in women with a history of childhood sexual abuse. *Child Abuse Negl.* 2000;24(4):547–556

23. Jones DJ, Runyan DK, Lewis T, et al. Trajectories of childhood sexual abuse and early adolescent HIV/AIDS risk behaviors: the role of other maltreatment, witnessed violence, and child gender. *J Clin Child Adolesc Psychol.* 2010;39(5):667–680

24. Mosack KE, Randolph ME, Dickson-Gomez J, Abbott M, Smith E, Weeks MR. Sexual risk-taking among high-risk urban women with and without histories of childhood sexual abuse: mediating effects of contextual factors. *J Child Sex Abuse.* 2010;19(1):43–61

25. Arnow BA, Hart S, Scott C, Dea R, O'Connell L, Taylor CB. Childhood sexual abuse, psychological distress, and medical use among women. *Psychosom Med.* 1999;61(6):762–770

26. Topitzes J, Mersky JP, Reynolds AJ. Child maltreatment and adult cigarette smoking:

a long-term developmental model. *J Pediatr Psychol.* 2010;35(5):484–498

27. Khoury L, Tang YL, Bradley B, Cubells JF, Ressler KJ. Substance use, childhood traumatic experience, and posttraumatic stress disorder in an urban civilian population. *Depress Anxiety.* 2010;27(12):1077–1086

28. Najdowski CJ, Ullman SE. Prospective effects of sexual victimization on PTSD and problem drinking. *Addict Behav.* 2009;34(11):965–968

29. Kellogg ND; Committee on Child Abuse and Neglect, American Academy of Pediatrics. Clinical report: the evaluation of sexual behaviors in children. *Pediatrics.* 2009;124(3):992–998

30. Lowen D, Reece RM. *Visual Diagnosis of Child Abuse on CD-ROM,* 3rd ed. Elk Grove Village, IL: American Academy of Pediatrics; 2008

31. Finkel MA, Giardino AP, eds. *Medical Evaluation of Child Sexual Abuse: A Practical Guide,* 3rd ed. Elk Grove Village, IL: American Academy of Pediatrics; 2009

32. Reece RM, Christian C, eds. *Child Abuse: Medical Diagnosis and Management,* 3rd ed. Elk Grove Village, IL: American Academy of Pediatrics; 2008

33. Flaherty EG, Sege RD, Griffith J, et al; PROS network; NMAPedsNet. From suspicion of physical child abuse to reporting: primary care clinician decision-making. *Pediatrics.* 2008;122(3):611–619

34. Flaherty EG, Jones R, Sege R; Child Abuse Recognition Experience Study Research Group. Telling their stories: primary care practitioners' experience evaluating and reporting injuries caused by child abuse. *Child Abuse Negl.* 2004;28(9):939–945

35. American Academy of Pediatrics Committee on Child Abuse and Neglect. Guidelines for the evaluation of sexual abuse of children: subject review. *Pediatrics.* 1999;103(1):186–191

36. Young KL, Jones JG, Worthington T, Simpson P, Casey PH. Forensic laboratory evidence in sexually abused children and adolescents. *Arch Pediatr Adolesc Med.* 2006;160(6):585–588

37. Christian CW, Lavelle JM, De Jong AR, Loiselle J, Brenner L, Joffe M. Forensic evidence findings in prepubertal victims of sexual assault. *Pediatrics.* 2000;106(1 pt 1):100–104

38. Thackeray JD, Hornor G, Benzinger EA, Scribano PV. Forensic evidence collection and DNA identification in acute child sexual assault. *Pediatrics.* 2011;128(2):227–232

39. Girardet R, Bolton K, Lahoti S, et al. Collection of forensic evidence from pediatric

victims of sexual assault. *Pediatrics*. 2011; 128(2):233–238

40. Fajman N, Wright R. Use of antiretroviral HIV post-exposure prophylaxis in sexually abused children and adolescents treated in an inner-city pediatric emergency department. *Child Abuse Negl*. 2006;30(8): 919–927

41. Workowski KA, Berman S; Centers for Disease Control and Prevention (CDC). Sexually transmitted diseases treatment guidelines, 2010. *MMWR Recomm Rep*. 2010;59(RR-12):1–110

42. Lentsch KA, Johnson CF. Do physicians have adequate knowledge of child sexual abuse? The results of two surveys of practicing physicians, 1986 and 1996. *Child Maltreat*. 2000;5(1):72–78

43. Narayan AP, Socolar RR, St Claire K. Pediatric residency training in child abuse and neglect in the United States. *Pediatrics*. 2006;117(6):2215–2221

44. Starling SP, Heisler KW, Paulson JF, Youmans E. Child abuse training and knowledge: a national survey of emergency medicine, family medicine, and pediatric residents and program directors. *Pediatrics*. 2009;123(4). Available at: www.pediatrics. org/cgi/content/full/123/4/e595

45. Committee on Practice and Ambulatory Medicine. Policy statement: Use of chaperones during the physical examination of the pediatric patient. *Pediatrics*. 2011;127 (5):991–993

46. Braverman PK, Breech L; Committee on Adolescence. American Academy of Pediatrics. Clinical report: gynecologic examination for adolescents in the pediatric office setting. *Pediatrics*. 2010;126(3):583–590

47. Kaufman M; American Academy of Pediatrics Committee on Adolescence. Care of the adolescent sexual assault victim. *Pediatrics*. 2008;122(2):462–470

48. American College of Obstetricians and Gynecologists. ACOG Committee Opinion No. 463: Cervical cancer in adolescents: screening, evaluation, and management. *Obstet Gynecol*. 2010;116(2 pt 1):469–472

49. Adams JA, Kaplan RA, Starling SP, et al. Guidelines for medical care of children who may have been sexually abused. *J Pediatr Adolesc Gynecol*. 2007;20(3):163–172

50. Makoroff KL, Brauley JL, Brandner AM, Myers PA, Shapiro RA. Genital examinations for alleged sexual abuse of prepubertal girls: findings by pediatric emergency medicine physicians compared with child abuse trained physicians. *Child Abuse Negl*. 2002;26(12):1235–1242

51. Adams JA. Guidelines for medical care of children evaluated for suspected sexual abuse: an update for 2008. *Curr Opin Obstet Gynecol*. 2008;20(5):435–441

52. Adams JA, Harper K, Knudson S, Revilla J. Examination findings in legally confirmed child sexual abuse: it's normal to be normal. *Pediatrics*. 1994;94(3):310–317

53. Muram D. Child sexual abuse: relationship between sexual acts and genital findings. *Child Abuse Negl*. 1989;13(2):211–216

54. Kellogg ND, Menard SW, Santos A. Genital anatomy in pregnant adolescents: "normal" does not mean "nothing happened." *Pediatrics*. 2004;113(1 pt 1). Available at: www. pediatrics.org/cgi/content/full/113/1/e67

55. McCann J, Miyamoto S, Boyle C, Rogers K. Healing of nonhymenal genital injuries in prepubertal and adolescent girls: a descriptive study. *Pediatrics*. 2007;120(5): 1000–1011

56. McCann J, Miyamoto S, Boyle C, Rogers K. Healing of hymenal injuries in prepubertal and adolescent girls: a descriptive study. *Pediatrics*. 2007;119(5). Available at: www. pediatrics.org/cgi/content/full/119/5/e1094

57. Girardet RG, Lahoti S, Howard LA, et al. Epidemiology of sexually transmitted infections in suspected child victims of sexual assault. *Pediatrics*. 2009;124(1):79–86

58. Whaitiri S, Kelly P. Genital gonorrhoea in children: determining the source and mode of infection. *Arch Dis Child*. 2011;96(3):247–251

59. Bell TA, Stamm WE, Wang SP, Kuo CC, Holmes KK, Grayston JT. Chronic *Chlamydia trachomatis* infections in infants. *JAMA*. 1992;267(3):400–402

60. Hammerschlag MR, Alpert S, Rosner I, et al. Microbiology of the vagina in children: normal and potentially pathogenic organisms. *Pediatrics*. 1978;62(1):57–62

61. Hammerschlag MR, Guillén CD. Medical and legal implications of testing for sexually transmitted infections in children. *Clin Microbiol Rev*. 2010;23(3):493–506

62. Lindegren ML, Hanson IC, Hammett TA, Beil J, Fleming PL, Ward JW. Sexual abuse of children: intersection with the HIV epidemic. *Pediatrics*. 1998;102(4). Available at: www.pediatrics.org/cgi/content/full/102/4/ E46

63. Black CM, Driebe EM, Howard LA, et al. Multicenter study of nucleic acid amplification tests for detection of *Chlamydia trachomatis* and *Neisseria gonorrhoeae* in children being evaluated for sexual abuse. *Pediatr Infect Dis J*. 2009;28(7): 608–613

64. Brown HL, Fuller DD, Jasper LT, Davis TE, Wright JD. Clinical evaluation of affirm VPIII in the detection and identification of *Trichomonas vaginalis*, *Gardnerella vaginalis*, and *Candida* species in vaginitis/vaginosis. *Infect Dis Obstet Gynecol*. 2004;12(1):17–21

65. US Food and Drug Administration. *ORA Laboratory Procedure*, vol. II: *Methods. Method Verification and Validation. Version No 1.5*. Silver Spring, MD: US Food and Drug Administration; 2003

66. Bachmann LH, Johnson RE, Cheng H, et al. Nucleic acid amplification tests for diagnosis of *Neisseria gonorrhoeae* and *Chlamydia trachomatis* rectal infections. *J Clin Microbiol*. 2010;48(5):1827–1832

67. Schachter J, Moncada J, Liska S, Shayevich C, Klausner JD. Nucleic acid amplification tests in the diagnosis of chlamydial and gonococcal infections of the oropharynx and rectum in men who have sex with men. *Sex Transm Dis*. 2008;35(7):637–642

68. Giannini CM, Kim HK, Mortensen J, Mortensen J, Marsolo K, Huppert J. Culture of non-genital sites increases the detection of gonorrhea in women. *J Pediatr Adolesc Gynecol*. 2010;23(4): 246–252

69. Leventhal JM, Murphy JL, Asnes AG. Evaluations of child sexual abuse: recognition of overt and latent family concerns. *Child Abuse Negl*. 2010;34(5):289–295

70. Everson MD, Hunter WM, Runyon DK, Edelsohn GA, Coulter ML. Maternal support following disclosure of incest. *Am J Orthopsychiatry*. 1989;59(2):197–207

71. Cohen JA, Mannarino AP, Deblinger EM. *Treating Trauma and Traumatic Grief in Children and Adolescents*. New York, NY: Guilford Press; 2006

Pediatricians' Role in Preventing Child Maltreatment Fatalities: A Call to Action

Rachel P. Berger, MD, MPH[a], David Sanders, PhD[b], David Rubin, MD, MSCE[c]; Commission to Eliminate Abuse and Neglect Fatalities

The death of any child is a tragedy. When that death is caused by abuse or neglect, sorrow is often coupled with anger: How could this have happened? More importantly, was this preventable? A federal commission, the Commission to Eliminate Child Abuse and Neglect Fatalities (CECANF), is working to turn anger into action to stop these tragedies.[1]

At least 1500 children die every year at the hands of those who are supposed to care for and protect them. We say "at least" because we do not have reliable data about the number of deaths from child maltreatment. There is no national standard for counting these deaths, and the data about child fatalities come from multiple sources that do not coordinate or share data. Most experts, including the US Government Accountability Office, believe that child abuse and neglect (CAN) fatalities are significantly undercounted.[2,3]

Recognizing that even 1 death from CAN is 1 too many, Congress passed the Protect Our Kids Act that created CECANF in 2012.[4] CECANF, a 12-member panel appointed by the president and Congress, began its work in February 2014. Commissioners have 2 years to study the extent and causes of CAN fatalities and to submit a report to Congress that includes concrete recommendations for a national strategy to eliminate CAN fatalities.

In June 2014, CECANF began a series of public hearings across the country. Commissioners reached out to experts from a broad range of disciplines. Local legislators, child welfare leaders, law enforcement officials, federal policy experts, data experts, community leaders, tribal representatives, child and parent advocates, former foster children, and pediatricians have been among those who have testified and offered recommendations to the commission. Their testimony is available on the CECANF Web site.[1]

CAN FATALITIES AS A PUBLIC HEALTH CRISIS

After a child dies or almost dies from abuse or neglect, the lay press and others often focus on what child protective services (CPS) should have done or not done. The reality is that a significant proportion of children are known to CPS before the incident that led to their death or near-death. Part of the reason is that child maltreatment fatalities occur

[a]Department of Pediatrics, University of Pittsburgh School of Medicine, Pittsburgh, Pennsylvania; [b]Casey Family Programs, Seattle, Washington; and [c]Department of Pediatrics, Perelman School of Medicine at the University of Pennsylvania and PolicyLab, The Children's Hospital of Philadelphia, Philadelphia, Pennsylvania

Dr Berger contributed to the conception of this piece and drafted the article; Drs Sanders and Rubin contributed to the interpretation of the data contained in the piece and revised the piece critically for important intellectual content; and all authors approved the final manuscript as submitted.

www.pediatrics.org/cgi/doi/10.1542/peds.2015-1776

DOI: 10.1542/peds.2015-1776

Accepted for publication Aug 12, 2015

Address correspondence to Rachel P. Berger, MD, MPH, Children's Hospital of Pittsburgh of UPMC, 4401 Penn Ave, Pittsburgh, PA 15224. E-mail: rachel.berger@chp.edu

PEDIATRICS (ISSN Numbers: Print, 0031-4005; Online, 1098-4275).

FINANCIAL DISCLOSURE: Dr Berger's salary is partially paid for by the Commission to Eliminate Child Abuse and Neglect Fatalities. The other authors have indicated they have no financial relationships relevant to this article to disclose.

FUNDING: No external funding.

POTENTIAL CONFLICT OF INTEREST: The authors have indicated they have no potential conflicts of interest to disclose.

predominantly in young children whose first contact with CPS may be the fatality itself; in 2013, nearly three-quarters of child maltreatment fatalities were in children <3 years of age. Almost half of all deaths were in children <1 year old.[5] Testimony provided to CECANF has emphasized that the factors leading to a CAN fatality are complex and that prevention cannot come from any single agency. CAN fatalities and near-fatalities are a public health crisis, not just a CPS crisis.

Most families in which there is a CAN fatality are known to some system. Almost all children are born in a hospital and are therefore known to the medical system because a pediatrician examined them in the newborn nursery and an insurance company paid for the delivery. Law enforcement may know families with a history of domestic violence, the behavioral health system may be involved for parental mental illness, and the education system is aware of families with preschool- or school-aged children. Finally, community and faith organizations are often aware of neighborhood families in crisis. The need for all these systems to work together to eliminate CAN fatalities has been discussed at length by CECANF.

Difficulty sharing information between the agencies listed here can lead to critical information being held in silos and not being available to on-the-ground CPS caseworkers, pediatricians, law enforcement personnel, or other social service providers. If agencies cannot or do not share information, it is difficult to protect children. Although the Health Insurance Portability and Accountability Act explicitly allows physicians to provide child abuse–related information to CPS, it does not allow CPS to share information with the very physicians who have raised concerns and provide medical care to the child. The American Academy of Pediatrics

recently submitted testimony to the commission and emphasized the importance of communication between CPS and pediatricians for identification, treatment, and prevention of future abuse and recommended "strong and funded health care liaisons with the child welfare system" to ensure a "coordinated approach to preventing and treating child abuse and neglect."[6] Importantly, there is now precedent for legislation to mandate this type of information sharing. Senate Bill 27, which recently passed in Pennsylvania, established formal 2-way communications between certified medical practitioners and CPS during child abuse investigations and in circumstances that affect the medical health of the child.[7]

The number of infants and young children who nearly die of CAN, often called near-fatalities, have also been discussed by the CECANF because causes and etiologic characteristics of near-fatalities closely mirrors those of fatalities; strategies designed to prevent CAN fatalities therefore will probably also prevent near-fatalities.[8] Twenty states review near-fatality cases in a way that is similar to Child Death Review teams. Dr Joanne Wood, a pediatrician at Children's Hospital of Philadelphia, testified before the CECANF about near-fatalities and the pediatrician's role in the diagnosis and evaluation of these cases.[9]

LOOKING AHEAD AND A CALL TO ACTION

The CECANF must submit its recommendations to the president and Congress by early 2016. In the time between now and then, >1500 children will die of abuse or neglect. That is more children than will die during this time from all childhood cancers.[10] Success in the treatment of pediatric cancer came when multiple groups came together in a unified front. It is time to create that type of

unified front to prevent CAN fatalities and near-fatalities. The importance of the medical system, specifically pediatricians, in this effort cannot be overemphasized. Because children who die of abuse or neglect are often young, physicians may be the only people outside the family who routinely see them. Multiple pediatricians[9,11,12] testified to the CECANF that pediatricians want to be part of a multidisciplinary approach to accomplish this goal. There are many ways for pediatricians to do so, including following the progress of CECANF, submitting testimony via the CECANF Web site, participating in child death review and near-fatality review teams, encouraging states to collect data about near-fatalities, continuing to collaborate with local and state CPS agencies, advocating for legislation that removes the barriers to sharing information, and finding out where the need is for physician expertise in the community. But as we await the outcomes of such advocacy, there are more immediate opportunities for action. As health care systems move toward integration of services for families, including with the community services, simply screening parents and children for depression or adverse childhood experiences and telling them to seek care if screened positive is not enough. Rather, we will be increasingly accountable to provide more direct links to services in behavioral health for both parents and children, whether through direct partnership with providers or more efficient processes of referral. If pediatricians can engage with community providers in a more fundamental way, we will be further along the road toward building a safe and healthy future for children.

ACKNOWLEDGMENTS

We thank Joanne Edgar and Janet Fromkin, MD, for their help preparing this piece.

REFERENCES

1. Commission to Eliminate Child Abuse and Neglect Fatalities (CECANF) Web site. Available at: https://eliminatechildabusefatalities.sites.usa.gov/

2. US Government Accountability Office. Strengthening national data on child fatalities could aid in prevention. Report to the chairman, Committee on Ways and Means, House of Representatives. Available at: www.gao.gov/new.items/d11599.pdf

3. Child abuse and neglect deaths in America. 2012. Available at: www.everychildmatters.org/storage/documents/pdf/reports/can_report_august2012_final.pdf

4. The Protect Our Kids Act of 2012. Available at: www.gpo.gov/fdsys/pkg/PLAW-112publ275/pdf/PLAW-112publ275.pdf

5. Children's Bureau (Administration on Children, Youth and Families, Administration for Children and Families) of the US Department of Health and Human Services. Child maltreatment 2013. Available at: www.acf.hhs.gov/sites/default/files/cb/cm2013.pdf

6. Hassink S. American Academy of Pediatrics testimony submitted to the Commission to Eliminate Child Abuse and Neglect Fatalities. 2015. Available at: https://www.aap.org/en-us/advocacy-and-policy/federal-advocacy/Documents/AAPCECANFComments.pdf

7. Improving the exchange of child abuse information among medical practitioners and county agencies 2013–2014. Available at: www.legis.state.pa.us/CFDOCS/billInfo/billInfo.cfm?syear=2013&sInd=0&body=S&type=B&bn=27

8. Sanders D. Why do we study near fatalities? Available at: https://eliminatechildabusefatalities.sites.usa.gov/2015/03/10/why-do-we-study-near-fatalities/

9. Wood J. What do we know about near fatalities that could assist in preventing fatalities? 2014. Available at: https://eliminatechildabusefatalities.sites.usa.gov/files/2014/08/CECANF-VT-Mtg_Presentations_-10-23-and-10-24-14.pdf

10. American Cancer Society. Cancer in children. 2012. Available at: www.cancer.org/Cancer/CancerinChildren/DetailedGuide/cancer-in-children-key-statistics. Accessed June 5, 2015

11. Palusci V. Child maltreatment fatalities: evidence-based counting and prevention. 2014. Available at: https://eliminatechildabusefatalities.sites.usa.gov/files/2014/05/MI-slides-final_rev-9-16-14.pdf

12. Wells K. Assessing present and prospective child safety: a view from the health services venue. 2014. Available at: https://eliminatechildabusefatalities.sites.usa.gov/files/2014/06/Combined-Denver-slides.pdf

Critical Elements in the Medical Evaluation of Suspected Child Physical Abuse

Kristine A. Campbell, MD, MSc, Lenora M. Olson, PhD, Heather T. Keenan, MDCM, PhD

BACKGROUND: Previous research has described variability in medical evaluation of suspected abuse. The objective of this study was to identify, through expert consensus, required and highly recommended elements of a child abuse pediatrics (CAP) evaluation for 3 common presentations of suspected physical abuse in children aged 0 to 60 months.

METHODS: Twenty-eight CAPs recruited from 2 national organizations formed the expert panel for this modified Delphi Process. An initial survey was developed for each presentation based on demographics, history of present illness, past medical, family and social history, laboratory, radiology, and consultation elements present in at least 10% of CAP consultations collected for a larger study. CAPs ranked each element on a 9-point scale then reviewed and discussed summary results through a project blog over 3 rounds. Required and highly recommended elements were defined as elements ranked as 9 and 8, respectively, by ≥75% of experts after the final round.

RESULTS: From 96 elements in the initial surveys, experts identified 30 Required elements and 37 Highly Recommended elements for CAP evaluation of intracranial hemorrhage, 21 Required and 33 Highly Recommended elements for CAP evaluation of long bone fracture, and 18 Required and 16 Highly Recommended elements for CAP evaluation of isolated skull fracture.

CONCLUSIONS: This guideline reflects expert consensus and provides a starting point for development of child abuse assessment protocols for quality improvement or research. Additional research is required to determine whether this guideline can reduce variability and/or improve reliability in the evaluation and diagnosis of child physical abuse.

University of Utah, Department of Pediatrics, Salt Lake City, Utah

Dr Campbell contributed substantially to conceptualization and design of the study, acquired and analyzed the data, and drafted the manuscript; Dr Olson contributed substantially to conceptualization and design of the study and critically revised the manuscript; Dr. Keenan conceptualized and designed the study, and critically revised the manuscript; and all authors approved the final manuscript as submitted.

www.pediatrics.org/cgi/doi/10.1542/peds.2014-4192

DOI: 10.1542/peds.2014-4192

Accepted for publication Apr 15, 2015

Address correspondence to Kristine A. Campbell, MD, MSc, Department of Pediatrics, University of Utah, 295 Chipeta Way, PO Box 581289, Salt Lake City, UT 84158. E-mail: kristine.campbell@hsc.utah.edu

PEDIATRICS (ISSN Numbers: Print, 0031-4005; Online, 1098-4275).

WHAT'S KNOWN ON THIS SUBJECT: Previous research has described important variability in the medical evaluation of suspected child physical abuse. This variability may contribute to bias and reduce reliability in the medical diagnosis of abuse.

WHAT THIS STUDY ADDS: A panel of child abuse pediatricians participated in a Delphi Process, defining critical elements for the medical evaluation of suspected physical abuse in children. Results can be used to reduce practice variability that may contribute to potential bias in evaluation.

ARTICLE

Every year, health care providers in the United States report >150 000 children to local Child Protective Services (CPS) agencies. More than 4500 children are hospitalized with injuries due to physical abuse every year.[1,2] Medical evaluation of suspected child physical abuse presents a unique challenge to physicians, requiring consideration of a broad differential, attention to detailed injury history, testing for occult injury, and difficult questions related to social risk factors often overlooked in the setting of acute trauma. Over the past decade, the American Academy of Pediatrics has published a series of practice recommendations for the medical evaluation of suspected child physical abuse based on expert opinion and literature review.[3-7] The strength of evidence supporting these recommendations remains limited, however, and may contribute to variability in diagnostic evaluations.

In the absence of a perpetrator confession or eyewitness report, there is no single clinical finding that is pathognomonic for child physical abuse. The differential diagnosis for potentially abusive injuries is narrowed only through the iterative process of exclusion of alternate diagnoses that may account for the injury seen (eg, accidental injury, bleeding disorders, or metabolic bone disease) and identification of occult injuries that support a pattern of abuse (eg, healing fractures, retinal hemorrhages, or abdominal trauma). Ultimately, the diagnosis of abuse relies on summation of these different evaluations rather than confirmation of the diagnosis against an accepted gold standard. The absence of a clear end point for this process creates uncertainty about when there is sufficient medical evidence to discontinue diagnostic evaluations and accept a diagnosis of abuse.[8] This uncertainty may be magnified by the implicit legal consequences of an abuse diagnosis. Previously published recommendations reflect this

uncertainty by providing a broad catalog of historical, laboratory, and radiographic data to be considered by physicians in the evaluation of suspected abuse.[2-7] Without unbiased cohort data to specify critical elements of this diagnostic evaluation, a "pick-and-choose" application of these recommendations may lead to practice variability, contributing to both over- and underevaluation of children with injuries concerning for abuse.[9-12]

In this setting of uncertainty, consensus of expert opinion can provide credible guidance for physicians involved in the medical evaluation of suspected abuse.[13] We used a formal process of consensus guideline development to identify key history, laboratory, radiographic, and consultation elements in the initial medical evaluation of abuse. The goal for this project was to describe required and highly recommended elements of a medical evaluation for 3 common presentations of suspected child physical abuse in children aged 0 to 60 months.

METHODS

Study Design

A modified Delphi method was used to develop consensus guidelines for the initial medical evaluation of suspected child physical abuse. The Delphi method relies on an iterative process of individual survey of expert opinion, statistical summary of survey responses, and group feedback of summary statistics to achieve convergence of expert opinion for the management of a specific clinical condition.[13-15] For this project, a blog was developed and maintained by the investigators to allow experts to complete Web-based surveys and to view statistical summaries of survey results. Experts were invited to participate in an anonymous discussion of survey results through the blog between

survey rounds. This study was reviewed and approved by the Institutional Review Board of the University of Utah.

Experts

A national panel of child abuse pediatricians (CAPs) originally recruited for a larger study related to risk perception in the evaluation of child physical abuse served as experts for this project. CAPs were recruited through the listservs of 2 professional associations: the Ray E. Helfer Society, an honorary society of physicians identified as leaders in prevention, diagnosis, treatment, and research related to child abuse and neglect, and the Section on Child Abuse and Neglect of the American Academy of Pediatrics (AAP), a self-selected society of AAP Fellows with interest in the recognition and care of child abuse and neglect.[16,17] To be eligible to participate, interested CAPs were required to have 5 years in pediatric practice postresidency, have obtained board certification in pediatrics, spend at least 50% of their clinical time evaluating possible child abuse cases including physical abuse, and be at an institution with an institutional review board. Twenty-eight of 32 CAPs participating in the original risk perception study formed the expert panel for this Delphi process. Panelists were primarily female (82%), Caucasian, non-Hispanic (75%), and highly experienced, with most participants reporting at least 10 years of CAP practice (61%).

Injury Types

We evaluated the medical assessment of 3 injury types frequently associated with suspected child physical abuse in children 0 to 60 months of age: intracranial hemorrhage, long bone fracture, and skull fracture.

Survey Development

To develop an initial survey regarding critical elements in the initial medical evaluation of suspected child physical abuse, we reviewed child abuse consultation notes submitted for the larger study. In the larger study, CAPs submitted completed clinical notes for physical abuse consultations selected at random from their own practice. Each expert deidentified his or her consultation notes and entered the original text into a secure, Web-based interface using a standard medical format. Laboratories, radiologic studies, and subspecialty consultations requested by the expert on initial evaluation were indicated through a checkbox process in the same interface.[18]

To identify an initial set of elements referenced in the medical evaluation of suspected child physical abuse, 1 author (KAC) reviewed 96 consultation notes (1 consultation note for each of 3 injury types evaluated by each of the 32 original participants). Elements of demographics, history of present illness, past medical history, family, and social history were coded based on a line-by-line reading of the consultation notes. Elements were described as "present" or "absent" for each note reviewed. For example, a note beginning with the sentence "Patient is a 6-month boy seen after a fall from a changing table at 6:15 this morning" would be coded present for the elements of child age, gender, injury mechanism, and injury timing. The element of child race, coded as present in previously reviewed consultations, would be absent unless identified elsewhere in this note. Pertinent negatives, when explicitly documented, were coded as present. A consultation noting, "History of injury has been consistent throughout hospitalization" would be coded present for the element "discrepancies in history," whereas a consultation note that did not address historical (in)consistencies would be coded absent for this element.

The initial survey included any text element present in >10% of all

consultations reviewed, and any laboratory or radiologic studies present in >10% of consultations for each injury type. Elements of past medical history and radiologic studies were stratified by child age in the survey (<6 months, 6–11 months, 12–23 months, and 24–60 months). A single "floor" element was included in each survey to test whether experts would rank any item as "not recommended" or "inappropriate." Due to investigator oversight, subspecialty consultations were not included in the original surveys. Questions related to subspecialty evaluations requested for diagnostic purposes (rather than treatment) in >10% of consultations for each injury type were added to a final survey round only. Using this approach, we identified 96 possible elements in the CAP evaluations of suspected child physical abuse for intracranial hemorrhage, long bone fracture, and skull fracture (Table 1).

Surveys

These elements, stratified by age when appropriate, formed the initial Web-based surveys distributed to the expert panel. Experts ranked the importance of each element using a 9-point Likert scale, with the following language provided to anchor individual responses:

1 (Inappropriate): This element should not be included in a CAP evaluation under almost any circumstances.

2–4: Presence of this element is not usual practice but remains within accepted practice.

5 (Optional): Presence of this element in a CAP evaluation is neither expected nor inappropriate.

6–8: Presence of this element is expected, but a CAP evaluation is not incomplete if it is absent.

9 (Required): Presence of this element is critical to a CAP evaluation.

A link to each survey was embedded within the study blog. All survey data

were collected and managed using REDCap (Research Electronic Data Capture), a secure, Web-based application designed to support data capture for research studies.[19]

Summary

Summary statistics for each element were calculated after each survey to describe group opinion. We constructed box plots with graphic and numeric median values, interquartile ranges, and adjacent values using Stata 12.1 (College Station, TX).

Feedback

Summarized results were posted to the blog after the first and second round of surveys. After reviewing these results, we asked experts to participate in a moderated discussion through the blog based on the following questions:

1. Were you surprised by the survey results?

2. Did you disagree with survey results?

3. How did results make you think about your own consultations?

Participation in the discussion was not required. Experts who followed the discussion without comment submission were not tracked.

Iteration

After each round, elements with complete statistical agreement and no discussion comments suggesting disagreement were removed from the survey to minimize participant burden. Elements suggested by at least 2 participants through free-text comments or blog discussion were added to the survey. After revision, links were posted on the blog to begin the subsequent cycle of survey, summary, and feedback.

Consensus Guideline Development

There is no universally recognized threshold to define consensus within a Delphi process.[13] On the basis of the study goal of identifying critical elements in the initial medical evaluation of child physical abuse, we relied on a conservative definition of consensus. "Required" and "Highly Recommended" elements were defined as critical elements ranked as 9 and 8, respectively, by ≥75% of participating experts after the final round of survey, summary, and feedback. We also identified "Inappropriate" elements, defined as elements ranked as 1 by ≥75% of participating experts after the final survey. Online discussion comments provided insight into the decision-making reflected in the process of consensus development.

RESULTS

All 28 participating experts completed 3 survey cycles, and half of the experts ($n = 14$) submitted 42 comments during discussions. There were no significant differences between participants who submitted comments and those who did not. Median rankings were generally stable over 3 survey rounds, increasing by 1 point for 17 elements and decreasing by 1 to 2 points for 21 elements across the 3 clinical scenarios.

From 96 surveyed elements, experts identified 30 Required elements and 37 Highly Recommended elements for the medical evaluation for suspected abuse in a patient presenting with intracranial hemorrhage. The expert panel also agreed on 21 Required and 33 Highly Recommended elements for the medical evaluation of suspected abuse in a patient presenting with long bone fracture, and 18 Required and 16 Highly Recommended elements for the medical evaluation of suspected abuse in a patient presenting with skull fracture (Table 2). Only the floor element ("identification of the most likely perpetrator") was identified as "Inappropriate" for all clinical scenarios.

TABLE 1 Elements included in Delphi Method Surveys Based on Presence of the Element in at Least 10% of Child Abuse Consultation Notes or Round 1 Feedback From Expert Panel

Domain	Element
Demographics	Child age
	Child gender
	Child race/ethnicity
	Sources of information
History of presenting illness or injury	Injury history
	Symptom timeline of injury/illness
	Caregiver at time of injury/illness
	Outside or prehospital care
	Caregivers treatment of or response to injury/illness
	Discrepancies in medical history
	Most likely perpetrator[a]
Prenatal and perinatal history responses stratified by age	Prenatal care of mother
	Prenatal trauma, such as car collision or stair fall
	Prenatal alcohol or drug exposure
	Prenatal nutrition, including vitamins
	Planning of pregnancy
	Use of assisted reproductive technologies/in vitro fertilization
	Estimated gestational age
	Birth weight and/or height
	Birth history or complications, such as instrumentation or shoulder dystocia
	Perinatal care, including vitamin K
	Perinatal discharge timing
	Perinatal illness, such as sepsis
	Perinatal jaundice or hyperbilirubinemia
	Umbilical oozing, delayed umbilical separation, or other umbilical concerns
	Gastroesophageal reflux
	Newborn state screening results
Developmental and dietary history responses stratified by age	Developmental stage (rolling, crawling, cruising, or walking)
	Child temperament or personality traits
	Sleep hygiene (sleep patterns, location of sleep)
	Developmental concerns of parents
	Child diet (formula vs breastfed, vitamins, picky eater)
Past medical history	Surgery or circumcision
	Easy bleeding or bruising
	Fracture or bony abnormality
	Dental malformation or abnormality
	Hair abnormalities (texture, fragility, or appearance)
	Hearing deficits
	Seizures or spells
	Complex or chronic disease
	Recurrent vomiting
	Bruises, rashes, or skin concerns
	Growth trajectory
	Well-child care
	Known primary care provider
	Immunization history
	Previous injuries
	Previous hospitalization or emergency care
	Medication usage
Family history	Bleeding or clotting problems
	Easy fracture or bony fragility
	Symptoms of osteogenesis imperfects (eg, blue sclera, hearing loss, short stature)
	Genetic or metabolic disorders
	Collagen disorders
	Seizures or neurologic disorders
	Developmental delay or mental retardation

TABLE 1 Continued

Domain	Element
Social history	Childhood death
	Mental illness
	Description of all child care settings
	Employment of caregivers
	Preferred language of caregivers
	Marital status of caregivers
	Parenting difficulties identified by caregivers
	Drug or alcohol abuse by caregiver
	Previous CPS involvement in household
	Abuse or neglect of child
	Abuse or neglect of caregiver
	History of legal problems or incarceration of caregivers
	Family country of origin[b]
	Economic stresses in household[b]
Laboratory studies	Complete blood count
	Basic metabolic panel
	Coagulation screening (PT/PTT/INR)
	Hepatic transaminases (alanine transaminase/aspartate aminotransferase)
	Pancreatic enzymes (amylase/lipase)
	Serum albumin
	Calcium/phosphorus
	Alkaline phosphatase
	Magnesium
	Urinalysis
	Von Willebrand's panel[c]
	Fibrinogen/D-dimer[c]
	Factors VIII, IX[c]
	Factor XIII[c]
	Urine organic acids/serum amino acids[c]
	Osteogenesis imperfecta testing[d]
	Parathyroid hormone[d]
	Vitamin 25 hydroxyvitamin-D[d,e]
Radiologic studies responses stratified by age	Head computed tomography
	Skeletal survey
	Neck and/or spine imaging
	Abdominal computed tomography
	Cranial magnetic resonance imaging[c]
	Focused extremity films[d]
	Focused skull series[e]
Consultations responses stratified by age	Pediatric ophthalmology[f]

All elements were included on initial survey for all injury types, with the exceptions noted in footnotes c, d, and e. PT/PTT/INR, prothrombin time/partial thromboplastin time/international normalized ratio.
[a] Included by investigators to test floor response of experts participating in Delphi.
[b] Added to survey after round 1 survey, summary, and feedback.
[c] Included on intracranial hemorrhage survey.
[d] Included on long bone fracture survey.
[e] Included on skull fracture survey.
[f] Added after round 2 survey, summary, and feedback.

Despite the statistical stability of expert opinion over survey rounds, online discussion of results reflected recent changes in CAP research and practice. One expert referenced a new AAP practice guideline, "The Factor XIII issue [ordering Factor XIII levels for intracranial hemorrhage] is interesting in light of the recently suggested heme workup paper in the setting of head trauma."[3] Another commented, "Ever since Dan Lindberg's study, I am getting liver enzymes on all my isolated fracture cases."[20] Some were surprised by practices recommended by other participants, including, "Neck imaging in children with head injury … is this something that everyone is already doing?"[21] Participants also considered the role of CAP evaluations in future research: "In regard to race/ethnicity, how great would it be for research if all CAP reports had this available. That is why I switched to a 9 [Required]."[9-11] Others disagreed, arguing, "with the possible exception of looking for a genetic disease/cause of bleeding for ICH cases, I do not think documentation of race is necessary or even 'recommended' in cases of child abuse."

The balance between over- and underevaluation was a common theme. One participant acknowledged, "I have varied feelings about obtaining a detailed social history with questions about risk factors. It's good to know this information, but will it bias my decision? Risk factors apply to populations rather than to individual cases." Others argued that identification of social risk was necessary for longitudinal care of children at high risk. One participant expressed disappointment "that many elements of the psychosocial history were not required. I wonder if it is because some clinicians are seeing these children only in the acute setting … [others are] in a position to make recommendations to CPS to address the psychosocial concerns." Finally, experts struggled with boundaries between clinical and forensic practice in CAP evaluations. Arguing in support of laboratory studies for unlikely diagnoses, one participant explained, "The number of labs ordered depends very much on the local environment and how vigorous the defense attorneys are. There are some I know that order everything on every kid they see as a preemptive strike. Once burned, twice shy."

DISCUSSION

Through a modified Delphi process, we developed consensus guidelines for required and highly recommended

TABLE 2 Required and Highly Recommended Elements in the Medical Evaluation for Suspected Child Abuse

Domain	Consensus	Injury type		
		Intracranial hemorrhage	Long bone fracture	Skull fracture
History of presenting illness	Required	Child age, source of history, injury history, symptom timeline, caregiver present at time of injury or illness	Child age, source of history, injury history, symptom timeline, caregiver present at time of injury or illness, caregiver response to symptoms, outside hospital or prehospital medical care	Child age, source of history, injury history, symptom timeline, caregiver present at time of injury or illness, caregiver response to symptoms, outside hospital or prehospital medical care
	Highly recommended	Caregiver response to symptoms, outside hospital or prehospital medical care, discrepancies in history	Discrepancies in history	Discrepancies in history
Past medical history	Required	Past injuries, surgeries, easy bleeding, seizures, skin concerns, special health care needs	Past injuries and fractures	Past injuries and fractures
	Highly recommended	Past Fractures, vomiting, growth pattern, known primary care provider, hospitalizations, medications	Dental concerns, hearing loss, skin concerns, growth pattern, hospitalizations, medications, special health care needs	Skin concerns, growth pattern, hospitalizations, special health care needs
Pre- and perinatal history (infants <6 mo of age unless otherwise specified)	Required	Estimated gestational age, birth complications, perinatal care (eg, vitamin K)	Estimated gestational age, birth complications	Birth complications
	Highly recommended	Prenatal care, prenatal injury, prenatal drug exposure, estimated gestational age,[a] birth weight, birth discharge timing, perinatal care (eg, vitamin K),[a] perinatal illness, neonatal state screen	Prenatal care, prenatal nutrition, estimated gestational age,[a] birth weight, perinatal illness	Prenatal care, prenatal injury, estimated gestational age, birth weight
Developmental history	Required	Developmental stage	Developmental stage	Developmental stage
	Highly recommended	Parental concerns for development	Parental concerns for development	Parental concerns for development
Dietary history	Required	N/A	Diet (eg, breast vs formula fed; vitamins given; picky eater)[b]	N/A
	Highly recommended	N/A	Diet (eg, breast vs formula fed; vitamins given; picky eater)[a,c,d]	N/A
Family history	Required	Easy bleeding or known bleeding disorder	Bone fragility, osteogenesis imperfecta	Bone fragility
	Highly recommended	Metabolic disorder, seizures, early childhood deaths, mental illness	Metabolic disorders, collagen disorders	Osteogenesis imperfecta, metabolic disorders, collagen disorders
Social history	Required	Description of child care settings	N/A	Description of child care settings, previous abuse/neglect of this child
	Highly recommended	Previous abuse/neglect of this child, intimate partner violence, caregiver history of abuse/neglect, past CPS involvement for household	Description of child care settings, previous abuse/neglect of this child, parenting difficulties, intimate partner violence, caregiver history of child abuse/neglect, past CPS involvement for household, past legal involvement of caregiver	Intimate partner violence, caregiver history of abuse/neglect, past CPS involvement for household

TABLE 2 Continued

Domain	Consensus	Injury type		
		Intracranial hemorrhage	Long bone fracture	Skull fracture
Laboratory	Required	Complete blood count, coagulation screening (PT/PTT), liver enzymes (ALT/AST)	N/A	N/A
	Highly recommended	Basic metabolic panel, pancreatic enzymes (amylase/lipase)	Alkaline phosphatase, calcium/phosphorous	N/A
Radiology	Required	Head CT,[a,b,c] skeletal survey[a,b,c]	Head CT,[b] skeletal survey[a,b,c]	Head CT,[a] skeletal survey[a]
	Highly recommended	Head CT,[d] brain MRI	Focused extremity	N/A
Consultations	Required	Pediatric ophthalmology[a,b]	N/A	N/A
	Highly recommended	Pediatric ophthalmology[c,d]	N/A	N/A

Expert consensus for evaluation of suspected physical abuse in children aged 0 to 60 mo unless indicated by footnotes. N/A, no elements were identified by expert consensus. ALT/AST, alanine transaminase/aspartate aminotransferase; CT, computed tomography; MRI, magnetic resonance imaging; PT/PTT, prothrombin time/partial thromboplastin time.

[a] In children aged 6–11 mo.
[b] In children aged <6 mo.
[c] In children aged 12–23 mo.
[d] In children aged 24–60 mo.

historical elements, laboratory studies, radiologic examinations, and subspecialty consultations for the initial medical evaluation of suspected child physical abuse in children 0 to 60 months of age presenting with intracranial hemorrhage, long bone fracture, or skull fracture. Panel discussions during guideline development reflect familiarity with published recommendations, awareness of emerging research, and mindfulness related to potential bias in the diagnostic evaluation of suspected child physical abuse.

The complexity involved in medical evaluation of suspected abuse is captured by the extensive historical information either required or highly recommended by the expert panel. Historical elements in the consensus guideline align substantially with available practice guidelines.[6] Although many of these elements are expected with any medical evaluation, other elements, such as source of history, caregiver present at the time of injury, caregiver's response to symptoms, and changes or discrepancies in the history provided, reflect the unique character of CAP evaluations. In contrast to traditional pediatric practice, CAPs recognize the potential misalignment of caregiver

and physician goals in reaching the "correct" diagnosis for a child. Broad inclusion of elements from the medical, developmental, and family history reflect the wide differential diagnosis entertained in cases of suspected abuse.

The laboratory studies, radiologic examinations, and subspecialty consultations identified as either required or highly recommended in the initial evaluation of suspected abuse are also consistent with published guidelines and reflective of recent research. In the setting of intracranial hemorrhage, screening studies for coagulation disorders and for occult abdominal trauma are required, whereas basic laboratory studies for bone health are required in cases of long bone fracture.[3,6,19,22,23] Similarly, radiologic recommendations are consistent with research supporting skeletal surveys for children under 2 years of age with suspected abusive head trauma or abusive long bone fracture but limited to children under 6 months of age presenting with skull fracture.[5,22,24,25] Discrepancies between this consensus guideline and previously published clinical practice recommendations may reflect changing or conflicting recommendations, as seen in the

discussions related to choices of laboratory tests for coagulation disorders and occult abdominal injury in children with suspected physical abuse, or a prioritization of elements identified as most critical to initial evaluation of an injury.

The expert panel did diverge importantly from published practice guidelines in identification of psychosocial elements critical to the initial medical evaluation of suspected abuse.[6,26] Few elements in the social history were required. Description of all child-care settings, required in the evaluation of intracranial hemorrhage and skull fracture, serves as a clarification of the source of the presenting history and whether other caregivers may have additional injury or symptom history. A past history of child abuse or neglect in the home, required only in cases of skull fracture, reflects research suggesting that this may serve as an effective risk indicator in initial evaluation of these children.[27] Almost all elements in the psychosocial history identified as highly recommended relate directly to the presence or absence of violence in the home, a risk factor for abuse as well as a potential injury mechanism.[28,29] Missing from the list of required and recommended elements are descriptions of caregiver mental health, substance abuse, pregnancy planning, and parent perceptions of child temperament or behavior, all of which have been recommended in clinical practice recommendations.[5,6] The importance of these psychosocial elements was a focus of discussion between survey rounds. Experts worried about narrowing a medical evaluation to exclude elements that might help to reduce future adversities for the child and family, yet acknowledged the potential for bias introduced by the psychosocial history.[9–12] The final consensus guideline reflects uncertainty regarding the reliability of these psychosocial factors in shaping early diagnostic decisions.

This study must be viewed in light of its limitations. Although drawn from national CAP listservs, the expert panel may not be representative of the wider CAP community. Consensus opinion does not reflect actual practice, which may vary across institution, provider, and patient.

Consensus opinion also may not be correct, and opinion may change as scientific truths emerge over time. This consensus guideline addresses only required and highly recommended elements in the initial evaluation of suspected abuse. It does not inform secondary evaluations in response to findings of occult injury or anomalous laboratory results and does not suggest that other elements should be excluded from any evaluation. Finally, sensitivity to potential medicolegal implications of a consensus guideline for medical evaluation of suspected physical abuse may have reduced the willingness of panel members to identify elements as either required or inappropriate. Panel discussions between survey rounds reflected each of these limitations.

As a new subspecialty, CAP providers have a unique opportunity to define appropriate practices that best balance the goals of traditional pediatrics with the emerging expectations of forensic evaluation.

Despite limitations, these consensus guidelines may provide a useful starting point for development of a checklist child abuse assessment protocol for quality improvement or research efforts in the future. Additional research is required to determine whether these consensus guidelines can reduce previously described variability, decrease potential bias, and/or improve reliability in the evaluation and diagnosis of child physical abuse.

ACKNOWLEDGMENTS

The authors thank all of the expert panelists for participating in this consensus guideline development process.

ABBREVIATIONS

AAP: American Academy of Pediatrics
CAP: child abuse pediatrician
CPS: Child Protective Services

FINANCIAL DISCLOSURE: Dr Campbell's institution receives financial compensation for expert witness testimony provided in cases of suspected child abuse for which she is subpoenaed to testify.

FUNDING: This research was supported by the Eunice Kennedy Shriver Institute of Child Health and Human Development of the National Institutes of Health grant number R01 HD061373 (principal investigator Dr Keenan). Study data were collected and managed using REDCap (Research Electronic Data Capture), hosted through the Center for Clinical and Translational Science at the University of Utah through CTSA grant number 5UL1RR025764-02.

POTENTIAL CONFLICT OF INTEREST: The authors have indicated they have no potential conflicts of interest to disclose.

REFERENCES

1. US Department of Health and Human Services, Administration for Children and Families, Administration on Children, Youth and Families, Children's Bureau. *Child Maltreatment 2012*. Published December 17, 2013. Available at: http://www.acf.hhs.gov/programs/cb/resource/child-maltreatment-2012. Accessed June 4, 2014

2. Leventhal JM, Gaither JR. Incidence of serious injuries due to physical abuse in the United States: 1997 to 2009. *Pediatrics*. 2012;130(5). Available at: www.pediatrics.org/cgi/content/full/130/5/e847

3. Anderst JD, Carpenter SL, Abshire TC; Section on Hematology/Oncology and Committee on Child Abuse and Neglect of the American Academy of Pediatrics. Evaluation for bleeding disorders in suspected child abuse. *Pediatrics*. 2013;131(4). Available at: www.pediatrics.org/cgi/content/full/131/4/e1314

4. Christian CW, Block R; Committee on Child Abuse and Neglect; American Academy of Pediatrics. Abusive head trauma in infants and children. *Pediatrics*. 2009;123(5):1409–1411

5. Flaherty EG, Perez-Rossello JM, Levine MA, Hennrikus WL; American Academy of Pediatrics Committee on Child Abuse and Neglect; Section on Radiology, American Academy of Pediatrics; Section on Endocrinology, American Academy of Pediatrics; Section on Orthopaedics, American Academy of Pediatrics; Society for Pediatric Radiology. Evaluating children with fractures for child physical abuse. *Pediatrics*. 2014;133(2). Available at: www.pediatrics.org/cgi/content/full/133/2/e477

6. Kellogg ND; American Academy of Pediatrics Committee on Child Abuse and Neglect. Evaluation of suspected child physical abuse. *Pediatrics*. 2007;119(6):1232–1241

7. Levin AV, Christian CW; Committee on Child Abuse and Neglect, Section on Ophthalmology. The eye examination in

the evaluation of child abuse [published correction appears in *Pediatrics*. 126(5): 1053]. *Pediatrics*. 2010;126(2):376–380

8. Moles RL, Asnes AG. Has this child been abused? Exploring uncertainty in the diagnosis of maltreatment. *Pediatr Clin North Am*. 2014;61(5):1023–1036

9. Lane WG, Rubin DM, Monteith R, Christian CW. Racial differences in the evaluation of pediatric fractures for physical abuse. *JAMA*. 2002;288(13):1603–1609

10. Wood JN, Hall M, Schilling S, Keren R, Mitra N, Rubin DM. Disparities in the evaluation and diagnosis of abuse among infants with traumatic brain injury. *Pediatrics*. 2010;126(3):408–414

11. Laskey AL, Stump TE, Perkins SM, Zimet GD, Sherman SJ, Downs SM. Influence of race and socioeconomic status on the diagnosis of child abuse: a randomized study. *J Pediatr*. 2012;160(6):1003–1008. e1001

12. Jenny C, Hymel KP, Ritzen A, Reinert SE, Hay TC. Analysis of missed cases of abusive head trauma. *JAMA*. 1999;281(7):621–626

13. Murphy MK, Black NA, Lamping DL, et al. Consensus development methods, and their use in clinical guideline development. *Health Technol Assess*. 1998;2(3):i–iv, 1–88

14. Hasson F, Keeney S, McKenna H. Research guidelines for the Delphi survey technique. *J Adv Nurs*. 2000;32(4): 1008–1015

15. Keeney S, Hasson F, McKenna HP. A critical review of the Delphi technique as a research methodology for nursing. *Int J Nurs Stud*. 2001;38(2):195–200

16. The Ray E. Helfer Society. Available at: http://www.helfersociety.org. Accessed September 10, 2014

17. American Academy of Pediatrics. Section on Child Abuse and Neglect (SOCAN). Child Abuse and Neglect. Available at: http://www2.aap.org/sections/childabuseneglect. Accessed September 10, 2014

18. Keenan HT, Campbell KA. Three models of child abuse consultations: a qualitative study of inpatient child abuse consultation notes [published online ahead of print December 4, 2014]. *Child Abuse Negl*. doi: 10.1016/j.chiabu.2014.11.009

19. REDCap. Research Electronic Data Capture. Available at: http://www.project-redcap.org. Accessed September 17, 2014

20. Lindberg D, Makoroff K, Harper N, et al; ULTRA Investigators. Utility of hepatic transaminases to recognize abuse in children. *Pediatrics*. 2009;124(2): 509–516

21. Brennan LK, Rubin D, Christian CW, Duhaime AC, Mirchandani HG, Rorke-Adams LB. Neck injuries in young pediatric homicide victims. *J Neurosurg Pediatr*. 2009;3(3):232–239

22. Section on Radiology; American Academy of Pediatrics. Diagnostic imaging of child abuse. *Pediatrics*. 2009;123(5):1430–1435

23. Lane WG, Dubowitz H, Langenberg P. Screening for occult abdominal trauma in children with suspected physical abuse. *Pediatrics*. 2009;124(6):1595–1602

24. Hansen KK, Campbell KA. How useful are skeletal surveys in the second year of life? *Child Abuse Negl*. 2009;33(5): 278–281

25. Laskey AL, Stump TE, Hicks RA, Smith JL. Yield of skeletal surveys in children ≤ 18 months of age presenting with isolated skull fractures. *J Pediatr*. 2013; 162(1):86–89

26. Leventhal JM. Thinking clearly about evaluations of suspected child abuse. *Clin Child Psychol Psychiatry*. 2000;5(1):139–147

27. Wood JN, Christian CW, Adams CM, Rubin DM. Skeletal surveys in infants with isolated skull fractures. *Pediatrics*. 2009; 123(2). Available at: www.pediatrics.org/cgi/content/full/123/2/e247

28. Christian CW, Scribano P, Seidl T, Pinto-Martin JA. Pediatric injury resulting from family violence. *Pediatrics*. 1997; 99(2):E8

29. Thackeray JD, Hibbard R, Dowd MD; Committee on Child Abuse and Neglect; Committee on Injury, Violence, and Poison Prevention. Intimate partner violence: the role of the pediatrician. *Pediatrics*. 2010;125(5):1094–1100

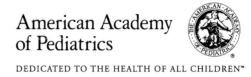

American Academy
of Pediatrics

DEDICATED TO THE HEALTH OF ALL CHILDREN™

The Evaluation of Suspected Child Physical Abuse

Cindy W. Christian, MD, FAAP, COMMITTEE ON CHILD ABUSE AND NEGLECT

abstract

Child physical abuse is an important cause of pediatric morbidity and mortality and is associated with major physical and mental health problems that can extend into adulthood. Pediatricians are in a unique position to identify and prevent child abuse, and this clinical report provides guidance to the practitioner regarding indicators and evaluation of suspected physical abuse of children. The role of the physician may include identifying abused children with suspicious injuries who present for care, reporting suspected abuse to the child protection agency for investigation, supporting families who are affected by child abuse, coordinating with other professionals and community agencies to provide immediate and long-term treatment to victimized children, providing court testimony when necessary, providing preventive care and anticipatory guidance in the office, and advocating for policies and programs that support families and protect vulnerable children.

INTRODUCTION

Each year in the United States, Child Protective Service (CPS) agencies investigate more than 2 million reports of suspected child maltreatment, 18% of which involve concerns of physical abuse.[1] After investigation, more than 650 000 children are substantiated as victims of maltreatment, and over 1500 child deaths are attributed to child abuse or neglect annually. The majority of these deaths (80%) occur in children who are under 4 years of age. Over recent years, official child welfare statistics suggest a consistent decline in child physical abuse rates, but because these reports represent only cases investigated and confirmed by state CPS agencies, these trends may reflect changes in reporting practices, investigation standards, and administrative or statistical procedures.[2] Indeed, the reported incidence of child physical abuse is dependent on the source of data. Results from the Fourth National Incidence Study, a congressionally mandated periodic study on child abuse that reports national incidence for reported and nonreported child maltreatment recognized by community professionals, showed a decline in physical abuse from 1993 to 2006.[3] In contrast, researchers examining hospitalization rates for physical abuse have shown either no significant

This document is copyrighted and is property of the American Academy of Pediatrics and its Board of Directors. All authors have filed conflict of interest statements with the American Academy of Pediatrics. Any conflicts have been resolved through a process approved by the Board of Directors. The American Academy of Pediatrics has neither solicited nor accepted any commercial involvement in the development of the content of this publication.

Clinical reports from the American Academy of Pediatrics benefit from expertise and resources of liaisons and internal (AAP) and external reviewers. However, clinical reports from the American Academy of Pediatrics may not reflect the views of the liaisons or the organizations or government agencies that they represent.

The guidance in this report does not indicate an exclusive course of treatment or serve as a standard of medical care. Variations, taking into account individual circumstances, may be appropriate.

All clinical reports from the American Academy of Pediatrics automatically expire 5 years after publication unless reaffirmed, revised, or retired at or before that time.

www.pediatrics.org/cgi/doi/10.1542/peds.2015-0356

DOI: 10.1542/peds.2015-0356

PEDIATRICS (ISSN Numbers: Print, 0031-4005; Online, 1098-4275).

recent changes[4] or recent increases in hospitalizations for physical abuse.[5,6] These studies likely represent more severe abuse and suggest that multiple data sources are needed to understand the scope and severity of the problem. Adult reports of childhood experiences indicate that physical abuse is more common than statistics reported from any pediatric data source. For example, data from the National Epidemiologic Survey on Alcohol and Related Conditions, a nationally representative sample of the adult US population, indicate that 17.6% of American adults are estimated to have been physically abused during childhood.[7] Regardless of the data source, physical abuse that is identified, reported to CPS, and investigated represents only a small percentage of the abuse that children experience.

DEFINITIONS

The recognition and reporting of physical abuse is influenced by variations in both legal and personal definitions of abuse. The Federal Child Abuse Prevention and Treatment Act provides minimum standards to the states for defining maltreatment, but each state defines child physical abuse within its own civil and criminal statutes. The act defines child abuse as "any recent act or failure to act on the part of a parent or caretaker which results in death, serious physical or emotional harm, sexual abuse or exploitation" or "an act or failure to act which presents an imminent risk of serious harm."[8] State laws defining physical abuse vary widely, and defining terms such as "risk of harm," "substantial harm," "substantial risk," or "reasonable discipline" may not be further clarified in state legislation. Some state statutes require "serious bodily injury" or "severe pain" to define abuse, and variability in state definitions ultimately contributes to widely variable rates of documented abuse across states.[1] States vary in their acceptance of corporal

punishment in schools, despite calls from the American Academy of Pediatrics for the abolishment of corporal punishment in schools by all states.[9] Personal, cultural, and professional experiences influence individual perceptions and definitions of abuse.[10] For example, when given hypothetical scenarios involving pediatric head trauma, pediatricians were more likely than pathologists to judge an event as abusive.[11] This finding may reflect differences in training, experience, and exposure to different populations of children. Ultimately, the variability in definitions influences consistent reporting practices across jurisdictions.

IMPACT OF PHYSICAL ABUSE ON PEDIATRIC AND ADULT HEALTH

Child maltreatment is a public health problem with lifelong health consequences for survivors and their families.[12] Adults who were maltreated as children have poor health outcomes, and there is accumulating evidence that early adverse childhood experiences are strong contributors to many adult diseases.[13-15] Both retrospective and prospective studies published in recent years have identified strong associations between cumulative traumatic childhood events including maltreatment, family dysfunction, and social isolation, and adult physical and mental health disease.[16-18] Few studies, however, have specifically examined the association between child physical abuse and child and adult health outcomes, in part, because many victims have suffered from more than 1 kind of maltreatment.[19,20]

Adults who self-report physical abuse when they were children are more likely as adults to report chronic physical and mental health conditions,[21] even when controlling for family background and additional adverse childhood experiences.[22] Adolescents who are victims of

physical abuse have high rates of depression, conduct disorder, drug abuse, and cigarette smoking.[23,24]

For some children, physical abuse results in permanent disability, affecting their lifelong health in profound ways. For example, victims of abusive head trauma (AHT) have high rates of neurologic disability, including sight and hearing impairment, epilepsy, cerebral palsy, and developmental and cognitive delay.[25-27] Abused children may suffer permanently disfiguring injuries. Victims of physical abuse in childhood are at risk for developing a variety of behavioral problems including conduct disorders, physically aggressive behaviors, depression, poor academic performance, and decreased cognitive functioning.[28-30]

There is emerging recognition that adverse childhood experiences, including physical abuse, influence biological adaptations associated with how the brain, neuroendocrine stress response, and immune system function.[31] In turn, these changes are associated with physical and behavioral health impairments decades later.[32] The recognition that social and environmental exposures early in life are associated with biological changes that influence health across generations necessitates that future efforts at improving the health of the population require interventions that limit exposure to adverse childhood experience and reduce toxic stress in young children.[33] Pediatricians have a unique opportunity to lead efforts addressing the social determinants of health, and prevention and early identification of child maltreatment, including physical abuse, is an important responsibility of the pediatrician in practice.

RISK FACTORS FOR CHILD PHYSICAL ABUSE

Child abuse is a highly complex phenomenon in which parent, child, and environmental characteristics interact to place children at risk[34] (Table 1). Child physical abuse affects children of all ages, ethnicities, and socioeconomic groups, although racial and socioeconomic factors influence reports to CPS.[35,36] Boys experience slightly higher rates of physical abuse than girls, and overall, adolescents are more likely than other children to receive injuries from physical abuse.[37] However, because of their small size and vulnerability, infants and toddlers are at highest risk of fatal and severe physical abuse.[38] Risk factors for infant abuse include maternal smoking, the presence of more than 2 siblings, low infant birth weight, and being born to an unmarried mother.[39] Children with disabilities are at high risk for physical, sexual, and emotional abuse.[40,41] Young, abused children who live in households with unrelated adults are at exceptionally high risk of fatal abuse,[42] and children previously reported to CPS are at significantly higher risk of both abusive and preventable accidental death compared with peers with similar sociodemographic characteristics.[43] Strong evidence exists for the association between poverty and child physical abuse, and children who live in poverty are overrepresented in both the child protective and foster care systems.[3] Military families are at risk for child maltreatment, particularly at times of deployment.[44,45]

Specific family and community preventive factors mitigate some of the risks, including parental resilience, parent knowledge of child development and parenting, concrete support in times of need, social connections, and a child's ability to form positive relationships.[46,47] The presence of safe, stable, nurturing relationships and environments prevent maltreatment and are essential for healthy childhood.

These risk and preventive factors, while important for guiding the development of prevention and intervention strategies, should be considered as broadly defined markers, rather than strong individual determinants of abuse.[48] Parents who have inappropriate developmental knowledge and expectations of their children, those who lack empathy for their children, those with harsh or inconsistent parenting practices, and those who reverse parent-child roles are also at risk for abusing their children.[49] Additional discussion related to risk and preventive factors for child maltreatment can be found in the American Academy of Pediatrics (AAP) clinical report on the pediatrician's role in child maltreatment prevention.[34]

MISSED OPPORTUNITIES FOR DIAGNOSING PHYSICAL ABUSE

Most injuries in children are not the result of abuse or neglect. Minor injuries in children are exceedingly common, and most childhood injuries do not require medical attention. Pediatric visits for injury are common, and millions of children are seen each year in emergency departments for injury.[50] Additionally, unusual accidental events happen to children and may result in injuries that are not characteristically seen from accidental causes.[51] Although anecdotal reports of fatal injury from short falls exist, fatal outcome from childhood falls is rare.[52] It has been estimated that the population-based risk of a short fall death for an infant or young child is <1 per 1 million young children per year.[53]

The identification of physical abuse can be difficult. Other than the perpetrator and the child, witnesses to the abuse are uncommon; perpetrators of the abuse infrequently admit to their actions; child victims are often preverbal and may be too severely injured or too frightened to disclose their abuse; and injuries can be nonspecific. Physicians are taught to rely on parents for accurate information about the child's history and may not be critical or skeptical of the information provided. Additionally, disbelieving parents or other relatives may intimidate or threaten physicians who raise concerns of abuse. These factors make it even more challenging to diagnose abuse.

Identifying suspected abuse and reporting reasonable suspicions to CPS can be one of the most challenging and difficult responsibilities for the pediatrician. Yet early identification and intervention to protect abused children have the potential to stop the abuse and secure the child's safety and mitigate toxic stress in victims; in some cases, early recognition of

TABLE 1 Factors and Characteristics That Place a Child at Risk for Maltreatment

Child	Parent	Environment (Community and Society)
Emotional/behavioral difficulties	Low self-esteem	Social isolation
Chronic illness	Poor impulse control	Poverty
Physical disabilities	Substance abuse/alcohol abuse	Unemployment
Developmental disabilities	Young maternal or paternal age	Low educational achievement
Preterm birth	Parent abused as a child	Single parent
Unwanted child	Depression or other mental illness	Nonbiologically related male living in the home
Unplanned pregnancy	Poor knowledge of child development or unrealistic expectations for child	Family or intimate partner violence
	Negative perception of normal child behavior	

Reproduced with permission from Flaherty et al.[34]

abuse can be life saving. There is evidence, however, that physicians miss opportunities for early identification and intervention.[54,55] This is especially true for infants and toddlers, who are at highest risk of life-threatening and fatal injuries at the hands of their caregivers.[56]

Proper management of minor but suspicious injuries provides an opportunity for early recognition and intervention to protect vulnerable children. Previous sentinel injuries, defined as inflicted injuries that are minor and recognized by physicians or parents before the recognition that the child has been abused, are common in abused infants but rare in those not abused.[54] For example, previous sentinel injuries are identified in 25% of abused infants and in one-third of those with AHT.[54,55] The majority of sentinel injuries are bruises, intraoral injuries, including frena tears, or fractures.[57-60]

Physicians sometimes underappreciate the significance of sentinel injuries or attribute them to noninflicted trauma, self-inflicted trauma, or medical disease.[54] Physicians may overlook injuries that are commonly considered accidental in ambulatory children but have higher specificity for abuse in young infants. Radiographs and other imaging, ordered for possible injury or for other complaints, may be misinterpreted, missing signs of trauma that are subtle or unique to the infant brain or skeleton.[61,62] When sentinel injuries raise the concern of abuse, the physician may be falsely reassured by a negative evaluation for additional occult injuries. Physicians may correctly identify an injury as suspicious but decide not to report their suspicion to child welfare for investigation.[63,64] CPS may fail to put in place adequate protection for children after suspected abuse is reported.[54] All of these factors contribute to increased morbidity and mortality for physically abused children.

CLINICAL PRESENTATIONS AND SETTINGS

Infants and children who have been abused may come to a pediatrician's attention in a variety of ways. An individual (mandated reporter or other adult) may identify and report a suspicious injury; individuals may report an abusive event they witnessed; a caregiver may observe symptoms related to an injury and bring the child for medical care but may be unaware that the child has been injured; a child or adolescent may disclose that he or she has been hurt in an abusive manner; abusers may seek medical attention because they believe an injury is severe.

The clinical approach to an infant or child with possible abusive injuries does not differ significantly from routine pediatric care. Abused children can present with a range of injuries, from minor to life-threatening. As with all patients, a severely injured child needs to be stabilized before further evaluation is undertaken. This initial evaluation may require a trauma response team and pediatric specialists in surgery, emergency medicine, and critical care. If the child presents to the pediatric office with a serious injury that requires further medical care in a specialty clinic or hospital setting, the physician may opt to gather the minimum information needed to report to CPS. Injuries suspicious for abuse or neglect are required by law to be reported to CPS. In many communities, especially those near academic pediatric centers, child abuse pediatricians are available for consultation and assistance with challenging cases, although as with other medical problems, many cases of maltreatment can be managed by the child's primary care pediatrician. The pediatrician may also refer the patient to a local community hospital to complete needed radiologic and laboratory evaluation. In some communities, hospital social workers are available to assist in making

referrals to CPS. If a physician is suspicious that the patient was maltreated, transferring the child to another physician or facility for medical care does not relieve the physician of his or her responsibility as a mandated reporter of suspected abuse.

MEDICAL HISTORY

Once the child is stabilized, a careful and well-documented history is an important element of the medical evaluation. Parents or other responsible caregivers can be asked to describe in detail events surrounding all reported injuries. The best approach is to allow the parent or other caregiver to provide a narrative without interruptions, so that the history is not influenced by the clinician's questions or interpretations. Clarifying questions can then follow. At times, it may be clinically helpful to interview each parent separately, although this is often not possible in the office setting. Information about the child's behavior before, during, and after the injury occurred, including the day's activities, events leading up to the injury, feeding times, and level of responsiveness, are important to collect. In cases of abuse, the exact timing of an injury may not be known, and information about the child's activities and wellness leading up to the medical visit is needed. Knowing when a child was last noted to be normally active and well-appearing may assist with identifying the timing of an injury. If there is no history of trauma provided, the physician can specifically ask whether the child may have sustained any trauma, and denials are helpful to record in the medical record. It is important to document descriptions of the reported mechanism of injury or injuries, onset and progression of symptoms, and the child's developmental capabilities. Few pediatricians are trained in forensic interviewing, and it is not the physician's responsibility to identify the perpetrator of the abuse or the exact details of an abusive event, but to recognize potential abuse, obtain a thorough medical and event history, initiate appropriate workup, and then refer the patient or involve the specialists who are expert in completing the medical evaluation and/or investigation.

School-aged children and adolescents may not disclose their abuse, even when their injuries strongly indicate abusive trauma. They may be afraid of repercussions or have feelings of loyalty to their abuser. They may be fearful of being removed from their family home and want to stay at home despite personal danger. Routine inquiry about physical, sexual, and other safety during adolescent health care visits may improve disclosure of abuse, and providing privacy and interviewing adolescents alone when they present with concerning injuries is an important feature of the adolescent evaluation.

Victims of significant trauma usually have observable changes in behavior, although exceptions exist. In young infants, changes in behavior can be difficult to assess by both parents and physicians. For example, children's behaviors after fracturing a bone are variable; in a recent study of accidental fractures in children less than 6 years of age, a notable minority of children with long-bone fractures did not cry or use their affected limb abnormally after injury, causing some delay in the seeking medical care.[65] Children with fatal head injuries are usually comatose immediately after the injury. However, on rare occasions, young victims of fatal head trauma may present with some level of neurologic alertness, although not normal, before death.[66,67] Some victims of AHT may have nonspecific symptoms for several hours or more before developing either seizures or coma, and others can present with nonspecific symptoms. Such symptoms may include reduced

activity, lethargy, irritability, poor feeding, vomiting, or apnea.[68,69] Documentation of historical details provided to the pediatrician can be important during later investigation of suspicious injuries.

Information can be gathered in a nonaccusatory but detailed manner. For example, asking the caregivers whether they have any concerns that someone might have harmed the child introduces a concern, without apportioning blame. Additional information that may be useful in the medical assessment of suspected physical abuse includes the following:

1. Standard history including medical, developmental, and social history;

2. Family history: especially of bleeding, bone disorders, and metabolic or genetic disorders;

3. Pregnancy history: wanted/unwanted, planned/unplanned, prenatal care, postnatal complications, postpartum depression, delivery in nonhospital settings;

4. Familial patterns of discipline;

5. Child temperament: whether the child is easy or difficult to care for; whether there is excessive crying in an infant; parents' expectations of the child's behaviors and development;

6. History of abuse to child, siblings, or parents and previous and/or present CPS involvement with the family;

7. Substance abuse by any caregivers or people living in the home; mental health problems of parents; past arrests, incarcerations, or interactions with law enforcement; and domestic violence (which may be necessary to ask of each parent or caregiver individually); and

8. Social and financial stressors and resources.

HISTORIES THAT SUGGEST CHILD ABUSE

Injuries are common in childhood; those sustained by ambulatory, active

children are often unwitnessed by caregivers. In such cases, parents can describe events surrounding the injury, but are unable to describe the precise mechanism of trauma. Verbal children can often provide their own history of trauma, which can be helpful in the evaluation. If the child can be interviewed, his or her demeanor can be noted during questioning. Some abused children display strong nonverbal cues of anxiety and reluctance when answering questions regarding potential abuse, because they are protective of their abuser or they fear retribution for "telling." Others may appear openly fearful of their abuser. However, some children hide their fear and emotions remarkably well. Such responses may be important to consider when a safety plan for the child is made.

In addition to a disclosure of abuse from a child or parent, there are histories that raise a concern for abusive trauma. These include histories in which

1. There is either no explanation or a vague explanation given for a significant injury;

2. There is an explicit denial of trauma in a child with obvious injury;

3. An important detail of the explanation changes in a substantive way;

4. An explanation is provided that is inconsistent with the pattern, age, or severity of the injury or injuries;

5. An explanation is given that is inconsistent with the child's physical and/or developmental capabilities;

6. There is an unexplained or unexpected notable delay in seeking medical care; or

7. Different witnesses provide markedly different explanations for the injury or injuries.

PHYSICAL EXAMINATION

An injury pattern is rarely pathognomonic for abuse or accident without careful consideration of the explanation provided, a thorough physical examination, and radiographic or laboratory analysis. In cases of rare accidental household injury leading to a severe or fatal outcome, investigation into the cause of the injury is often necessary, and reporting the injury for investigation is still warranted. In many states, parental consent is not needed to photograph abusive injuries or obtain radiographs or other needed studies in cases of suspected abuse.

Child abuse is sometimes diagnosed when a child is brought for evaluation and treatment of a specific injury, but some abusive injuries may be uncovered unexpectedly during a routine physical examination or an examination done for another reason. When injuries are identified during an examination, it is appropriate to ask the child (or parent, if the child is preverbal) how the injury occurred, and if significant, whether the child was seen for treatment of the injury.

If child abuse is suspected, based on history or physical examination findings, a thorough examination with the child undressed (in a gown) is necessary. The general examination of the child may reveal evidence of neglect, including malnutrition, extensive dental caries, untreated diaper dermatitis, or neglected wound care. It is important to carefully measure and plot all growth measures on a growth chart, and obtaining previous measurements can help gauge whether the growth velocity has been appropriate. Plotting growth parameters is important, because clinicians may miss significant growth failure in infants and children if the clinician relies only on clinical impression. Physical abuse and neglect are sometimes concurrent, and on occasion, children may be intentionally starved.[70,71] The head, eyes, ears, nose, and throat (HEENT) examination includes an inspection of the scalp for traumatic wounds or

traumatic alopecia. The mouth examination may reveal healing mucosal tears, dental trauma, or dental caries.[72,73] Careful examination of the frena in infants may reveal acute or healing injury. The skin examination may reveal bruises, lacerations, burns, bites, or other injuries that can be documented with the location, size, shape, and other details of the injury. Skin injury in unusual locations such as the pinna, the back of the ear, the hairline behind the ear, the buttocks, and thighs are seen in abused children and require attention during the physical examination. Adolescents may display defensive wounds on the hands, forearms, or other parts of the extremities, as they try to protect themselves from their abuser. Skin injuries can be documented in the medical record by written description, photograph, or both. The chest and abdomen may reveal injury, and a careful palpation of the legs, arms, feet, hands, ribs, and head may reveal acute or healing (callous) fractures. A complete neurologic assessment, including assessment of the anterior fontanelle, reflexes, cranial nerves, sensorium, and gross and fine motor abilities appropriate to the child's development and age, is important in the overall assessment. The child's alertness and demeanor may reflect the neurologic status and degree of discomfort and pain. Abnormalities may reflect current or past injuries to the central nervous system. Abused children may also have developmental disabilities because of deprivation in the home environment or other causes.

PHYSICAL EXAMINATION FINDINGS THAT SUGGEST ABUSE

Specific individual injuries and certain patterns of injury warrant careful consideration for abuse, although few single injuries are pathognomonic for abuse. Typically, the comparison of the provided mechanism, the age and development of the child, and the severity and age

or timing of the injury will identify those that require further investigation for abuse. Additionally, there are diseases that can be mistaken for child abuse, and testing to identify diseases in the differential diagnosis is sometimes required.[74] In some cases, this will require consultation with pediatric subspecialists. General physical examination findings that suggest abuse include the following:

1. ANY injury to a young, pre-ambulatory infant, including bruises, mouth injuries, fractures, and intracranial or abdominal injury;

2. Injuries to multiple organ systems;

3. Multiple injuries in different stages of healing;

4. Patterned injuries;

5. Injuries to nonbony or other un-usual locations, such as over the torso, ears, face, neck, or upper arms;

6. Significant injuries that are un-explained; and

7. Additional evidence of child neglect.

Skin Injuries

Bruises are the most common and readily visible injuries due to physical abuse but are missed as a sentinel injury in almost half of fatal and near-fatal abusive injuries.[54,63] Bruising may be the only external indicator of more serious internal injury.[75] There is ample evidence that evaluating bruising patterns in abused and nonabused children helps to identify specific ages, locations, and patterns of bruising that are highly correlated with child abuse.[76–81]

In children with bruising related to normal activity, the prevalence and mean number of bruises increases with age, and the majority of preschool-aged and schoolchildren have accidental bruises.[82] The commonest sites of bruising in nonabused, ambulatory children are to the knees and shins, and the vast majority of normal bruises are over bony prominences, including the forehead.[82]

Overall bruising patterns in abused children differ from those in nonabused children. The head and face are the most common sites of bruising in abused children,[83] and abused children tend to have more bruises identified at the time of diagnosis.[82] Abused children may have clustering of bruises, sometimes representing defensive injuries. Bruises may carry the imprint or negative image of an implement, such as seen with handprints or looped marks from extension cords. Bruises are notably rare in preambulatory infants. There is a strong correlation between bruising and mobility in infants and toddlers, and any bruising identified in a nonambulatory infant requires careful consideration and medical evaluation for possible abuse: "those who don't cruise, rarely bruise."[78] All parts of the body are vulnerable to bruising from abuse, and bruises to the torso, ears, or neck in children ≤4 years of age are predictive of abuse.[76] The mnemonic "TEN 4" is an easy way to identify bruises that are of concern for abuse:

- T: torso;

- E: ear;

- N: neck; and

- 4: in children less than or equal to 4 years of age and in ANY infant under 4 months of age.

The age of a bruise cannot be determined accurately.[84] Deep bruises may not be readily visible for several hours or in some cases, a few days. Areas that are painful to palpation may require repeat examination in 1 to 2 days, when the bruise may become apparent. Soft tissue swelling is associated with recent trauma and can persist for several days.

Many diseases are associated with bruises, including coagulopathies and vasculitides, and children who present with suspicious bruises may require screening for diseases that are included in the differential diagnosis of abuse. Additional discussion related to the evaluation of bleeding disorders in suspected child abuse can be found in the recently published AAP clinical and technical reports.[85,86]

Bite marks can be important evidence in cases of suspected child abuse. Bite marks are characterized by ecchymoses, abrasions, or lacerations that are found in an elliptical or ovoid pattern. Bite marks may have a central area of ecchymosis caused by either positive pressure from the closing of the teeth with disruption of small vessels or negative pressure caused by suction and tongue thrusting.[87] Bite marks can be inflicted by an adult, another child, an animal, or the patient. Identifying the perpetrator is determined by size, dentition characteristics within the wound, location of the wound, presence of puncture marks, arch form, and intercuspid distance. All of these characteristics may or may not be found in every bite mark. Dental professionals are invaluable resources for identifying wound patterns suspicious for bites. When in doubt, health care professionals may seek the advice of a dentist or forensic odontologist, if available, to assist in the evaluation. Photographing bite marks requires special techniques and resources and is not part of routine pediatric practice. For those who have access to professional medical photographers, multiple color photos, all including a known color and measurement index and taken perpendicular to each body plane, can be taken by using various exposures to facilitate adequate evidence collection. If a standard index, such as the American Board of Forensic Odontology No. 2 scale, is not available, any indexing item of known size and shape, such as a quarter or other coin, can be a suitable index for processing and analysis. Swabs of a fresh bite can be sent to a crime laboratory for DNA analysis, something occasionally done in the emergency department.

Although burns are common childhood injuries, only a minority are associated with abuse. Inflicted burns tend to be more severe, in part because they are often associated with delay in seeking medical care, and are more common in young children.[88] Scald burns, including immersions, are the most common cause of severe burns requiring hospitalization in children. Inflicted immersion burns characteristically have sharp lines of demarcation and often involve the genitals and the lower extremities in symmetric distributions.[89] These burns are often associated with soiling accidents or other behaviors that require cleaning the child and are seen most often in toddlers. Object contact burns are inflicted with hot solids, such as irons, radiators, stoves, or cigarettes. Burns inflicted with hot objects can be difficult to differentiate from accidental mechanisms, because both may be patterned, but inflicted contact burns are characteristically deep and leave a clear imprint of the hot instrument. The history, number of burns, and continuity of the burn pattern over curved body surfaces may indicate a greater probability of inflicted injury. Dermatologic and infectious diseases can mimic abusive burns, including toxin-mediated staphylococcal and streptococcal infections, impetigo, phytophotodermatitis, and chemical burns of the buttocks from senna-containing laxatives.[90] Inflicted burn injuries require the same treatment as any burn, but children with inflicted burns have a higher morbidity and longer hospital stays than children with accidental burns.[91]

Skeletal Injuries

Most fractures in childhood are the result of accidental trauma, and of the small percentage of fractures that result from abuse, most are found in infants.[92-94] Abused infants and children may present with skeletal trauma as their sentinel injury, and fractures are regularly identified by skeletal radiographs during the medical evaluation of suspected abuse as well as other conditions. The timely identification of skeletal injury can lead to earlier identification of abuse, sparing the victim further injury, which sometimes can be life-threatening.[62] Children with recent fractures are usually symptomatic, with crying, visible swelling, or refusal to use the affected area. On occasion, the child's symptoms are minimal, which can lead to a delay in seeking care.[65] When fractures are suspected, skin surfaces can be carefully examined for 'grab marks' that may indicate restraint or areas that were pulled or twisted to create the fracture. Absence of such bruising does not exclude a fracture or an abusive mechanism of injury. In fact, most fractures sustained by healthy children are not associated with bruising either at the time of presentation (only 10% with bruising) or within the first week (28% with bruising) after trauma.[95] Abusive fractures have been described in virtually every bone in the body, and any single fracture can be the result of accident or abuse. Skull fractures are common injuries in nonabused infants, and parietal and linear skull fractures are most common in both abuse and nonabuse.[96,97] Physical abuse is in the differential diagnosis for children with fractures in the following situations:

1. Fracture(s) in nonambulatory infants, especially in those without a clear history of trauma or a known medical condition that predisposes to bone fragility;

2. Children with multiple fractures;

3. Infants and children with rib fractures;

4. Infants and toddlers with midshaft humerus or femur fractures;

5. Infants and children with unusual fractures, including those of the scapula, classic metaphyseal lesions (CMLs) of the long bones, vertebrae, and sternum, unless explained by a known history of severe trauma or underlying bone disorder; and

6. The history of trauma does not explain the resultant fracture.

Some fractures in abused children, including rib fractures and CMLs, may not be clinically detectable, and a negative clinical examination does not preclude the need for a skeletal radiologic survey when inflicted trauma is suspected, particularly in children younger than 2 years.

Radiographic skeletal survey is the standard tool for detecting clinically unsuspected fractures in possible victims of child abuse (Table 2), and skeletal surveys should conform to American College of Radiology standards.[98] A recent analysis of more than 700 consecutive skeletal surveys performed at 1 children's hospital revealed occult skeletal trauma in 11% of those tested, influencing the diagnosis of abuse in more than half of the positive cases.[99] Race and socioeconomic status appear to influence a physician's practice in obtaining skeletal surveys when children present with skeletal trauma, leading to both over- and underreporting of abuse in different populations.[36,100] Repeating skeletal surveys 2 to 3 weeks after an initial

TABLE 2 Indications for Obtaining a Skeletal Survey

All children <2 y with obvious abusive injuries
All children <2 y with any suspicious injury, including
   Bruises or other skin injuries in nonambulatory infants;
   Oral injuries in nonambulatory infants; and
   Injuries not consistent with the history provided
Infants with unexplained, unexpected sudden death (consult with medical examiner/coroner first)
Infants and young toddlers with unexplained intracranial injuries, including hemorrhage and hypoxic-ischemic injury
Infants and siblings <2 y and household contacts of an abused child
Twins of abused infants and toddlers

presentation of suspected abuse improves diagnostic sensitivity and specificity for identifying skeletal trauma in abused infants.[101,102] Not all abusive fractures (eg, rib fractures and CMLs) are visible by radiograph initially, and prospective studies have shown that repeat skeletal imaging increases the number of fractures diagnosed by more than 25% in abuse victims.[101] Repeat skeletal surveys can identify fractures not visible on initial skeletal survey, assist in dating of injuries, clarify questionable findings, and alter the clinical diagnosis in equivocal cases.

Diseases and conditions that affect collagen and/or bone mineralization can be included in the differential diagnosis of skeletal trauma due to abuse; identifying these diseases or conditions reduces false accusations of abuse.[103] Vitamin and mineral deficiencies and genetic and infectious diseases may be considered in the differential diagnosis when appropriate.[104–107] Additional discussion related to the differential diagnosis of fractures and fracture evaluation in suspected child abuse can be found in the recently published AAP clinical report.[108]

Thoracoabdominal Injuries

Injuries to the chest are common in abuse, although clinically significant internal organ injury occurs less frequently. Most thoracic injuries are due to blows or crush injury to the chest and/or abdomen. Abusive injuries that involve the heart, including direct cardiac trauma and dysrhythmias, are rare. Commotio cordis, hemopericardium, myocardial contusions, and cardiac aneurysms and rupture have all been reported from abuse, as has shearing of the thoracic duct resulting in chylothorax.[109–113] Pulmonary injuries in abused children include contusions, lacerations resulting in pneumothorax, hemorrhagic effusions or pneumomediastinum, and pulmonary edema associated with suffocation or head trauma.[114,115] Rib fractures are strongly associated with physical abuse.[92] They are usually due to forceful squeezing of the chest, are often multiple, can be unilateral or bilateral, and can occur anywhere along the rib's arc.[94,116] Acute rib fractures may be associated with shallow breathing attributable to pain and splinting, or with irritability when the infant is picked up and moved. Acute rib fractures can be difficult to identify radiographically, and both oblique views of the ribs and follow-up skeletal surveys done 2 to 3 weeks after an initial evaluation increase the identification of inflicted rib fractures. Rib fractures in infants can be related to osteopenia of prematurity or other metabolic bone disease, and careful clinical correlation is always required.[117,118] Although cardiopulmonary resuscitation (CPR) remains an unusual cause of rib fractures,[119] changes in CPR technique in the past few years may increase the risk of anterior and lateral rib fractures from CPR in infants.[120,121]

Abdominal injury is a severe form of maltreatment and represents the second leading cause of mortality from physical abuse.[122] The highest rates of abusive abdominal trauma are seen in infants and toddlers.[123] Compared with children who sustain accidental abdominal trauma, victims of abuse tend to be younger, are more likely to have an injury to the hollow viscera, are more likely to have delayed presentations to medical care, and have a higher mortality rate.[124,125] Solid organ injuries, most often involving the liver, are more common overall in both accidental and abusive abdominal injury, but abused children are more likely to have accompanying hollow viscus injury.[124] Abdominal bruising often is not seen, even in children with severe or fatal abdominal injury.[126] Symptomatic children can present with signs of hemorrhage or peritonitis, but many children will not display overt findings, or their

abdominal trauma may be masked by other injuries. Screening laboratory tests, including liver and pancreatic enzyme levels, are important to obtain in all children who present with serious trauma, even if they do not display acute abdominal symptoms.[127,128] A urinalysis may also identify trauma to the urinary tract and kidneys. Radiographic studies, especially contrast-enhancing computed tomography (CT), are helpful in determining the types and severity of intra-abdominal trauma and are warranted when screening laboratory tests indicate possible abdominal trauma, in all cases of symptomatic injury, and most cases when the physical examination is unreliable because of the patient's age, presence of other injuries that may obfuscate the abdominal examination, or presence of accompanying head injury. Surgical consultation is required for children with inflicted abdominal injury.[114]

Head Injuries

Head trauma is the leading cause of child physical abuse fatality and occurs most commonly in infants.[129] Most fatal head injuries in infants and young children are the result of abuse.[130] Children with AHT may present for medical care with a false history of accidental trauma or with nonspecific symptoms related to their injuries. Several factors contribute to missed opportunities for AHT detection[55]: caregivers do not or cannot provide an accurate history of the injury to the physician, the presenting symptoms can be mild and nonspecific, and young infants are difficult to evaluate clinically, which makes accurate diagnosis impossible in some cases. On occasion, minor head injuries such as bruising or abrasions are discounted by physicians, developing macrocephaly goes unnoticed, or radiographs are misinterpreted. Racial and social biases may also contribute to misdiagnosis. Common erroneous diagnoses given to victims of AHT

include viral gastroenteritis, gastroesophageal reflux, colic, accidental head injury, and otitis media.[55]

Multiple mechanisms contribute to the cerebral, spinal, and cranial injuries that result from inflicted head injury to infants and young children, including both shaking and blunt impact.[131] Confessions from some perpetrators have highlighted the often repetitive nature of the abuse, and the crying of an infant as a common impetus for the violence.[69,132] Compared with children with severe accidental trauma, children with AHT are more likely to have subdural hemorrhage, retinal hemorrhages, and associated cutaneous, skeletal, and visceral injuries.[97,133–136] Inflicted injuries tend to occur in younger patients and result in higher mortality and longer hospital stays than does accidental head trauma.[97,129,137] Infants with intracranial injuries may have no neurologic symptoms and are sometimes identified during a medical evaluation for other suspicious injuries.[75,138] Because the potential morbidity of AHT is so great, infants who are being evaluated for abuse benefit from brain imaging, whether or not they have neurologic symptoms.

All infants and children with suspected AHT require cranial CT, MRI, or both.[139] For symptomatic children, CT of the head will identify abnormalities that require immediate surgical intervention and is preferred over MRI for identifying acute hemorrhage and skull fractures and scalp swelling from blunt injury. MRI is the optimal modality for assessing intracranial injury, including cerebral hypoxia and ischemia, and is used for all children with abnormal CT scans, asymptomatic infants with noncranial abusive injuries, and for follow-up of identified trauma.[140,141] Ultrasound is often used in the initial evaluation of macrocephaly in young infants and can identify large extra-axial cerebrospinal fluid collections. Any abnormal ultrasound study requires more sophisticated follow-up with MRI. Ultrasound is not sensitive for identifying small subdural collections and is not the test of choice in the emergency setting.

Retinal hemorrhages are common, but not universal, in victims of AHT.[142] Although seen on occasion in children with accidental injury, severe retinal hemorrhages are highly associated with abuse, particularly in young infants.[143] The extent and severity of retinal hemorrhages are also greater in abuse victims and correlate with the severity of acute neurologic symptoms.[136,144] Retinal hemorrhages are occasionally identified in nonabused critically ill children, primarily those with coagulopathy, leukemia, or severe accidental injury, and are distinguished from abuse by history and laboratory testing.[145,146] An examination by using indirect ophthalmoscopy is required in the evaluation of AHT, preferably by an ophthalmologist with pediatric or retinal experience. The ophthalmologist can provide documentation of the retinal hemorrhages by photography or detailed annotated drawings. Location, depth, and extent of retinal hemorrhages may distinguish between abusive and nonabusive causes of head trauma.[147] Hemorrhages that extend to the ora serrata and involve multiple layers of the retina are strongly associated with AHT. A fundoscopic examination is not an adequate screening test for intracranial findings, as neurologically asymptomatic infants rarely have retinal hemorrhages but may, in fact, have intracranial injury. Recent studies suggest that fundoscopic examination may not be necessary if examination and neuroimaging show no evidence of intracranial injury, since the likelihood of encountering retinal hemorrhages in those children is very low.[75,148]

Conditions that may be confused with AHT include accidental trauma; metabolic, genetic, and other diseases that are associated with vasculitis, coagulation defects, or cerebral atrophy; and primary coagulopathies.[149] Although most household trauma results in minor or no injury, on rare occasion, severe or fatal head injury has been reported.[53] In addition to searching for occult trauma in patients who present with such a history, or in infants and young children who present with unexplained intracranial hemorrhage and/or hypoxic ischemic cerebral injury, consideration of alternate explanations is often required. Investigation by child welfare or law enforcement can also help to distinguish accidental from abusive head injury, and reporting to CPS for investigation in all suspicious cases is advised.

DIAGNOSTIC TESTING AND DOCUMENTATION

When abuse is suspected as the cause of an injury, the clinician may conduct tests to screen for other injuries and/or underlying medical causes that can contribute to the finding or be considered in the differential diagnosis of abuse. The extent of diagnostic testing depends on several factors, including the severity of the injury, type of injury, and age and developmental level of the child. In general, the more severe the injury and younger the child, the more extensive is the need for diagnostic testing for other injuries. Table 3 is a summary of tests that may be used during a medical assessment for suspected abuse. Additionally, child abuse pediatricians and pediatric subspecialists can be consulted to assist with recommendations and questions.

When 1 child is identified as a suspected victim of abuse, siblings, other young children in the household, and other child contacts of the suspected abuser greatly benefit

from being assessed for injuries in a timely manner.[150] This assessment is especially important for twins, who are at substantial risk of injury, including occult fractures. The extent of the assessment depends on the child's age, symptoms, and signs; infants and toddlers may require more extensive testing, because symptoms and signs may be less useful in determining the presence of occult abusive injuries. A skeletal survey is extremely useful for children <2 years of age who are siblings or other household members of abused children, as occult fractures are detected in more than 10% of these children.[150]

Thorough medical documentation of the reported history and physical examination findings can be crucial to protecting and intervening early with children suspected of being abused. Careful documentation of visible injuries by written description, digital photographs, and/or body diagrams facilitates peer review as well as court testimony, when required. In some regions, investigators from law enforcement or CPS are trained to take forensic photographs. It is important to include diagnostic impressions in the medical record that address the likelihood of nonaccidental injury when child abuse is suspected. In cases with multiorgan, severe, or obvious injuries, abuse may be clear, and a strong diagnostic statement is warranted. Some injuries, while suspicious, are less diagnostic and may warrant further medical evaluation by a child abuse pediatrician, a specialist in pediatric radiology, neurology, orthopedics, surgery, or other specialties, and/or a CPS investigation. Medical records that reflect specific levels of concern, alternative diagnostic possibilities, and include the results of additional testing are important for later review and to assist CPS or police investigation. It is helpful to document reports to CPS and law enforcement in the medical record. If

TABLE 3 Diagnostic Tests That May Be Used in the Medical Assessment of Suspected Physical Abuse and Differential Diagnoses[a]

Type of Injury or Condition	Laboratory Testing	Radiologic Testing	Comments
Fractures[108]	• Bone health laboratory testing, including calcium, phosphorus, alkaline phosphatase • Consider 25-hydroxyvitamin D and PTH level • Consider serum copper, Vitamin C, and ceruloplasmin levels if child is at risk for scurvy or copper deficiency • Consider skin biopsy for fibroblast culture and/or venous blood for DNA analysis for osteogenesis imperfecta	Skeletal survey	• Repeat skeletal survey in 2 wk for high-risk cases • Single whole-body films are unacceptable • Bone scintigraphy may be used to complement the skeletal survey
Bruises[85,86]	Tests for hematologic disorders: CBC, platelets, PT, INR, aPTT, VWF antigen, VWF activity (ristocetin cofactor), factor VIII level, factor IX level	• Skeletal survey for nonambulatory infants with bruises and for infants and toddlers with suspicious bruising • Brain imaging for infants with suspicious bruising.	• Useful when bleeding disorder is a concern because of clinical presentation or family history • Consultation with pediatric hematologist for any abnormal screen or other concern
Abdominal trauma	• Liver enzyme tests: aspartate aminotransferase, alanine aminotransferase • Pancreatic enzymes: amylase, lipase; urinalysis	• CT of abdomen with contrast • Skeletal survey in children <2 y	• Screening abdominal laboratory tests are helpful in diagnosing occult abdominal injury in young abuse victims • IV contrast should be used for CT scan and is preferable to PO[135]
Head trauma	• CBC with platelets, PT/INR/aPTT; factor VIII level, factor IX level, fibrinogen, d-dimer • Review newborn screen • Consider urine organic acids to screen for GA1	• CT scan: head[b] • MRI of head and spine • Skeletal survey	• MRI may provide better dating of intracranial injuries than CT • MRI more sensitive than CT for subtle intracranial injuries in patients with normal CT and abnormal neurologic examinations • Diffusion-weighted imaging may show extent of parenchymal injury early in course • MRI more sensitive than plain radiographs and CT for detecting cervical spine fractures/injury • CT, and three-dimensional spiral CT enhance detection of skull fractures
Cardiac injury	Cardiac enzymes: troponin, creatine kinase with muscle and brain subunits (CK-MB); troponin		

aPTT, activated partial thromboplastin time; CBC, complete blood cell count; CK-MB, creatine kinase MB band; GA1, glutaric aciduria type I; INR, international normalized ratio; IV, intravenous; PO, oral; PT, prothrombin time; PTH, parathyroid hormone; VWF, von Willebrand factor.

[a] Tests can be ordered judiciously and in consultation with the appropriate genetics, hematology, radiology, and child abuse specialists. Careful consideration of the patient's history, age, and clinical findings guide selection of the appropriate tests.

[b] CT scan may provide clinically relevant information more expeditiously than MRI in some facilities.

a child has sustained a serious injury because he or she was left unsupervised in a dangerous environment, the physician can report suspected neglect or inappropriate adult supervision to CPS; this includes injuries sustained while under the care of an intoxicated adult.[151]

TREATMENT

Once medical assessment and stabilization are achieved and a report has been made to investigative agencies, the physician can continue to be an advocate for the child, helping to see that the child receives necessary follow-up services. The child's primary care physician, if not already involved, should be notified, and CPS can assist the family in complying with the plan of care. These services may include referral not only to appropriate medical providers but also often to mental health providers for an evaluation because of the psychological effect of abuse or neglect on the young child, the siblings, and the nonoffending caregiver. Because adult intimate partner violence, drug abuse, and other adult stressors commonly co-occur with child abuse, family members may require timely medical and mental health assistance.

THE ROLE OF THE PEDIATRICIAN

Pediatricians are in a unique position to recognize abuse and protect victims, especially young children,

children with disabilities, and other children who are isolated in some way from regular contact with the public. The management of child abuse is one of the most challenging and unsettling responsibilities in pediatric practice, and pediatricians often struggle to balance their roles as family and child advocates.[63,64] Child abuse is common, however, and the morbidity significant, which is why identifying, promptly reporting, and managing cases of suspected abuse can be so important to the health and safety of children.

Duty to Report Child Abuse

This report has provided a general overview of child physical abuse. As with all medical diagnoses, successful management begins with awareness and attention to detail in clinical practice. When the history or physical examination reveals suspicious injuries, and the pediatrician has a reasonable suspicion that a child has been abused, a report to CPS for further investigation is mandated by law. Mandatory reporting laws do not require certainty, and failure to make a report can result in civil or criminal penalties for the physician, or most dire, additional injury or death of a child.[49] All state laws provide some type of immunity for good-faith reporting, although laws vary slightly between states. Many states have laws that permit physicians to evaluate children who are suspected victims of abuse, to conduct tests, and to take photographs of children's injuries without parental consent. In practice, parents are informed of testing, radiographs, and photographs that will be taken, and parental refusal is uncommon. Pediatricians can look to specific state laws for additional guidance if these issues arise.

Child abuse cases can be difficult to evaluate, and input from a trusted colleague, senior clinician, or medical specialists can be helpful. If the pediatrician is uncertain about whether to report a suspicion to CPS,

consultation with pediatric specialists in child abuse, radiology, orthopedics, neurology, surgery, and other specialties can be a valuable resource. Arranging hospitalization for a child who requires additional medical testing and/or protection is often required, allows for additional consultation and observation, and should be considered medically necessary by third-party payers.

Many hospitals and communities have developed teams of child abuse pediatricians and other professionals who specialize in the assessment of suspected abuse.[152] Involving such teams early in the process can improve accurate and comprehensive assessments and information sharing among the medical and nonmedical disciplines involved.[153] Other regions do not have specialized child abuse teams, but do have physicians with expertise in child abuse.

Once the decision has been made to report a concern of physical abuse to CPS, it is important to discuss the report with the child's parent(s). This is one of the most difficult discussions a pediatrician may have in clinical practice, but an honest conversation will allow for more open communication during and after the ensuing investigation. In this conversation, it can be helpful to raise concern about an injury, while not apportioning blame, and inform the parent that because of the nature and circumstances of the injury, a report for further investigation is mandated by law. Although some families may abandon the pediatrician's practice after a report is made, it is important not to abandon the family at the time of the report. An investigation of possible abuse is a time of crisis for a family, and a supportive physician can be of great assistance to the child and nonoffending parent(s) and family members. In addition, most cases of child physical abuse result from family stress, and state CPS agencies typically provide useful family support in these cases. These

supports may range from day care vouchers to in-home therapy. Only a minority of children reported to CPS enter the foster care system, and these cases are carefully overseen by the court system. Thus, it is rare that a physician report alone leads to removal of children from their biological parents.

The physician's cooperation with CPS investigations is necessary to improve decision-making by investigators. Health Insurance Portability and Accountability Act (HIPAA) rules allow disclosure of protected health information to CPS without legal guardian authorization when the physician has made a mandatory report, but state laws differ regarding the release of health information to investigators under other circumstances and after investigations are complete.[154] Because CPS and law enforcement investigators do not typically have a medical background or training, the pediatrician's interpretation of the child's injuries in straightforward language that allows for a meaningful conversation with the investigators is needed for proper investigation, decision-making, and protection of the child. The physician may be required to write a summary statement of his or her findings and to testify in civil or criminal trial proceedings. Additional information on testifying in civil and criminal legal proceedings can be found in an AAP policy statement on the subject.[155]

Prevention

Child abuse prevention is important but difficult and requires efforts that are broad and sustained. The pediatrician, as a trusted advisor to parents, caregivers, and families about health, development, and discipline, can play an important role in abuse prevention by assessing caregivers' strengths and deficits, providing education to enhance parenting skills, connecting families with supportive community resources that address parent and family needs, and promoting evidence-based parenting practices that are nurturing and positive.[34] Pediatricians can serve as effective advocates for funding and implementation of evidence-based prevention programs in their communities, as well as at the state and national level. Pediatricians can also partner with home-visiting and parenting programs in their community. Finally, recognizing abuse and intervening on behalf of an abused child can save a life and can protect a vulnerable child from a lifetime of negative consequences.

SUMMARY

To protect children who are victims of physical abuse,

1. Pediatricians can be alert for injuries that raise suspicion of abuse but may be overlooked by unsuspecting physicians, including
   a. ANY injury to a nonmobile infant, including bruises, oral injuries, or fractures;
   b. Injuries in unusual locations, such as over the torso, ears or neck;
   c. Patterned injuries;
   d. Injuries to multiple organ systems;
   e. Multiple injuries in different stages of healing; and
   f. Significant injuries that are unexplained.

2. Pediatricians can consider the possibility of trauma in young infants who present with non-specific symptoms of possible head trauma, including unexplained vomiting, lethargy, irritability, apnea, or seizures, and consider head imaging in their evaluation.

3. A skeletal survey for any child <2 years old with suspicious injuries can identify occult injuries that may exist in abused children and is very useful in the evaluation of suspected abuse.

4. Brain imaging may identify injury in abused infants, even in those who are not overtly symptomatic.

5. Examining siblings and household contacts of abused children often reveals injuries to those children; those under 2 years old benefit from a skeletal survey.

6. Consultation with colleagues, child abuse pediatricians, and other pediatric specialists to assist in the evaluation of difficult cases is very helpful.

7. Pediatricians are mandated reporters of suspected abuse, and reports to CPS are required by law when the physician has a reasonable suspicion of abuse. Transferring a child's care to another physician or hospital does not relieve the pediatrician of his or her reporting responsibilities.

8. Pediatricians may need to hospitalize children with suspicious injuries for medical evaluation, treatment, and/or protection.

9. Thorough documentation in medical records and effective communication with nonmedical investigators in child protection may improve outcomes of investigations and protect vulnerable children.

LEAD AUTHOR

Cindy W. Christian, MD, FAAP

COMMITTEE ON CHILD ABUSE AND NEGLECT, 2013-2014

Cindy W. Christian, MD, FAAP, Chairperson
James E. Crawford-Jakubiak, MD, FAAP
Emalee G. Flaherty, MD, FAAP
John M. Leventhal, MD, FAAP
James L. Lukefahr, MD, FAAP
Robert D. Sege, MD, PhD, FAAP

LIAISONS

Harriet MacMillan, MD — *American Academy of Child and Adolescent Psychiatry*
Catherine M. Nolan, MSW, ACSW — *Administration for Children, Youth, and Families*
Linda Anne Valley, PhD — *Centers for Disease Control and Prevention*

STAFF

Tammy Piazza Hurley

REFERENCES

1. US Department of Health and Human Services, Administration for Children and Families, Administration on Children, Youth and Families, Children's Bureau. Child maltreatment 2011. Available at: http://www.acf.hhs.gov/programs/cb/research-data-technology/statistics-research/child-maltreatment. Accessed August 25, 2014

2. Finkelhor D, Jones L. Have Sexual Abuse and Physical Abuse Declined Since the 1990s? Durham, NH: Crimes Against Children Research Center; 2012. Available at: http://www.unh.edu/ccrc/pdf/CV267_Have%20SA%20%20PA%20Decline_FACT%20SHEET_11-7-12.pdf. Accessed August 25, 2014

3. Sedlak AJ, Mettenburg J, Basena M, et al. *Fourth National Incidence Study of Child Abuse and Neglect (NIS–4): Report to Congress, Executive Summary.* Washington, DC: US Department of Health and Human Services, Administration for Children and Families; 2010

4. Farst K, Ambadwar PB, King AJ, et al. Trends in hospitalization rates and severity of injuries from abuse in young children, 1997-2009. *Pediatrics.* 2013; 131(6). Available at: www.pediatrics.org/cgi/content/full/131/6/e1796

5. Leventhal JM, Gaither JR. Incidence of serious injuries due to physical abuse in the United States: 1997 to 2009. *Pediatrics.* 2012;130(5). Available at: www.pediatrics.org/cgi/content/full/130/5/e847

6. Berger RP, Fromkin JB, Stutz H, et al. Abusive head trauma during a time of increased unemployment: a multicenter analysis. *Pediatrics.* 2011;128(4): 637–643

7. Afifi TO, Mather A, Boman J, et al. Childhood adversity and personality disorders: results from a nationally representative population-based study. *J Psychiatr Res.* 2011;45(6):814–822

8. The Child Abuse Prevention and Treatment Act (CAPTA) Reauthorization Act of 2010, Public Law 111-320, (42 USC 5106a). Available at: www.acf.hhs.gov/programs/cb/laws_policies/cblaws/capta/capta2010.pdf. Accessed August 25, 2014

9. American Academy of Pediatrics, Committee on School Health. Corporal

punishment in schools. *Pediatrics.* 2000;106(2):343

10. Ferrari AM. The impact of culture upon child rearing practices and definitions of maltreatment. *Child Abuse Negl.* 2002;26(8):793–813

11. Laskey AL, Sheridan MJ, Hymel KP. Physicians' initial forensic impressions of hypothetical cases of pediatric traumatic brain injury. *Child Abuse Negl.* 2007;31(4):329–342

12. Middlebrooks JS, Audage NC. *The Effects of Childhood Stress on Health Across the Lifespan.* Atlanta, GA: Centers for Disease Control and Prevention, National Center for Injury Prevention and Control; 2008

13. Norman RE, Byambaa M, De R, Butchart A, Scott J, Vos T. The long-term health consequences of child physical abuse, emotional abuse, and neglect: a systematic review and meta-analysis. *PLoS Med.* 2012;9(11):e1001349

14. Shonkoff JP, Boyce WT, McEwen BS. Neuroscience, molecular biology, and the childhood roots of health disparities: building a new framework for health promotion and disease prevention. *JAMA.* 2009;301(21): 2252–2259

15. Gilbert R, Widom CS, Browne K, Fergusson D, Webb E, Janson S. Burden and consequences of child maltreatment in high-income countries. *Lancet.* 2009;373(9657):68–81

16. Hillis SD, Anda RF, Dube SR, Felitti VJ, Marchbanks PA, Marks JS. The association between adverse childhood experiences and adolescent pregnancy, long-term psychosocial consequences, and fetal death. *Pediatrics.* 2004;113(2): 320–327

17. Caspi A, Harrington H, Moffitt TE, Milne BJ, Poulton R. Socially isolated children 20 years later: risk of cardiovascular disease. *Arch Pediatr Adolesc Med.* 2006;160(8):805–811

18. Schilling EA, Aseltine RH Jr, Gore S. Adverse childhood experiences and mental health in young adults: a longitudinal survey. *BMC Public Health.* 2007;7:30

19. Edwards VJ, Holden GW, Felitti VJ, Anda RF. Relationship between multiple forms of childhood maltreatment and adult mental health in community

respondents: results from the adverse childhood experiences study. *Am J Psychiatry.* 2003;160(8):1453–1460

20. Flaherty EG, Thompson R, Litrownik AJ, et al. Adverse childhood exposures and reported child health at age 12. *Acad Pediatr.* 2009;9(3):150–156

21. Shaw BA, Krause N. Exposure to physical violence during childhood, aging, and health. *J Aging Health.* 2002; 14(4):467–494

22. Springer KW, Sheridan J, Kuo D, Carnes M. Long-term physical and mental health consequences of childhood physical abuse: results from a large population-based sample of men and women. *Child Abuse Negl.* 2007;31(5): 517–530

23. Kaplan SJ, Pelcovitz D, Salzinger S, et al. Adolescent physical abuse: risk for adolescent psychiatric disorders. *Am J Psychiatry.* 1998;155(7):954–959

24. Hussey JM, Chang JJ, Kotch JB. Child maltreatment in the United States: prevalence, risk factors, and adolescent health consequences. *Pediatrics.* 2006; 118(3):933–942

25. Jayawant S, Parr J. Outcome following subdural haemorrhages in infancy. *Arch Dis Child.* 2007;92(4):343–347

26. Bonnier C, Nassogne MC, Saint-Martin C, Mesples B, Kadhim H, Sébire G. Neuroimaging of intraparenchymal lesions predicts outcome in shaken baby syndrome. *Pediatrics.* 2003;112(4): 808–814

27. Hymel KP, Makoroff KL, Laskey AL, Conaway MR, Blackman JA. Mechanisms, clinical presentations, injuries, and outcomes from inflicted versus noninflicted head trauma during infancy: results of a prospective, multicentered, comparative study. *Pediatrics.* 2007;119(5):922–929

28. Kolko DJ. Characteristics of child victims of physical violence: research findings and clinical implications. *J Interpers Violence.* 1992;7(2): 244–276

29. Perez CM, Widom CS. Childhood victimization and long-term intellectual and academic outcomes. *Child Abuse Negl.* 1994;18(8):617–633

30. Fergusson DM, Boden JM, Horwood LJ. Exposure to childhood sexual and physical abuse and adjustment in early

adulthood. *Child Abuse Negl.* 2008;32(6): 607–619

31. Johnson SB, Riley AW, Granger DA, Riis J. The science of early life toxic stress for pediatric practice and advocacy. *Pediatrics.* 2013;131(2):319–327

32. Shonkoff JP. Building a new biodevelopmental framework to guide the future of early childhood policy. *Child Dev.* 2010;81(1):357–367

33. Garner AS, Shonkoff JP; Committee on Psychosocial Aspects of Child and Family Health; Committee on Early Childhood, Adoption, and Dependent Care; Section on Developmental and Behavioral Pediatrics. Early childhood adversity, toxic stress, and the role of the pediatrician: translating developmental science into lifelong health. *Pediatrics.* 2012;129(1). Available at: www.pediatrics.org/cgi/content/full/129/1/e224

34. Flaherty EG, Stirling J Jr; American Academy of Pediatrics. Committee on Child Abuse and Neglect. Clinical report—the pediatrician's role in child maltreatment prevention. *Pediatrics.* 2010;126(4):833–841

35. Wulczyn F. Epidemiological perspectives on maltreatment prevention. *Future Child.* 2009;19(2):39–66

36. Lane WG, Rubin DM, Monteith R, Christian CW. Racial differences in the evaluation of pediatric fractures for physical abuse. *JAMA.* 2002;288(13):1603–1609

37. Finkelhor D, Turner HA, Shattuck A, Hamby SL. Violence, crime, and abuse exposure in a national sample of children and youth: an update. *JAMA Pediatr.* 2013;167(7):614–621

38. Child Welfare Information Gateway. Child abuse and neglect fatalities 2012: statistics and interventions. Available at: https://www.childwelfare.gov/pubs/factsheets/fatality.cfm. Accessed August 25, 2014

39. Wu SS, Ma CX, Carter RL, et al. Risk factors for infant maltreatment: a population-based study. *Child Abuse Negl.* 2004;28(12):1253–1264

40. Sullivan PM, Knutson JF. Maltreatment and disabilities: a population-based epidemiological study. *Child Abuse Negl.* 2000;24(10):1257–1273

41. Hibbard RA, Desch LW; American Academy of Pediatrics Committee on

Child Abuse and Neglect; American Academy of Pediatrics Council on Children With Disabilities. Maltreatment of children with disabilities. *Pediatrics*. 2007;119(5):1018–1025

42. Schnitzer PG, Ewigman BG. Child deaths resulting from inflicted injuries: household risk factors and perpetrator characteristics. *Pediatrics*. 2005;116(5). Available at: www.pediatrics.org/cgi/content/full/116/5/e687

43. Putnam-Hornstein E. Report of maltreatment as a risk factor for injury death: a prospective birth cohort study. *Child Maltreat*. 2011;16(3):163–174

44. Gibbs DA, Martin SL, Kupper LL, Johnson RE. Child maltreatment in enlisted soldiers' families during combat-related deployments. *JAMA*. 2007;298(5):528–535

45. Rentz ED, Marshall SW, Loomis D, Casteel C, Martin SL, Gibbs DA. Effect of deployment on the occurrence of child maltreatment in military and nonmilitary families. *Am J Epidemiol*. 2007;165(10):1199–1206

46. Horton C. Protective Factors Literature Review: Early Care and Education Programs and the Prevention of Child Abuse and Neglect. Washington, DC: Center for the Study of Social Policy; 2003. Available at: www.cssp.org/reform/strengthening-families/resources/body/LiteratureReview.pdf. Accessed August 25, 2014

47. Sege R, Linkenbach J. Essentials for childhood: promoting healthy outcomes from positive experiences. *Pediatrics*. 2014;133(6). Available at: www.pediatrics.org/cgi/content/full/133/6/e1489

48. Cadzow SP, Armstrong KL, Fraser JA. Stressed parents with infants: reassessing physical abuse risk factors. *Child Abuse Negl*. 1999;23(9):845–853

49. Asnes AG, Leventhal JM. Managing child abuse: general principles. *Pediatr Rev*. 2010;31(2):47–55

50. Merrill CT, Owens PL, Stocks C. Pediatric Emergency Department Visits in Community Hospitals from Selected States, 2005. HCUP Statistical Brief #52. Rockville, MD: Agency for Healthcare Research and Quality; 2008. Available at: www.hcupus.ahrq.gov/reports/statbriefs/sb52.pdf. Accessed August 25, 2014

51. Scheidler MG, Shultz BL, Schall L, Vyas A, Barksdale EM Jr. Falling televisions: the hidden danger for children. *J Pediatr Surg*. 2002;37(4):572–575

52. Lantz PE, Couture DE. Fatal acute intracranial injury, subdural hematoma, and retinal hemorrhages caused by stairway fall. *J Forensic Sci*. 2011;56(6):1648–1653

53. Chadwick DL, Bertocci G, Castillo E, et al. Annual risk of death resulting from short falls among young children: less than 1 in 1 million. *Pediatrics*. 2008;121(6):1213–1224

54. Sheets LK, Leach ME, Koszewski IJ, Lessmeier AM, Nugent M, Simpson P. Sentinel injuries in infants evaluated for child physical abuse. *Pediatrics*. 2013;131(4):701–707

55. Jenny C, Hymel KP, Ritzen A, Reinert SE, Hay TC. Analysis of missed cases of abusive head trauma. *JAMA*. 1999;281(7):621–626

56. King WK, Kiesel EL, Simon HK. Child abuse fatalities: are we missing opportunities for intervention? *Pediatr Emerg Care*. 2006;22(4):211–214

57. Thackeray JD. Frena tears and abusive head injury: a cautionary tale. *Pediatr Emerg Care*. 2007;23(10):735–737

58. Petska HW, Sheets LK, Knox BL. Facial bruising as a precursor to abusive head trauma. *Clin Pediatr (Phila)*. 2013;52(1):86–88

59. Pierce MC, Smith S, Kaczor K. Bruising in infants: those with a bruise may be abused. *Pediatr Emerg Care*. 2009;25(12):845–847

60. Feldman KW. The bruised premobile infant: should you evaluate further? *Pediatr Emerg Care*. 2009;25(1):37–39

61. Oral R, Yagmur F, Nashelsky M, Turkmen M, Kirby P. Fatal abusive head trauma cases: consequence of medical staff missing milder forms of physical abuse. *Pediatr Emerg Care*. 2008;24(12):816–821

62. Ravichandiran N, Schuh S, Bejuk M, et al. Delayed identification of pediatric abuse-related fractures. *Pediatrics*. 2010;125(1):60–66

63. Flaherty EG, Sege RD, Griffith J, et al; PROS network; NMAPedsNet. From suspicion of physical child abuse to reporting: primary care clinician decision-making. *Pediatrics*. 2008;122(3):611–619

64. Jones R, Flaherty EG, Binns HJ, et al; Child Abuse Reporting Experience Study Research Group. Clinicians' description of factors influencing their reporting of suspected child abuse: report of the Child Abuse Reporting Experience Study Research Group. *Pediatrics*. 2008;122(2):259–266

65. Farrell C, Rubin DM, Downes K, Dormans J, Christian CW. Symptoms and time to medical care in children with accidental extremity fractures. *Pediatrics*. 2012;129(1). Available at: www.pediatrics.org/cgi/content/full/129/1/e128

66. Willman KY, Bank DE, Senac M, Chadwick DL. Restricting the time of injury in fatal inflicted head injuries. *Child Abuse Negl*. 1997;21(10):929–940

67. Arbogast KB, Margulies SS, Christian CW. Initial neurologic presentation in young children sustaining inflicted and unintentional fatal head injuries. *Pediatrics*. 2005;116(1):180–184

68. Haviland J, Russell RI. Outcome after severe non-accidental head injury. *Arch Dis Child*. 1997;77(6):504–507

69. Starling SP, Patel S, Burke BL, Sirotnak AP, Stronks S, Rosquist P. Analysis of perpetrator admissions to inflicted traumatic brain injury in children. *Arch Pediatr Adolesc Med*. 2004;158(5):454–458

70. Block RW, Krebs NF; American Academy of Pediatrics Committee on Child Abuse and Neglect; American Academy of Pediatrics Committee on Nutrition. Failure to thrive as a manifestation of child neglect. *Pediatrics*. 2005;116(5):1234–1237

71. Kellogg ND, Lukefahr JL. Criminally prosecuted cases of child starvation. *Pediatrics*. 2005;116(6):1309–1316

72. American Academy of Pediatrics Committee on Child Abuse and Neglect; American Academy of Pediatric Dentistry; American Academy of Pediatric Dentistry Council on Clinical Affairs. Guideline on oral and dental aspects of child abuse and neglect. *Pediatr Dent*. 2008-2009-2009;30(7 suppl):86–89

73. Maguire S, Hunter B, Hunter L, Sibert JR, Mann M, Kemp AM; Welsh Child

Protection Systematic Review Group. Diagnosing abuse: a systematic review of torn frenum and other intra-oral injuries. *Arch Dis Child.* 2007;92(12): 1113–1117

74. Hymel KP, Boos S. Conditions mistaken for child physical abuse. In: Reece RM, Christian CW, eds. *Child Abuse Medical Diagnosis and Management.* 3rd ed. Elk Grove Village, IL: American Academy of Pediatrics; 2009:227–255

75. Rubin DM, Christian CW, Bilaniuk LT, Zazyczny KA, Durbin DR. Occult head injury in high-risk abused children. *Pediatrics.* 2003;111(6 pt 1):1382–1386

76. Pierce MC, Kaczor K, Aldridge S, O'Flynn J, Lorenz DJ. Bruising characteristics discriminating physical child abuse from accidental trauma. *Pediatrics.* 2010;125(1):67–74

77. Maguire S, Mann MK, Sibert J, Kemp A. Are there patterns of bruising in childhood which are diagnostic or suggestive of abuse? A systematic review. *Arch Dis Child.* 2005;90(2): 182–186

78. Sugar NF, Taylor JA, Feldman KW; Puget Sound Pediatric Research Network. Bruises in infants and toddlers: those who don't cruise rarely bruise. *Arch Pediatr Adolesc Med.* 1999;153(4): 399–403

79. Carpenter RF. The prevalence and distribution of bruising in babies. *Arch Dis Child.* 1999;80(4):363–366

80. Labbé J, Caouette G. Recent skin injuries in normal children. *Pediatrics.* 2001;108(2):271–276

81. Dunstan FD, Guildea ZE, Kontos K, Kemp AM, Sibert JR. A scoring system for bruise patterns: a tool for identifying abuse. *Arch Dis Child.* 2002;86(5):330–333

82. Kemp AM, Maguire SA, Nuttall D, Collins P, Dunstan F. Bruising in children who are assessed for suspected physical abuse. *Arch Dis Child.* 2014;99(2): 108–113

83. Cairns AM, Mok JY, Welbury RR. Injuries to the head, face, mouth and neck in physically abused children in a community setting. *Int J Paediatr Dent.* 2005;15(5):310–318

84. Maguire S, Mann MK, Sibert J, Kemp A. Can you age bruises accurately in children? A systematic review. *Arch Dis Child.* 2005;90(2):187–189

85. Anderst JD, Carpenter SL, Abshire TC; Section on Hematology/Oncology and Committee on Child Abuse and Neglect of the American Academy of Pediatrics. Evaluation for bleeding disorders in suspected child abuse. *Pediatrics.* 2013; 131(4). Available at: www.pediatrics. org/cgi/content/full/131/4/e1314

86. Carpenter SL, Abshire TC, Anderst JD; Section on Hematology/Oncology and Committee on Child Abuse and Neglect of the American Academy of Pediatrics. Evaluating for suspected child abuse: conditions that predispose to bleeding. *Pediatrics.* 2013;131(4). Available at: www.pediatrics.org/cgi/content/full/ 131/4/e1357

87. Kellogg N; American Academy of Pediatrics Committee on Child Abuse and Neglect. Oral and dental aspects of child abuse and neglect. *Pediatrics.* 2005;116(6):1565–1568

88. Purdue GF, Hunt JL, Prescott PR. Child abuse by burning—an index of suspicion. *J Trauma.* 1988;28(2): 221–224

89. Maguire S, Moynihan S, Mann M, Potokar T, Kemp AM. A systematic review of the features that indicate intentional scalds in children. *Burns.* 2008;34(8):1072–1081

90. Leventhal JM, Griffin D, Duncan KO, Starling S, Christian CW, Kutz T. Laxative-induced dermatitis of the buttocks incorrectly suspected to be abusive burns. *Pediatrics.* 2001;107(1):178–179

91. Thombs BD. Patient and injury characteristics, mortality risk, and length of stay related to child abuse by burning: evidence from a national sample of 15,802 pediatric admissions. *Ann Surg.* 2008;247(3):519–523

92. Leventhal JM, Martin KD, Asnes AG. Incidence of fractures attributable to abuse in young hospitalized children: results from analysis of a United States database. *Pediatrics.* 2008;122(3): 599–604

93. Day F, Clegg S, McPhillips M, Mok J. A retrospective case series of skeletal surveys in children with suspected non-accidental injury. *J Clin Forensic Med.* 2006;13(2):55–59

94. Kemp AM, Dunstan F, Harrison S, et al. Patterns of skeletal fractures in child abuse: systematic review. *BMJ.* 2008; 337:a1518

95. Mathew MO, Ramamohan N, Bennet GC. Importance of bruising associated with paediatric fractures: prospective observational study. *BMJ.* 1998; 317(7166):1117–1118

96. Wood JN, Christian CW, Adams CM, Rubin DM. Skeletal surveys in infants with isolated skull fractures. *Pediatrics.* 2009;123(2). Available at: www. pediatrics.org/cgi/content/full/123/2/ e247

97. Reece RM, Sege R. Childhood head injuries: accidental or inflicted? *Arch Pediatr Adolesc Med.* 2000;154(1): 11–15

98. American College of Radiology, Society for Pediatric Radiology. ACR-SPR practice guideline for skeletal surveys in children. Reston, VA: American College of Radiology; 2011. Available at: www.acr.org/~/media/ACR/Documents/ PGTS/guidelines/Skeletal_Surveys.pdf. Accessed August 25, 2014

99. Duffy SO, Squires J, Fromkin JB, Berger RP. Use of skeletal surveys to evaluate for physical abuse: analysis of 703 consecutive skeletal surveys. *Pediatrics.* 2011;127(1). Available at: www. pediatrics.org/cgi/content/full/127/1/e47

100. Lane WG, Dubowitz H. What factors affect the identification and reporting of child abuse-related fractures? *Clin Orthop Relat Res.* 2007;461(461): 219–225

101. Kleinman PK, Nimkin K, Spevak MR, et al. Follow-up skeletal surveys in suspected child abuse. *AJR Am J Roentgenol.* 1996;167(4):893–896

102. Zimmerman S, Makoroff K, Care M, Thomas A, Shapiro R. Utility of follow-up skeletal surveys in suspected child physical abuse evaluations. *Child Abuse Negl.* 2005;29(10):1075–1083

103. Bishop N, Sprigg A, Dalton A. Unexplained fractures in infancy: looking for fragile bones. *Arch Dis Child.* 2007;92(3):251–256

104. Shore RM, Chesney RW. Rickets: part II. *Pediatr Radiol.* 2013;43(2):152–172

105. Marquardt ML, Done SL, Sandrock M, Berdon WE, Feldman KW. Copper deficiency presenting as metabolic bone disease in extremely low birth weight, short-gut infants. *Pediatrics.* 2012;130(3). Available at: www. pediatrics.org/cgi/content/full/130/3/ e695

106. Byers PH, Krakow D, Nunes ME, Pepin M; American College of Medical Genetics. Genetic evaluation of suspected osteogenesis imperfect (OI). *Genet Med.* 2006;8(6):383–388

107. Taylor MN, Chaudhuri R, Davis J, Novelli V, Jaswon MS. Childhood osteomyelitis presenting as a pathological fracture. *Clin Radiol.* 2008;63(3):348–351

108. Flaherty EG, Perez-Rossello JM, Levine MA, Hennrikus WL; American Academy of Pediatrics Committee on Child Abuse and Neglect; Section on Radiology, American Academy of Pediatrics; Section on Endocrinology, American Academy of Pediatrics; Section on Orthopedics, American Academy of Pediatrics; Society for Pediatric Radiology. Evaluating children with fractures for child physical abuse. *Pediatrics.* 2014;133(2). Available at: www.pediatrics.org/cgi/content/full/133/2/e477

109. Denton JS, Kalelkar MB. Homicidal commotio cordis in two children. *J Forensic Sci.* 2000;45(3):734–735

110. Baker AM, Craig BR, Lonergan GJ. Homicidal commotio cordis: the final blow in a battered infant. *Child Abuse Negl.* 2003;27(1):125–130

111. Karpas A, Yen K, Sell LL, Frommelt PC. Severe blunt cardiac injury in an infant: a case of child abuse. *J Trauma.* 2002;52(4):759–764

112. Cohle SD, Hawley DA, Berg KK, Kiesel EL, Pless JE. Homicidal cardiac lacerations in children. *J Forensic Sci.* 1995;40(2):212–218

113. Guleserian KJ, Gilchrist BF, Luks FI, Wesselhoeft CW, DeLuca FG. Child abuse as a cause of traumatic chylothorax. *J Pediatr Surg.* 1996;31(12):1696–1697

114. Larimer EL, Fallon SC, Westfall J, Frost M, Wesson DE, Naik-Mathuria BJ. The importance of surgeon involvement in the evaluation of non-accidental trauma patients. *J Pediatr Surg.* 2013;48(6):1357–1362

115. Rubin D, McMillan C, Helfaer M, Christian CW. Pulmonary edema associated with child abuse: case reports and review of the literature. *Pediatrics.* 2001;108(3):769–775

116. Bulloch B, Schubert CJ, Brophy PD, Johnson N, Reed MH, Shapiro RA. Cause and clinical characteristics of rib fractures in infants. *Pediatrics.* 2000;105(4). Available at: www.pediatrics.org/cgi/content/full/105/4/e48

117. Lucas-Herald A, Butler S, Mactier H, McDevitt H, Young D, Ahmed SF. Prevalence and characteristics of rib fractures in ex-preterm infants. *Pediatrics.* 2012;130(6):1116–1119

118. Carroll DM, Doria AS, Paul BS. Clinical-radiological features of fractures in premature infants—a review. *J Perinat Med.* 2007;35(5):366–375

119. Maguire S, Mann M, John N, Ellaway B, Sibert JR, Kemp AM; Welsh Child Protection Systematic Review Group. Does cardiopulmonary resuscitation cause rib fractures in children? A systematic review. *Child Abuse Negl.* 2006;30(7):739–751

120. Reyes JA, Somers GR, Taylor GP, Chiasson DA. Increased incidence of CPR-related rib fractures in infants—is it related to changes in CPR technique? *Resuscitation.* 2011;82(5):545–548

121. Matshes EW, Lew EO. Two-handed cardiopulmonary resuscitation can cause rib fractures in infants. *Am J Forensic Med Pathol.* 2010;31(4):303–307

122. Barnes PM, Norton CM, Dunstan FD, Kemp AM, Yates DW, Sibert JR. Abdominal injury due to child abuse. *Lancet.* 2005;366(9481):234–235

123. Lane WG, Dubowitz H, Langenberg P, Dischinger P. Epidemiology of abusive abdominal trauma hospitalizations in United States children. *Child Abuse Negl.* 2012;36(2):142–148

124. Wood J, Rubin DM, Nance ML, Christian CW. Distinguishing inflicted versus accidental abdominal injuries in young children. *J Trauma.* 2005;59(5):1203–1208

125. Maguire SA, Upadhyaya M, Evans A, et al. A systematic review of abusive visceral injuries in childhood—their range and recognition. *Child Abuse Negl.* 2013;37(7):430–445

126. Cooper A, Floyd T, Barlow B, et al. Major blunt abdominal trauma due to child abuse. *J Trauma.* 1988;28(10):1483–1487

127. Lindberg DM, Shapiro RA, Blood EA, Steiner RD, Berger RP; ExSTRA Investigators. Utility of hepatic transaminases in children with concern for abuse. *Pediatrics.* 2013;131(2):268–275

128. Lane WG, Dubowitz H, Langenberg P. Screening for occult abdominal trauma in children with suspected physical abuse. *Pediatrics.* 2009;124(6):1595–1602

129. Keenan HT, Runyan DK, Marshall SW, Nocera MA, Merten DF, Sinal SH. A population-based study of inflicted traumatic brain injury in young children. *JAMA.* 2003;290(5):621–626

130. Gill JR, Goldfeder LB, Armbrustmacher V, Coleman A, Mena H, Hirsch CS. Fatal head injury in children younger than 2 years in New York City and an overview of the shaken baby syndrome. *Arch Pathol Lab Med.* 2009;133(4):619–627

131. Christian CW, Block R; Committee on Child Abuse and Neglect; American Academy of Pediatrics. Abusive head trauma in infants and children. *Pediatrics.* 2009;123(5):1409–1411

132. Adamsbaum C, Grabar S, Mejean N, Rey-Salmon C. Abusive head trauma: judicial admissions highlight violent and repetitive shaking. *Pediatrics.* 2010;126(3):546–555

133. Kemp AM, Jaspan T, Griffiths J, et al. Neuroimaging: what neuroradiological features distinguish abusive from non-abusive head trauma? A systematic review. *Arch Dis Child.* 2011;96(12):1103–1112

134. Piteau SJ, Ward MG, Barrowman NJ, Plint AC. Clinical and radiographic characteristics associated with abusive and nonabusive head trauma: a systematic review. *Pediatrics.* 2012;130(2):315–323

135. Feldman KW, Bethel R, Shugerman RP, Grossman DC, Grady MS, Ellenbogen RG. The cause of infant and toddler subdural hemorrhage: a prospective study. *Pediatrics.* 2001;108(3):636–646

136. Binenbaum G, Mirza-George N, Christian CW, Forbes BJ. Odds of abuse associated with retinal hemorrhages in children suspected of child abuse. *J AAPOS.* 2009;13(3):268–272

137. Fujiwara T, Okuyama M, Miyasaka M. Characteristics that distinguish abusive from nonabusive head trauma among young children who underwent head computed tomography in Japan. *Pediatrics.* 2008;122(4). Available at:

www.pediatrics.org/cgi/content/full/122/4/e847

138. Laskey AL, Holsti M, Runyan DK, Socolar RR. Occult head trauma in young suspected victims of physical abuse. *J Pediatr.* 2004;144(6):719–722

139. Section on Radiology; American Academy of Pediatrics. Diagnostic imaging of child abuse. *Pediatrics.* 2009;123(5):1430–1435

140. Ichord RN, Naim M, Pollock AN, Nance ML, Margulies SS, Christian CW. Hypoxic-ischemic injury complicates inflicted and accidental traumatic brain injury in young children: the role of diffusion-weighted imaging. *J Neurotrauma.* 2007;24(1):106–118

141. Sieswerda-Hoogendoorn T, Boos S, Spivack B, Bilo RA, van Rijn RR. Abusive head trauma part II: radiological aspects. *Eur J Pediatr.* 2012;171(4):617–623

142. Levin AV. Retinal hemorrhage in abusive head trauma. *Pediatrics.* 2010;126(5):961–970

143. Vinchon M, de Foort-Dhellemmes S, Desurmont M, Delestret I. Confessed abuse versus witnessed accidents in infants: comparison of clinical, radiological, and ophthalmological data in corroborated cases. *Childs Nerv Syst.* 2010;26(5):637–645

144. Binenbaum G, Christian CW, Ichord RN, et al. Retinal hemorrhage and brain injury patterns on diffusion-weighted magnetic resonance imaging in children with head trauma. *J AAPOS.* 2013;17(6):603–608

145. Agrawal S, Peters MJ, Adams GG, Pierce CM. Prevalence of retinal hemorrhages in critically ill children. *Pediatrics.* 2012;129(6). Available at: www.pediatrics.org/cgi/content/full/129/6/e1388

146. Adams GG, Agrawal S, Sekhri R, Peters MJ, Pierce CM. Appearance and location of retinal haemorrhages in critically ill children. *Br J Ophthalmol.* 2013;97(9):1138–1142

147. Morad Y, Kim YM, Armstrong DC, Huyer D, Mian M, Levin AV. Correlation between retinal abnormalities and intracranial abnormalities in the shaken baby syndrome. *Am J Ophthalmol.* 2002;134(3):354–359

148. Greiner MV, Berger RP, Thackeray JD, Lindberg DM; Examining Siblings to Recognize Abuse (ExSTRA) Investigators. Dedicated retinal examination in children evaluated for physical abuse without radiographically identified traumatic brain injury. *J Pediatr.* 2013;163(2):527–531

149. Sirotnak A. Medical disorders that mimic abusive head trauma. In: Frasier L, Rauth-Farley K, Alexander R, Parrish R, Upshaw Downs JC, eds. *Abusive Head Trauma in Infants and Children.* St Louis, MO: GW Medical Publishing; 2006:191–226

150. Lindberg DM, Shapiro RA, Laskey AL, Pallin DJ, Blood EA, Berger RP; ExSTRA Investigators. Prevalence of abusive injuries in siblings and household contacts of physically abused children. *Pediatrics.* 2012;130(2):193–201

151. Hymel KP; Committee on Child Abuse and Neglect. When is lack of supervision neglect? *Pediatrics.* 2006;118(3):1296–1298

152. Children's Hospital Association. Defining the children's hospital role in child maltreatment. 2nd ed. Washington, DC: Children's Hospital Association; 2011. Available at: www.childrenshospitals.net/childabuseguidelines. Accessed August 25, 2014

153. Anderst J, Kellogg N, Jung I. Is the diagnosis of physical abuse changed when Child Protective Services consults a Child Abuse Pediatrics subspecialty group as a second opinion? *Child Abuse Negl.* 2009;33(8):481–489

154. Committee on Child Abuse and Neglect. Policy statement—Child abuse, confidentiality, and the health insurance portability and accountability act. *Pediatrics.* 2010;125(1):197–201

155. Committee on Medical Liability and Risk Management. Policy statement—Expert witness participation in civil and criminal proceedings. *Pediatrics.* 2009;124(1):428–438

Sentinel Injuries in Infants Evaluated for Child Physical Abuse

AUTHORS: Lynn K. Sheets, MD,[a,b] Matthew E. Leach, MD,[c] Ian J. Koszewski, MD,[d] Ashley M. Lessmeier, BS,[a] Melodee Nugent, MA,[a] and Pippa Simpson, PhD[a]

[a]Medical College of Wisconsin, Milwaukee, Wisconsin; [b]Children's Hospital of Wisconsin, Milwaukee, Wisconsin; [c]St Louis University School of Medicine, St Louis, Missouri; and [d]University of Wisconsin Hospital and Clinics, Madison, Wisconsin

KEY WORDS
abuse, bruising, infants, maltreatment, screening, abusive head trauma

ABBREVIATIONS
AHT—abusive head trauma
CHW—Children's Hospital of Wisconsin
CPT—Child Protection Team

Dr Sheets conceptualized and designed the study, assisted in data abstraction, drafted the initial article, and approved the final article as submitted. Dr Sheets had full access to all the data in the study and takes responsibility for the integrity of the data and the accuracy of the data analysis. As second-year medical students at the Medical College of Wisconsin, Drs Leach and Koszewski and Ms Lessmeier performed chart abstraction in the abusive head trauma, non–abusive head trauma definite abuse, and control/intermediate substudies, respectively, entered data into the database, edited the article, and approved the final article as submitted. Ms Nugent and Dr Simpson assisted with study design and power calculations, performed data analysis, wrote the statistical components of the article, edited the article, and approved the final article as submitted.

www.pediatrics.org/cgi/doi/10.1542/peds.2012-2780

doi:10.1542/peds.2012-2780

Accepted for publication Dec 11, 2012

Address correspondence to Lynn K. Sheets, MD, Children's Hospital of Wisconsin, Child Advocacy and Protection Services, C615, PO Box 1997, Milwaukee, WI 53201. E-mail: lsheets@chw.org

PEDIATRICS (ISSN Numbers: Print, 0031-4005; Online, 1098-4275).

Copyright © 2013 by the American Academy of Pediatrics

FINANCIAL DISCLOSURE: Dr Sheets has provided paid expert testimony for prosecution and defense attorneys in cases of alleged child physical maltreatment; the other authors have indicated they have no financial relationships relevant to this article to disclose.

FUNDING: Funding for the medical student summer research stipends and for data analysis by Quantitative Health Sciences was provided by the Child Abuse Prevention Fund of Children's Hospital of Wisconsin, the Wisconsin Children's Trust Fund, and the Department of Pediatrics at the Medical College of Wisconsin.

WHAT'S KNOWN ON THIS SUBJECT: Although it is known that relatively minor abusive injuries sometimes precede more severe physical abuse, the prevalence of these previous injuries in infants evaluated for abuse was not known.

WHAT THIS STUDY ADDS: A history of bruising or oral injury in a precruising infant evaluated for abuse should heighten the level of suspicion because these injuries are common in abused infants and rare in infants found not to be abused.

abstract

OBJECTIVE: Relatively minor abusive injuries can precede severe physical abuse in infants. Our objective was to determine how often abused infants have a previous history of "sentinel" injuries, compared with infants who were not abused.

METHODS: Case-control, retrospective study of 401, <12-month-old infants evaluated for abuse in a hospital-based setting and found to have definite, intermediate concern for, or no abuse after evaluation by the hospital-based Child Protection Team. A sentinel injury was defined as a previous injury reported in the medical history that was suspicious for abuse because the infant could not cruise, or the explanation was implausible.

RESULTS: Of the 200 definitely abused infants, 27.5% had a previous sentinel injury compared with 8% of the 100 infants with intermediate concern for abuse (odds ratio: 4.4, 95% confidence interval: 2.0–9.6; $P < .001$). None of the 101 nonabused infants (controls) had a previous sentinel injury ($P < .001$). The type of sentinel injury in the definitely abused cohort was bruising (80%), intraoral injury (11%), and other injury (7%). Sentinel injuries occurred in early infancy: 66% at <3 months of age and 95% at or before the age of 7 months. Medical providers were reportedly aware of the sentinel injury in 41.9% of cases.

CONCLUSIONS: Previous sentinel injuries are common in infants with severe physical abuse and rare in infants evaluated for abuse and found to not be abused. Detection of sentinel injuries with appropriate interventions could prevent many cases of abuse. *Pediatrics* 2013;131:701–707

Infancy is a time of high risk for maltreatment.[1] Early detection of subtle injuries from abuse in young infants might identify those who are at risk for suffering more serious abusive injuries.[2–7] Child physical abuse prevention efforts have focused on risk reduction through educational interventions such as home visitation, parenting programs, and coping with infant crying.[8] Given the high social and financial costs of infant physical abuse,[2] prevention efforts such as improved recognition of the earliest signs of physical abuse before the abuse escalates would be beneficial. Relatively minor injuries, such as frenulum tears or bruising in precruising infants (infants unable to pull to a stand and walk while holding onto something), may be the first indication to a caregiver or medical provider of child physical abuse.[3–7] Minor injuries other than superficial abrasions are uncommon in normal, precruising infants[9–11] and, when they occur, should raise a concern for abuse.[10] In an illustrative case from our institution, a 2-month-old infant was admitted to the hospital after suddenly becoming limp and unresponsive at home. He had subdural hemorrhages, extensive retinal hemorrhages, and acute and healing fractures. Ultimately, he was diagnosed with abusive head trauma (AHT). Two weeks before admission, his mother had noticed a bruise on his cheek (Fig 1). If the mother had sought medical attention for the bruise, the subsequent AHT might have been prevented, assuming the medical provider could establish the appropriate diagnosis. Failure to recognize and take action when relatively minor, suspicious injuries occur may have devastating consequences for the infant and family.

Despite the known association between intraoral injuries and bruising in precruising infants with later, more serious abuse,[3–7] it is not known how many infants evaluated for abuse have a previous history of relatively minor, suspicious injuries. We termed these previous injuries sentinel injuries. The purpose of this study was to determine what percentage of definitely abused infants evaluated by a hospital-based Child Protection Team (CPT) had a history of a sentinel injury and compare them to: (1) those infants with intermediate concerns for abuse and (2) those infants evaluated for abuse but found to not be abused, termed "controls."

METHODS

This study was a retrospective, case-control study of 401 infants <12 months of age evaluated by the hospital-based, interdisciplinary CPT at Children's Hospital of Wisconsin (CHW) between March 2001 and October 2011. The study analyzed 4 nonconcurrent cohorts of 100 infants each, in separate substudies (with the exception of 101 control infants). In each substudy, cases were selected for inclusion consecutively from the CPT log of all comprehensive CPT consults. Comprehensive CPT consults at CHW have been performed in a consistent manner for at least the past 10 years and have routinely included a complete medical history, physical examination, and

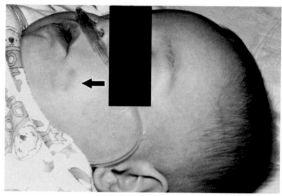

FIGURE 1
Illustrative example of sentinel injury: a 2-month-old infant with unexplained cheek bruising, likely from abuse.

appropriate diagnostic studies. Comprehensive consults were defined as those for which a medical history and physical examination were performed by the CPT pediatrician and a consultation report was produced that provided an opinion about the level of concern for abuse. Controls were infants evaluated for abuse and found to not be abused.

Description of Substudies

The 4 study cohorts, spanning different time frames (Fig 2), were classified by CPT level of concern for abuse: definite abuse by AHT (March 2001–February 2008), definite abuse with non-AHT injuries (includes abusive abdominal trauma, fractures, and burns, July 2002–March 2009), intermediate concern for abuse (July 2006–October 2011), and no concern for abuse (March 2007–February 2011). The cohort with no concern for abuse served as the control. The AHT and non-AHT definite-abuse cohorts consisted of infants with CPT consultation reports containing phrases such as "with reasonable medical certainty" and "diagnostic." For the intermediate concern and control cohorts, the level of suspicion 7-point scale developed by Lindberg et al[12] was used during chart abstraction to categorize infants into cohorts. Infants in the intermediate

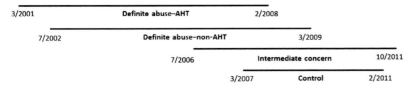

FIGURE 2
Case ascertainment intervals of each substudy. The case ascertainment interval for each of the 4 substudies is demonstrated. Institutional review board (IRB) approval is the last date of each line.

level of concern cohort (levels 3–5) were those whose CPT reports contained phrases such as "concerning but not diagnostic" and "somewhat concerning." The CPT reports for infants in the control cohort (Lindberg levels 1 and 2) contained phrases such as "consistent with history," "explained by underlying condition," and "no concern for abuse." Consensus about the abuse level of certainty ranking by 2 of the authors was required to include a case in each cohort: AHT (L.K.S. and M. E.L.), non-AHT abuse (L.K.S. and I.J.K.), and intermediate-concern and control cohorts (L.K.S. and A.M.L.). Infants were excluded from all cohorts if the CPT consultation was not comprehensive.

Data Abstraction

Basic demographic data for each subject were recorded, including gender, ethnicity (as classified by the subject's parent/guardian), and subject's age at the time of admission. Developmental information regarding mobility at the time of the sentinel injury was noted. The CHW institutional review board approved each of the 4 substudies. The research team reviewed all available records, including all medical records, the primary care physician's records, child protective service reports, and law enforcement reports. Medical records were specifically reviewed for any history of previous injuries such as bruising, intraoral injuries, or other injuries, excluding superficial abrasions. The reported location of previous bruising was categorized as head (forehead, ear, or other areas of the face), extremity, or trunk. Examples of

intraoral injury include frenulum injury or contusion of the tongue.

Classification of Injuries

A previous injury was defined as a sentinel injury if it was reported to have been visible to at least 1 parent before the events leading to the current admission and was suspicious for abuse because the child was not able to cruise or there was an implausible explanation offered. Occult injuries, such as healing rib fractures not diagnosed until the CPT consult, were not classified as sentinel injuries because they are not visible. For example, in the illustrative case of the 2-month-old infant with AHT who had a history of a cheek bruise and had healing rib fractures diagnosed at the time of the CPT evaluation, only the bruise seen 2 weeks before admission would be considered a sentinel injury. Details of each previous injury, including the type of injury, who was reportedly aware of the injury, the age of the child at time of injury, the location on the body, the circumstances of the injury, and the time to resolution were recorded when that information was available. Vague recollections of nonspecific marks, such as a "red mark" after bumping the head, were not included. When there was a history that a medical provider knew about an injury, we attempted to ascertain whether the provider suspected abuse and what action was taken.

Statistical Analysis

Percentages of sentinel injuries in the 4 cohorts were compared; odds ratios

and 95% confidence intervals were calculated when feasible. Because some percentages were 0, odds ratios could not be calculated. χ^2 Tests were performed for categorical variables. Owing to nonnormality of continuous variables, the nonparametric Mann–Whitney test was performed. The cutoff level for significance was set at $P = .05$. Statistical analyses were performed by using SPSS version 20 (IBM SPSS Statistics, IBM Corporation, Armonk, NY). There were no missing patients in each consecutive series.

RESULTS

Across the 4 cohorts, subjects did not differ with respect to gender ($P = .76$) or age ($P = .06$) (Table 1). Of the 401 subjects, male infants (63%) outnumbered female infants (37%). There were more African-American infants and fewer infants classified as Hispanic/other in the non-AHT definite abuse cohort than in the other 3 cohorts ($P \leq .001$). There were 15 deaths in the AHT cohort, none in the definitely abused, non-AHT cohort, 1 nonabusive death in the intermediate concern cohort, and 2 natural deaths in the control cohort ($P \leq .001$).

There were 63 infants with a history of sentinel injury: 30 of 100 (30%) in the AHT cohort, 25 of 100 (25%) in the non-AHT abuse cohort, 8 of 100 (8%) in the intermediate-concern cohort, and 0 of 101 in the control cohort (Fig 3). Of the 200 infants who were definitely abused (combined AHT and non-AHT cohorts), 55 (27.5%) had a sentinel injury. Of those, 80% had a bruise, 11% had an intraoral injury, and 7% had a fracture. Some definitely abused infants had >1 sentinel injury either within 1 reported episode or during different episodes. In the 55 definitely abused infants with sentinel bruising, there were 66 sentinel bruises in various locations: bruising of the head (face, forehead, and ear) accounted for 41 of 66

TABLE 1 Demographics of Study Subjects, by Presence or Absence of a History of Sentinel Injury

	Definite Abuse				Intermediate Concern		Control	
	AHT		Non-AHT Abuse					
	SI	No SI	SI	No SI	SI	No SI	SI	No SI
	N (%)	N (%)	N (%)	N (%)	N (%)	N (%)	N = 0	N (%)
Race/ethnicity, N (%)[a]								
White	17 (57)	28 (40)	12 (48)	23 (31)	5 (63)	43 (47)	—	38 (37)
African American	1 (3)	18 (26)	9 (36)	39 (52)	1 (13)	27 (29)	—	33 (33)
Hispanic	3 (10)	20 (28)	2 (8)	6 (8)	—	16 (18)	—	14 (14)
Mixed/other	9 (30)	4 (6)	2 (8)	7 (9)	2 (24)	6 (6)	—	11 (11)
Unknown	—	—	—	—	—	—	—	5 (5)
Gender, N (%)								
Male	16 (53)	51 (73)	15 (60)	48 (64)	7 (88)	53 (58)	—	62 (62)
Female	14 (47)	19 (27)	10 (40)	27 (36)	1 (12)	39 (42)	—	39 (39)
Median age, mo	3.8	4.0	4.0	4.0	5.0	5.0	—	4.0
Age range	0.8–11.5	0.5–11.0	1.0–11.5	0.7–11.5	2.0–10.0	0.5–11.0	—	0.1–11.0
Total SI/total	30/100		25/100		8/100		0/101	

[a] SI versus no SI is only significant for AHT × race, P < .001. AHT, abusive head trauma; SI, sentinel injury.

sentinel bruises (62.1%), followed in frequency by extremity bruising (14 of 66, 21.2%) and bruising of the trunk (11 of 66, 16.7%). Of the 8 infants with sentinel injuries in the intermediate-concern cohort, 7 (87.5%) had a history of bruising and 1 (12.5%) had a poorly explained subluxation of the radial head. Definitely abused infants were more likely to have a history of a sentinel injury than infants with intermediate concerns (odds ratio: 4.4, 95% confidence interval: 2.0–9.6; P < .001). Unlike infants in the other cohorts, none of the infants in the control cohort had a previous sentinel injury (P < .001). The initial medical findings that prompted the CPT consultations in the 101 control infants were ultimately diagnosed as accidental injury in 83 (83%), medical mimic in 11 (11%), and a normal variant mistaken for an injury in 6 (6%).

In 23 of the 55 (41.9%) definite-abuse cases with sentinel injury, the parent reported that a medical provider was aware of the injury. Not all of these cases could be confirmed because outside medical records were not always available. In 10 of these 23 cases (43.5%), medical providers suspected abuse, and in 13 (56.5%), there was no evidence suggesting the providers suspected abuse. In some cases for which the provider records were available and abuse was not suspected, the injury was simply noted as a finding on examination, or the injury was diagnosed as accidental, self-inflicted, or a condition unrelated to injury. Some medical providers who suspected abuse made reports to authorities, but the children were not protected, whereas others suspected abuse but concluded there was no abuse because no other injuries were found on the work-up.

Because of the risk of circular reasoning, we analyzed consultation reports to determine if a history of a sentinel injury increased the level of concern for abuse at the time of the initial CPT evaluation. None of the cases of definite abuse were classified as definite abuse because of a sentinel injury. There were no cases in the intermediate-concern cohort in which the level of concern was increased from a low level (levels 1 and 2) to an intermediate level (levels 3-5) on the basis of a history of a sentinel injury. There was 1 case in the intermediate level that had an enhanced level of concern because of a sentinel injury; however, the sentinel injury did not increase the level of concern to definite abuse.

The ages at the time of CPT evaluation and at sentinel injury are depicted by cohort in Fig 3. In the definite-abuse cohorts, these ages were separated by a median of 1 month (range, 1 day to 7.3 months). Of the 52 abused infants for whom the age at first sentinel injury was known, 37 (71%) manifested the sentinel injury at or before 3 months of age, and 52 (94%) at or before 7 months of age.

DISCUSSION

Our study suggests that when an infant is evaluated for possible abuse, a history of a sentinel injury should heighten the concern for abuse. Infants who are not yet cruising have bruises on well-child physical examinations in 0% to 2.2% of cases, according to published research.[9–11] When a bruise is present, it should be considered as potentially sentinel for physical abuse if there is no predisposing disorder or plausible explanation.[5] We found that in the medical history, parents' reports of sentinel injuries are common in abused infants and are rare in infants evaluated for abuse and found to not be abused.

The findings from our study also suggest that in 27.5% of cases of definite physical abuse, there may be escalating and repeated violence toward the infant instead of a single event of momentary loss of control by an angry or frustrated caregiver. The link between early abusive injury and later severe injury is further corroborated by our finding of an intermediate prevalence of sentinel injuries in the cohort in which abuse was suspected but not definitively diagnosed. It is likely that this cohort contains both abused and nonabused infants. Other researchers have demonstrated serial abuse of infants with missed opportunities for prevention.[2–4,6–8] Some abused infants may present for medical care but are missed because their symptoms are mistaken for other

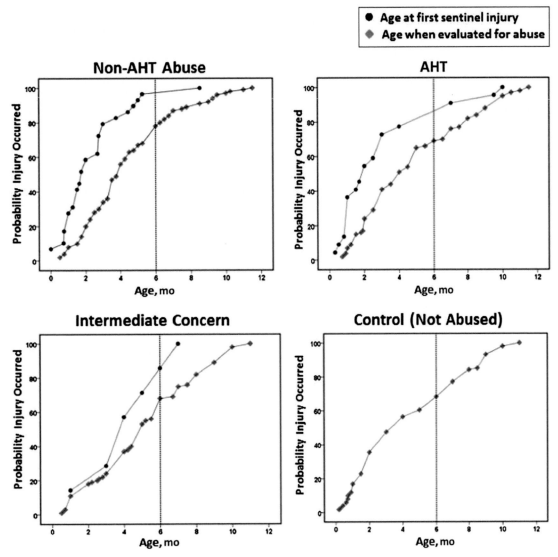

FIGURE 3
Probability of sentinel injury by age in 4 cohorts.

disease processes.[8] Other studies in which researchers examined perpetrator confessions or the presence of other injuries in abused children demonstrate that abuse is often chronic by the time it is definitively diagnosed.[13,14] We are unaware of any published study that describes how often parents report a history of bruising in precruising infants. Our study adds to the literature by showing that there is a high prevalence of caregiver-reported, visible, relatively minor injuries that are concerning for abuse in infants who later suffer abu-

sive injuries, and that a substantial number of these sentinel injuries are known to a medical provider. Appropriate child abuse screening and intervention at the first concern of child physical abuse, such as a history or physical finding of sentinel injury, might prevent many abusive injuries.

Early detection of sentinel injuries and effective evaluation and intervention will require educating caregivers of young infants, child protective service workers, and medical providers about the significance of sentinel injuries. Parents, relatives, public health nurses,

home visitors and day care providers should be taught to recognize that bruising and intraoral injuries in precruising infants are unexpected and should prompt medical evaluation. Investigators such as child welfare workers should understand the significance of a bruise and other "minor" injuries in precruising infants as potentially serious and possibly concerning for abuse. Medical providers also play a significant role in child protection. The history of a sentinel injury should prompt a medical provider in any setting to consider abuse and should heighten the suspicion for abuse in an infant with an injury of indeterminate etiology. In our study, for most sentinel injuries known to a medical provider, there was no evidence from the available records that the medical provider seriously considered abuse. In these cases, the medical provider did not seem to fully recognize the importance of the injury. For example, an intraoral injury was either diagnosed as self-inflicted (eg, "patient scratched self with fingernail" or "chewed on own tongue") or was medically treated without seeking an explanation. In another case, an ankle bruise was noted at a well-baby visit, but the history of the infant "vigorously kicking the crib" was accepted as a plausible cause.

Even in cases in which abuse was considered, medical providers performed an abuse work-up after noticing bruising but seemed to lessen their suspicion of abuse when findings from the work-up indicated no other injuries. A sentinel injury can be the first and only abusive injury. Reporting the sentinel injury to child protective services is appropriate in many cases in which there is no plausible explanation, even when there are no additional occult injuries found. The purpose of the child abuse medical evaluation, such as a computed tomographic scan of the head and skeletal survey, is to detect occult injuries rather than to rule out abuse. A child abuse evaluation that does not show injuries beyond the sentinel injury is different from a negative sepsis evaluation; the former represents additional injury surveillance, and the latter represents

medically ruling out a diagnostic consideration. Educational efforts with medical providers should include this important distinction.

With an estimated $210,000 lifetime cost estimate for each case of child physical abuse,[15] prevention of further abuse through early detection and effective intervention has the potential of producing significant financial savings. Our findings suggest that improved detection and management of minor injuries in precruising infants has the potential of preventing up to 27.5% of abuse cases evaluated at a tertiary care children's hospital. Not only should the examination finding of a poorly explained bruise or intraoral injury in a precruising infant raise a concern about abuse, but our study also suggests that simply a history of such injury, particularly in infants being evaluated for abuse, should heighten the concern about abuse. The reliability of using a history of sentinel injuries in screening for abuse requires further exploration.

There are several potential limitations to this study. First, classification of injuries as sentinel relied on the documented histories from parents and is potentially flawed by recall errors and intentional omissions. Recall bias would be expected to affect all 4 cohorts equally, because each infant's evaluation began with a CPT consult for a concerning injury. Furthermore, we relied on documented medical histories that are also affected by thoroughness in medical history-taking and documentation. Given that we only classified a reported injury as

a sentinel injury if there was a clear, detailed description provided, we likely undercounted the number of sentinel injuries. Second, our retrospective review would miss fatally abused infants who never presented to the hospital. It is unknown if these cases are different than those included in our study. Third, during chart abstraction, there is a possibility that injuries were misclassified as either sentinel injuries or accidental injuries. Fourth, variations in practice over time and between medical providers could have affected our results. Finally, there is a risk of circular reasoning because the presence of a sentinel injury in the medical history could heighten the level of concern for abuse. This limitation was addressed through additional analysis, as noted previously.

CONCLUSIONS

Many definitely abused infants have a history of minor injuries that occurred before cruising, whereas such injuries are rare in infants evaluated for abuse and found to not be abused. Improved recognition of previous sentinel injuries combined with appropriate interventions would improve secondary prevention of abuse.

ACKNOWLEDGMENTS

We thank our prevention partners, the Child Abuse Prevention Fund of Children's Hospital of Wisconsin and the Wisconsin Children's Trust Fund, for funding and the Medical College of Wisconsin Injury Research Center for their support of summer research students.

REFERENCES

1. US Department of Health and Human Services, Administration for Children and Families, Administration on Children, Youth and Families, Children's Bureau. (2011). *Child Maltreatment 2010*. Available at: www.acf. hhs.gov/programs/cb/stats_research/index. htm#can. Accessed February 13, 2013

2. Jenny C, Hymel KP, Ritzen A, Reinert SE, Hay TC. Analysis of missed cases of abusive head trauma. *JAMA.* 1999;281(7):621–626

3. Thackeray JD. Frena tears and abusive head injury: a cautionary tale. *Pediatr Emerg Care.* 2007;23(10):735–737

4. Oral R, Yagmur F, Nashelsky M, Turkmen M, Kirby P. Fatal abusive head trauma cases:

consequence of medical staff missing milder forms of physical abuse. *Pediatr Emerg Care*. 2008;24(12):816–821

5. Feldman KW. The bruised premobile infant: should you evaluate further? *Pediatr Emerg Care*. 2009;25(1):37–39

6. Pierce MC, Smith S, Kaczor K. Bruising in infants: those with a bruise may be abused. *Pediatr Emerg Care*. 2009;25(12):845–847

7. Petska HW, Sheets LK, Knox BL. Facial bruising as a precursor to abusive head trauma. *Clin Pediatr*. 2013;52(1):86–88

8. Jenny C. Preventing head trauma from abuse in infants. *CMAJ*. 2009;180(7):703–704

9. Wedgwood J. Childhood bruising. *Practitioner*. 1990;234(1490):598–601

10. Sugar NF, Taylor JA, Feldman KW; Puget Sound Pediatric Research Network. Bruises in infants and toddlers: those who don't cruise rarely bruise. *Arch Pediatr Adolesc Med*. 1999;153(4):399–403

11. Labbé J, Caouette G. Recent skin injuries in normal children. *Pediatrics*. 2001;108(2):271–276

12. Lindberg DM, Lindsell CJ, Shapiro RA. Variability in expert assessments of child physical abuse likelihood. *Pediatrics*. 2008;121(4). Available at: www.pediatrics.org/content/121/4/e945

13. Alexander R, Crabbe L, Sato Y, Smith W, Bennett T. Serial abuse in children who are shaken. *Am J Dis Child*. 1990;144(1):58–60

14. Adamsbaum C, Grabar S, Mejean N, Rey-Salmon C. Abusive head trauma: judicial admissions highlight violent and repetitive shaking. *Pediatrics*. 2010;126(3):546–555

15. Fang X, Brown DS, Florence CS, Mercy JA. The economic burden of child maltreatment in the United States and implications for prevention. *Child Abuse Negl*. 2012;36(2):156–165

Testing for Abuse in Children With Sentinel Injuries

Daniel M. Lindberg, MD[a,b], Brenda Beaty, MPH[c], Elizabeth Juarez-Colunga, PhD[c,d], Joanne N. Wood, MD, MSHP[e], Desmond K. Runyan, MD, DrPH[a]

OBJECTIVE: Child physical abuse is commonly missed, putting abused children at risk for repeated injury and death. Several so-called sentinel injuries have been suggested to be associated with high rates of abuse, and to imply the need for routine testing for other, occult traumatic injuries. Our objective was to determine rates of abuse evaluation and diagnosis among children evaluated at leading children's hospitals with these putative sentinel injuries.

METHODS: This is a retrospective secondary analysis of the Pediatric Health Information System database. We identified 30 355 children with putative sentinel injuries. We measured rates of abuse diagnosis and rates of testing commonly used to identify occult injuries.

RESULTS: Among all visits for children <24 months old to Pediatric Health Information System hospitals, the rate of abuse diagnosis was 0.17%. Rates of abuse diagnosis for children with at least 1 putative sentinel injury ranged from 3.5% for children <12 months old with burns to 56.1% for children <24 months with rib fractures. Rates of skeletal survey and other testing that can identify occult traumatic injury were highly variable between centers and for different injuries.

CONCLUSIONS: Several putative sentinel injuries are associated with high rates of physical abuse. Among eligible children with rib fracture(s), abdominal trauma, or intracranial hemorrhage, rates of abuse were more than 20%. Future work is warranted to test whether routine testing for abuse in these children can improve early recognition of abuse.

abstract

[a]Kempe Center for the Prevention and Treatment of Child Abuse and Neglect, Denver, Colorado; [b]Department of Emergency Medicine, School of Medicine, and [c]Adult and Child Center for Health Outcomes Research and Delivery Science, University of Colorado, Denver Colorado; [d]Department of Biostatistics and Informatics, Colorado School of Public Health, Aurora, Colorado; and [e]Children's Hospital of Philadelphia, Department of Pediatrics, Perelman School of Medicine at the University of Pennsylvania, Philadelphia, Pennsylvania

Dr Lindberg conceptualized and designed the study, participated in data analysis, drafted the initial manuscript. Ms Beaty participated in study design and led the data analysis. Drs Juarez-Colunga and Wood participated in study design and data analysis. Dr Runyan participated in study conceptualization and design. Drs Juarez-Colunga, Wood, and Runyan, and Ms Beaty reviewed and revised the manuscript, and approved the final manuscript as submitted. Dr Lindberg has had access to all study data and takes responsibility for the study as a whole.

www.pediatrics.org/cgi/doi/10.1542/peds.2015-1487

DOI: 10.1542/peds.2015-1487

Accepted for publication Aug 4, 2015

Address correspondence to Daniel M. Lindberg, MD, 12401 E 17th Ave, Mailstop B215, Aurora, CO 80045. E-mail: daniel.lindberg@ucdenver.edu

PEDIATRICS (ISSN Numbers: Print, 0031-4005; Online, 1098-4275).

WHAT'S KNOWN ON THIS SUBJECT: Several injuries have been suggested to be disproportionately associated with abuse in young children, but rates of abuse among children with these injuries are not currently known.

WHAT THIS STUDY ADDS: Abuse is diagnosed commonly in children with sentinel injuries, including the majority of children <24 months with rib fractures.

ARTICLE

Child physical abuse is common, with more than 119 000 victims, 600 deaths, and $124 billion in total costs annually in the United States.[1-5] It is also commonly missed by health care providers. Approximately 30% of abusive head trauma and 20% of abusive fractures are missed initially, putting children at risk for ongoing abuse.[6-8] Several diagnostic studies (eg, skeletal survey [SS], neuroimaging, hepatic transaminases, and retinal examination) can identify occult abusive injuries and improve abuse recognition and diagnosis.[9-15] However, use of these studies has been shown to be widely variable, and to be affected by practice setting, race, and socioeconomic status.[16,17] Twice as many children with high-risk injuries are recognized as abused in children's hospitals than in general hospitals,[18] and abusive fractures are 7 times more likely to be missed in general emergency departments (EDs) than in pediatric EDs.[7] Even among leading children's hospitals, testing of children with high-risk injuries ranges from 40% to 90%.[19]

In the absence of objective, validated measures of abuse likelihood, the decision to undertake screening often depends on an individual provider's gestalt about the likelihood of abuse. One source of testing variability may be the subjective nature of several factors that may affect this gestalt. Factors such as affect, eye contact, and the amount of detail in an offered history have been suggested to be important in estimating the likelihood of abuse, though they are difficult to measure objectively and their reliability, sensitivity, and specificity have not been reported.[20,21]

An alternative, more objective approach would be to routinely screen those children who are found to have injuries most associated with abuse. Several such sentinel injuries have been suggested on the basis of case reports and retrospective analyses of cohorts of abused

children.[22-24] However, these studies have not been able to estimate the likelihood of abuse in children with these injuries because they have not identified the denominator of children presenting with these injuries. One large analysis of the association between fractures and abuse was able to overcome this challenge, but was limited to children who were admitted to the hospital.[25]

Our goal was to determine which putative sentinel injuries are most associated with physical abuse. We performed a secondary analysis of children who were seen in the ED or inpatient wards of leading children's hospitals by using the Pediatric Health Information System (PHIS) database. We determined rates of recognized abuse among children with putative sentinel injuries.

METHODS

Data Source

This was a retrospective analysis of data from the PHIS database for patients seen in the ED, observation, and/or inpatient setting from January 1, 2004, through December 31, 2011. We included data from the 18 institutions with continuous valid data submission throughout this period. PHIS is an administrative database that contains inpatient, ED, ambulatory surgery, and observation data from 43 leading not-for-profit, tertiary care pediatric hospitals in the United States. These hospitals are affiliated with the Children's Hospital Association (Shawnee Mission, KS), a business alliance of children's hospitals. Data quality and reliability are assured through a joint effort between the Children's Hospital Association and participating hospitals. The data warehouse function for PHIS is managed by Thomson Reuters (Ann Arbor, MI). No patient-specific clinical data exist in the database. This project was determined to be exempt from review

as human subjects research by the Colorado Multiple Institutional Review Board.

Study Population

From the published literature, we identified putative sentinel injuries and the ages at which children with each injury are thought to be at increased risk for abuse (Table 1). For example, although bruises are extremely common in older children, they are strongly associated with abuse in children <6 months old.[26,27] Children with at least one candidate injury were identified on the basis of *International Classification of Diseases, Ninth Revision, Clinical Modification* (ICD-9-CM) codes. We excluded children with a previous diagnosis of physical abuse during the data abstraction period and children whose injuries were diagnosed after a motor vehicle collision (as determined by the presence of ICD-9-CM codes: E810–E845) because these patients are rarely thought to be victims of abuse.[28] We excluded visits with Medicare Severity-Diagnosis Related Group code 795 (normal newborn). Because children who were transferred from another center may have had testing completed before arrival to the PHIS center, and because they may represent a population with different likelihood of abuse, patients who were noted to have been transferred were excluded from the main study cohort and were analyzed separately.

We determined how frequently SS, neuroimaging (computed tomography [CT] or MRI), and hepatic transaminases were obtained for children with each putative sentinel injury, and how frequently abuse was diagnosed. Performance of testing was determined by using clinical transaction code (CTC) procedure codes (skeletal survey 427811, neuroimaging–head CT 417051; brain CT 411051; neuro/head MRI 417052; head arteriography MRI 471052; or brain MRI 411052, hepatic

TABLE 1 Putative Sentinel Injuries

Candidate Injuries	Age at Risk, mo	ICD-9-CM Codes	Source
Bruising	<6	920–924	Harper et al[27]; Sugar et al[26]
Burns	<6	940–949	DeGraw et al[36]; Hicks and Stolfi[37]
Oropharyngeal injury	<6	873.6–873.7	Thackeray[22]; Maguire[38]
Femur/humerus fracture	<12	812, 820–821	Leventhal et al[25]; Scherl[39]; Strait[40]
Radius/ulna/tibia/fibula fracture	<12	813, 823, 824	Leventhal et al[25]; John[41]
Isolated skull fracture	<12	800–804[a]	Deye et al[42]; Wood[33]; Laskey[43]
Intracranial hemorrhage	<12	800–801, 803–804, 851–853[a]	Wood[17]; Trokel[18]; Kemp[44]
Rib fracture(s)	<24	807.0, 807.1, 807.4	Rubin et al[12]; Maguire[45]
Abdominal trauma	<24	863–869	Lindberg et al[9,46]; Trokel[28]
Genital injury	<24	922.4, 878	Carpenter[47]
Subconjunctival hemorrhage	<24	372.72	Sheets et al[24]; DeRidder[48]

[a] ICD-9 codes that signify skull fracture with intracranial hemorrhage (eg, 804.2) were included in the group with intracranial hemorrhage, not with subjects who have isolated skull fractures.

transaminases–liver profile 310400; 14-test chem profile 310114; critical care panel 300171; other multichem panel 310129; general health profile 300140; aspartate aminotransferase (AST) 315060; or alanine aminotransferase (ALT) 315020). No participating center used codes for skeletal survey, unspecified technique 427800 or skeletal survey, other specified technique 427899. A diagnosis of abuse was defined by the assignment of any of the following ICD-9-CM codes, which have been used previously to identify recognized abuse from within the PHIS cohort (995.50, 995.54, 995.55, 995.59, E960–E967, E968.0–E968.3, and E968.5–E968.9).[19]

Rates of abuse testing and diagnose were computed by using descriptive

statistics. Correlation between rates of abuse diagnosis and rates of SS was computed by using linear regression. All analyses were performed by using SAS 9.4 (SAS Institute, Inc., Cary, NC).

RESULTS

From 2004 to 2011, 18 participating hospitals in the PHIS database with continuously submitted data had 4 131 177 patient visits for children <24 months old, excluding normal newborn deliveries. Among all patient visits, 7062 (0.17%) were associated with a diagnosis of abuse. Rates of abuse diagnoses for all patient visits in children <24 months old for each hospital ranged from 0.04% to 0.46%.

After excluding injuries documented during visits transferred from

another facility (n = 2747), there were 34 565 putative sentinel injuries identified at 30 766 visits (0.7% of all visits) among 30 355 children <24 months old. These visits formed the main study cohort.

The number of patient visits with each putative sentinel injury and demographic characteristics of subjects is shown in Table 2. The large majority of subjects (89.8%) had only 1 putative sentinel injury identified. Two putative sentinel injuries were identified in 7.6% and 2.6% had 3 to 6 injuries identified. For the 4 100 411 patient visits in which no sentinel injury was identified, abuse was diagnosed in 1414 (0.03%).

Rates of abuse diagnosis and testing commonly used to identify occult injury for each sentinel injury are shown in Table 3. Rates of abuse diagnosis ranged from 3.5% for children <6 months old with burns to 56.1% for children <24 months old with rib fractures. Among all centers, 14 138 visits (46.0%) with identified putative sentinel injuries included SS; 21 094 (68.6%) included neuroimaging, and 7651 (24.9%) had hepatic transaminases obtained. Testing varied widely between centers for all injuries and all testing modalities (Table 3). Among infants with skull fractures, the rate of SS between centers ranged from just over 20% of patients, to as high as 74%.

TABLE 2 Demographic Characteristics of Subjects With Sentinel Injuries

Candidate Injury[a]	n	Age in Months, Median (Interquartile Range)	Boy, %	White, %	Hispanic, %
Age <6 mo					
Bruise(s)	7906	3 (1–4)	54.1	33.2	17.1
Burn(s)	1218	3 (1–4)	54.7	18.7	13.4
Oropharyngeal injury	295	3 (1–4)	60.3	27.5	13.2
Age <12 mo					
Femur/humerus fracture	4587	6 (3–8)	52.5	28.0	14.0
Radius/ulna/tibia/fibula fracture	3692	8 (5–10)	52.7	29.5	17.5
Isolated skull fracture[b]	6433	5 (2–8)	59.3	36.9	17.8
Intracranial hemorrhage	5829	3 (1–6)	58.8	32.9	16.0
Age <24 mo					
Rib fracture(s)	1633	3 (2–6)	60.4	27.9	13.0
Abdominal trauma	837	11 (3–18)	57.6	23.2	13.0
Genital injury	535	15 (7–19)	58.7	36.5	12.3
Subconjunctival hemorrhage	1600	7 (3–15)	51.8	25.5	18.8

[a] Subjects identified as having been transferred from another health care facility excluded.
[b] Isolated skull fracture implies that there was no ICD-9 code for intracranial hemorrhage. It does not preclude the identification of injuries in other body areas.

TABLE 3 Rates of Abuse Diagnosis and Testing for Children With Putative Sentinel Injuries

Candidate Injury	% With Abuse Diagnosis, Mean (Range)	% With Skeletal Survey, Mean (Range)	% With Neuroimaging, Mean (Range)	% With Hepatic Transaminases, Mean (Range)
Age <6 mo				
Bruise(s)	8.3 (1.1–21.3)	20.0 (5.4–30.8)	44.0 (19.9–60.1)	14.9 (2.5–24.0)
Burn(s)	3.5 (0–6.9)	13.1 (0–23.3)	15.7 (4.8–29.4)	15.9 (0–44.1)
Oropharyngeal injury	17.0 (0–41.7)	31.9 (11.1–62.5)	39.3 (11.1–62.5)[a]	26.1 (7.1–40.0)
Age <12 mo				
Femur/humerus fracture	18.9 (7.1–51.4)	59.8 (40.9–82.0)	63.8 (43.3–84.7)	35.2 (9.8–71.2)
Radius/ulna/tibia/fibula fracture	19.2 (3.5–49.3)	42.8 (25.0–78.9)	45.1 (25.5–78.9)	25.7 (6.0–64.8)
Isolated skull fracture	4.3 (0.3–11.8)	40.6 (21.5–74.3)	79.6 (66.6–95.4)	19.8 (1.3–47.8)
Intracranial hemorrhage	26.3 (10.7–42.9)	59.0 (42.3–81.6)	89.3 (75.8–96.9)	49.6 (15.9–71.4)
Age <24 mo				
Rib fracture(s)	56.1 (11.5–71.6)	81.5 (69.2–94.9)	90.6 (78.2–98.6)	73.1 (11.5–87.7)
Abdominal trauma	24.5 (0–47.4)	31.9 (18.2–57.9)	58.7 (36.4–75.7)	74.3 (35.8–91.8)
Genital injury	12.3 (0–21.4)	18.5 (0–40.0)	20.0 (0–45.0)	16.5 (39.5–89.5)
Subconjunctival hemorrhage	8.6 (0–22.0)	14.3 (5.9–36.6)	19.7 (10.9–38.2)	14.7 (0–35.4)

Rates are percentages after excluding visits noted to be transfers from another institution.

[a] Ranges for SS and neuroimaging are identical because the 2 institutions with the highest and lowest rates of testing in this group obtained neuroimaging in all children who received SS.

The rate of abuse diagnosis for each putative sentinel injury correlated with the rate of SS completion (R^2 = 0.679) with high rates of SS generally associated with high rates of abuse diagnosis. However, children with fracture(s) of the skull, femur, or humerus were disproportionately more likely to have SS, whereas patients with subconjunctival hemorrhage, genital injury, or abdominal injury were disproportionately less likely, relative to the rate of abuse diagnosis (Fig 1).

Among 32 858 total patient visits, 2092 (6.4%) were noted to have been transferred from another institution. A large majority of visits (26 402 85.8%) was coded as having other or unknown source of admission. A diagnosis of abuse was more likely among children noted to have been transferred from another center: unadjusted odds ratio = 3.63 (95% confidence interval: 3.28–4.01). Odds of having a SS performed were also higher: unadjusted odds ratio = 2.67 (95% confidence interval: 2.44–2.92).

DISCUSSION

Among young children found to have putative sentinel injuries without a motor vehicle collision at leading children's hospitals, rates of diagnosed abuse were high. Rib fractures were by far the most concerning for abuse, with intracranial hemorrhage and abdominal injury also associated with abuse in more than 20% of cases. Children with burns and isolated skull fractures had the lowest rates of abuse diagnoses, though rates were still high relative to the baseline risk for children without putative sentinel injuries.

The American Academy of Pediatrics considers the radiographic SS to be "mandatory" for children with concern for abuse; this recommendation is echoed by the American College of Radiology.[29,30] In our population where all children were <24 months of age, the decision to obtain SS might be taken as 1 surrogate measure of whether there was a concern for abuse that rose to the level of evaluation. The observed correlation between rates of abuse diagnosis and rates of SS is consistent with the ideas that (1) SS is more likely to be ordered when concern for abuse is higher and (2) concern for abuse is likely to increase if SS identifies additional, occult fractures in a child with a sentinel injury. However, the likelihood of abuse does not account for all the variability in SS use, either between centers, or from injury to injury. These data suggest that SS use should be increased for children with abdominal injury, subconjunctival hemorrhage, or genital injury.

Overall rates of abuse diagnosis were also highly variable (range, 0.04%–0.46%) between centers. We suggest several reasons for this variability. First, it is possible that true rates of abuse are actually highly variable between centers on the basis of characteristics of the population the hospital serves or on referral patterns. Alternatively, it is possible that the recognition of abuse differed between hospitals. Finally, it is possible that recognition of abuse was similar between centers, but ICD-9 coding of abuse suspicion differed systematically between centers.[31] Systematic undercoding for abuse by some centers would result in underestimating the significance of putative sentinel injuries and overestimating the variability between centers.

Children who were noted to have been transferred from another institution were significantly more likely to undergo SS and to be diagnosed with abuse. This is consistent with the hypothesis that children with traumatic injuries are more likely to be transferred to the pediatric referral centers that participate in the PHIS database when

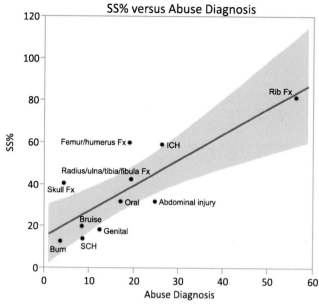

FIGURE 1
Rate of abuse diagnosis and SS completion for each putative sentinel injury. Skull fracture and femur or humerus fractures had higher rates of SS completion relative to rates of abuse diagnoses, whereas genital and abdominal injuries had lower rates. Fx, fracture; ICH, intracranial hemorrhage; SCH, subconjunctival hemorrhage.

there is some concern for abuse. It is also possible that abused children are more likely to present initially to nonpediatric centers, or that the difference could be explained by other characteristics of transferred children (age, injury type) that correlate with abuse likelihood. Children may also have had testing that we did not identify if they were transferred out from a PHIS center to another institution. Because all centers are tertiary referral centers, we suspect that the number of such subjects is small.

Our study is subject to several limitations. ICD-9 codes have been shown to have variable and limited sensitivity for abuse.[31,32] Because a final determination of any traumatic injury's etiology may come after a child is discharged from the hospital, it is possible that many children ultimately determined to have been abused were not identified by our search. The relatively lower rate of abuse diagnosis in young infants with bruises is consistent with this possibility. Sugar et al[26] demonstrated that <1% of healthy

infants <6 months old had any bruising, and when such bruised infants are evaluated for abuse, rates of additional injuries and abuse diagnoses have been reported at 50%.[27] However, the rate of abuse that we identified in children with burns or isolated skull fractures seems more consistent with previous work.[33-37] This limitation might be especially relevant for children without any identified putative sentinel injuries who might only be finally diagnosed as abused after hospital discharge. If this is true, rates of abuse would increase for children with and without putative sentinel injuries, but our estimate of the relative increase in abuse prevalence among children with putative sentinel injuries would be inflated.

Furthermore, these administrative data may have poor sensitivity to detect all diagnostic procedures that were performed in each subject. For example, among subjects coded as having intracranial hemorrhage, neuroimaging was identified in only 89.3%, whereas it would seem that

neuroimaging would be needed to establish the diagnosis for 100% of cases. This could be explained if ICD-9 codes for intracranial hemorrhage were incorrectly applied to children with subgaleal hematoma or other injuries that could be diagnosed without neuroimaging, or if we failed to identify children who were transferred from another institution after neuroimaging had been obtained. This latter possibility seems especially likely given the high rate of children coded as other or unknown for the source of admission. These limits of our administrative data imply that true rates of testing may be higher than our estimates, but would not affect the variability we identify between sites and injuries unless there is also systematic regional variability in the testing practices of referring hospitals. Because children with concern for abuse are more likely than other children with sentinel injuries to be transferred to PHIS centers, inaccuracies in coding transfers could artificially inflate the rates of abuse for children with putative sentinel injuries.

Although CTC procedure codes are relatively consistent for SS and neuroimaging, it is likely that there is more variability in coding for hepatic transaminases. Although some hospitals may include AST and ALT in a "14-test chem profile" (CTC code 310114), others may only include them in "critical care panel" (CTC code 300171) or another such panel. Further, it is possible that some hospitals obtained hepatic transaminases as part of a panel that was obtained to check other laboratory data, or from routine ordering, and not to test for additional abusive injuries. We attempted to include all CTC codes that might have included AST/ALT to use the maximum estimate of testing prevalence. If CTC codes were not accurate, and if this inaccuracy was systematically associated with different centers, our estimates of the variability in ordering of hepatic transaminases would be inflated.

Although SS is primarily done for occult injury evaluation, neuroimaging and hepatic transaminase testing may be undertaken either to identify occult injuries or those with clear or subtle signs. We are not able to determine the reasons that testing was undertaken. If rates of clinically apparent injuries differed systematically between centers, this would account for some of the variability in testing that we identified.

Whereas our use of the term sentinel injury applied to children in whom abuse was diagnosed on the index visit, other authors have used the term to refer to children who are subsequently diagnosed with recurrent abuse on a future visit. Whether the risk of abuse is in the immediate, near, or long-term, we feel that the core attribute of a sentinel injury is that it should prompt the clinician to consider the possibility of physical abuse, and in most cases to undertake testing for additional occult injuries.

True sentinel injuries would present without other clinically apparent injuries or history of abuse. We were not able to determine the presenting injury for any given child, nor whether a child's sentinel injury was accompanied by other obvious signs of abuse, such as a history of witnessed assault. It is therefore possible that the putative sentinel injuries that are most likely to have been identified in the course of an abuse evaluation (eg, rib fractures)

would have inflated rates of abuse. However, for the large majority of patient visits, only a single putative sentinel injury was identified, suggesting at least that these injuries were not only the least noticeable injuries in children with obvious polytrauma. We therefore believe that the high rates of abuse among children with the listed injuries create a strong presumption that abuse should be carefully considered when these injuries are identified.

Similarly, because we are not able to identify the reason for presentation, children who present with clear evidence of a sentinel injury are grouped with children whose injuries were only identified after testing prompted for less specific complaints. It has been well-described that abused children frequently present with subtle signs and symptoms, and that the history may be incomplete or misleading.[6,22,23] Therefore, although rates of abuse diagnoses were vanishingly low in patients without a putative sentinel injury, our results should not be interpreted to discourage abuse evaluations when sentinel injuries are not obvious.

Several methods could be used to increase testing and decrease variability for children with putative sentinel injuries. These and other data could be included in physician training and in the development of clinical guidelines and pathways that address abuse evaluations. In centers with access to subspecialty child abuse pediatricians, the presence of a putative sentinel injury could be considered an indication for

subspecialty consultation to determine the plan for occult injury testing. Finally, these data could form the basis for electronic clinical decision support prompting clinicians to consider occult injury testing for children with putative sentinel injuries.

CONCLUSIONS

Previous work has revealed that physical abuse is commonly missed. Our data reveal an overall high rate of diagnosed abuse, but tremendous variability in evaluation and diagnosis of abuse across hospitals and injury categories. Together, these facts suggest that increased, routine, or protocolized testing for children with these injuries can identify other children with abuse that might otherwise be missed. These results support future trials of protocolized evaluations for children with these putative sentinel injuries.

ACKNOWLEDGMENT

We are grateful to Meghan Birkholz for assistance with data extraction from the PHIS database.

ABBREVIATIONS

CT: computed tomography
ED: emergency department
ICD-9-CM: *International Classification of Diseases, Ninth Revision, Clinical Modification*
PHIS: Pediatric Health Information System
SS: skeletal survey

FINANCIAL DISCLOSURE: Dr Wood's and Dr Runyan's institutions have received payment for expert witness court testimony that each has provided in cases of suspected child abuse for which they have been subpoenaed to testify; Dr Lindberg, Ms Beaty, and Dr Juarez-Colunga have indicated they have no financial relationships relevant to this article to disclose.

FUNDING: No external funding.

POTENTIAL CONFLICT OF INTEREST: Dr Lindberg has provided paid expert testimony in cases of alleged child maltreatment; the other authors have indicated they have no potential conflicts of interest to disclose.

REFERENCES

1. Sedlak AJ, Mettenburg J, Besena M, et al. Fourth National Incidence Study of Child Abuse and Neglect (NIS-4): Report to Congress. Washington, DC: Department of Health and Human Services; 2010

2. Florence C, Brown DS, Fang X, Thompson HF. Health care costs associated with child maltreatment: impact on Medicaid. *Pediatrics*. 2013;132(2):312–318

3. US Department of Health and Human Services Administration for Children and Families. Child Maltreatment 2013. In: Administration on Children Youth and Families, ed. Washington, DC: Children's Bureau; 2015

4. Russo CA, Hambrick MM, Owens PL. Hospital Stays Related to Child Maltreatment, 2005. HCUP Statistical Brief #49. Rockville, MD: Agency for Healthcare Research and Quality; 2008

5. Fang X, Brown DS, Florence CS, Mercy JA. The economic burden of child maltreatment in the United States and implications for prevention. *Child Abuse Negl*. 2012;36(2):156–165

6. Jenny C, Hymel KP, Ritzen A, Reinert SE, Hay TC. Analysis of missed cases of abusive head trauma. *JAMA*. 1999;281(7):621–626

7. Ravichandiran N, Schuh S, Bejuk M, et al. Delayed identification of pediatric abuse-related fractures. *Pediatrics*. 2010;125(1):60–66

8. Sieswerda-Hoogendoorn T, Bilo RA, van Duurling LL, et al. Abusive head trauma in young children in the Netherlands: evidence for multiple incidents of abuse. *Acta Paediatr*. 2013;102(11):e497–e501

9. Lindberg D, Makoroff K, Harper N, et al; ULTRA Investigators. Utility of hepatic transaminases to recognize abuse in children. *Pediatrics*. 2009;124(2):509–516

10. Lindberg DM, Shapiro RA, Blood EA, Steiner RD, Berger RP; ExSTRA investigators. Utility of hepatic transaminases in children with concern for abuse. *Pediatrics*. 2013;131(2):268–275

11. Laskey AL, Holsti M, Runyan DK, Socolar RR. Occult head trauma in young suspected victims of physical abuse. *J Pediatr*. 2004;144(6):719–722

12. Rubin DM, Christian CW, Bilaniuk LT, Zazyczny KA, Durbin DR. Occult head injury in high-risk abused children. *Pediatrics*. 2003;111(6 pt 1):1382–1386

13. Kleinman PK, Blackbourne BD, Marks SC, Karellas A, Belanger PL. Radiologic contributions to the investigation and prosecution of cases of fatal infant abuse. *N Engl J Med*. 1989;320(8):507–511

14. Kleinman PL, Kleinman PK, Savageau JA. Suspected infant abuse: radiographic skeletal survey practices in pediatric health care facilities. *Radiology*. 2004;233(2):477–485

15. Greiner MV, Berger RP, Thackeray JD, Lindberg DM; Examining Siblings to Recognize Abuse (ExSTRA) Investigators. Dedicated retinal examination in children evaluated for physical abuse without radiographically identified traumatic brain injury. *J Pediatr*. 2013;163(2):527–531

16. Lane WG, Dubowitz H. What factors affect the identification and reporting of child abuse-related fractures? *Clin Orthop Relat Res*. 2007;461(461):219–225

17. Wood JN, Hall M, Schilling S, Keren R, Mitra N, Rubin DM. Disparities in the evaluation and diagnosis of abuse among infants with traumatic brain injury. *Pediatrics*. 2010;126(3):408–414

18. Trokel M, Waddimba A, Griffith J, Sege R. Variation in the diagnosis of child abuse in severely injured infants [published correction appears in *Pediatrics*. 2006;118(3):1324]. *Pediatrics*. 2006;117(3):722–728

19. Wood JN, Feudtner C, Medina SP, Luan X, Localio R, Rubin DM. Variation in occult injury screening for children with suspected abuse in selected US children's hospitals. *Pediatrics*. 2012;130(5):853–860

20. Kellogg ND; American Academy of Pediatrics Committee on Child Abuse and Neglect. Evaluation of suspected child physical abuse. *Pediatrics*. 2007;119(6):1232–1241

21. Louwers EC, Korfage IJ, Affourtit MJ, et al. Effects of systematic screening and detection of child abuse in emergency departments. *Pediatrics*. 2012;130(3):457–464

22. Thackeray JD. Frena tears and abusive head injury: a cautionary tale. *Pediatr Emerg Care*. 2007;23(10):735–737

23. Oral R, Yagmur F, Nashelsky M, Turkmen M, Kirby P. Fatal abusive head trauma cases: consequence of medical staff missing milder forms of physical abuse. *Pediatr Emerg Care*. 2008;24(12):816–821

24. Sheets LK, Leach ME, Koszewski IJ, Lessmeier AM, Nugent M, Simpson P. Sentinel injuries in infants evaluated for child physical abuse. *Pediatrics*. 2013;131(4):701–707

25. Leventhal JM, Martin KD, Asnes AG. Incidence of fractures attributable to abuse in young hospitalized children: results from analysis of a United States database. *Pediatrics*. 2008;122(3):599–604

26. Sugar NF, Taylor JA, Feldman KW; Puget Sound Pediatric Research Network. Bruises in infants and toddlers: those who don't cruise rarely bruise. *Arch Pediatr Adolesc Med*. 1999;153(4):399–403

27. Harper N, Feldman K, Sugar N, Anderst J, Lindberg D; ExSTRA Investigators. Occult injury in bruised infants: a multisite analysis. Helfer Society Annual Meeting; March 25–28, 2012; Austin, TX

28. Trokel M, DiScala C, Terrin NC, Sege RD. Blunt abdominal injury in the young pediatric patient: child abuse and patient outcomes. *Child Maltreat*. 2004;9(1):111–117

29. Kleinman PK, Di Pietro MA, Brody AS, et al; Section on Radiology; American Academy of Pediatrics. Diagnostic imaging of child abuse. *Pediatrics*. 2009;123(5):1430–1435

30. American College of Radiology. ACR appropriateness criteria: suspected physical abuse–child. Reston, VA: American College of Radiology; 2009

31. Hooft AM, Asnes AG, Livingston N, et al. Identifying physical abuse in 4 children's hospitals: accuracy of ICD codes. Annual Meeting of the Helfer Society; 2014; Annapolis, MD

32. Hooft A, Ronda J, Schaeffer P, Asnes AG, Leventhal JM. Identification of physical abuse cases in hospitalized children: accuracy of International Classification of Diseases codes. *J Pediatr*. 2013;162(1):80–85

33. Wood JN, Christian CW, Adams CM, Rubin DM. Skeletal surveys in infants with isolated skull fractures. *Pediatrics*. 2009;123(2). Available at: www.pediatrics.org/cgi/content/full/123/2/e247

34. Deye KP, Berger RP, Lindberg DM; ExSTRA Investigators. Occult abusive injuries in infants with apparently isolated skull fractures. *J Trauma Acute Care Surg.* 2013;74(6):1553–1558

35. Laskey AL, Stump TE, Hicks RA, Smith JL. Yield of skeletal surveys in children ≤ 18 months of age presenting with isolated skull fractures. *J Pediatr.* 2013; 162(1):86–89

36. Degraw M, Hicks RA, Lindberg D; Using Liver Transaminases to Recognize Abuse (ULTRA) Study Investigators. Incidence of fractures among children with burns with concern regarding abuse. *Pediatrics.* 2010; 125(2). Available at: www.pediatrics.org/cgi/content/full/125/2/e295

37. Hicks RA, Stolfi A. Skeletal surveys in children with burns caused by child abuse. *Pediatr Emerg Care.* 2007;23(5): 308–313

38. Maguire S, Hunter B, Hunter L, Sibert JR, Mann M, Kemp AM. Diagnosing abuse: a systematic review of torn frenum and other intra-oral injuries. *Archives of disease in childhood.* 2007;92(12): 1113–1117

39. Scherl SA, Miller L, Lively N, Russinoff S, Sullivan CM, Tornetta P, 3rd. Accidental and nonaccidental femur fractures in children. *Clinical orthopaedics and related research.* 2000(376):96–105

40. Strait RT, Siegel RM, Shapiro RA. Humeral fractures without obvious etiologies in children less than 3 years of age: when is it abuse? *Pediatrics.* 1995;96(4 Pt 1): 667–671

41. John SD, Moorthy CS, Swischuk LE. Expanding the concept of the toddler's fracture. *Radiographics: a review publication of the Radiological Society of North America, Inc.* 1997;17(2):367–376

42. Deye K, Lindberg D, for the ExSTRA Investigators. Screening for Occult Injuries in Children with Apparently Isolated Skull Fractures. Helfer Society Annual Meeting, March 25–28, 2012; Austin, TX

43. Laskey AL, Stump TE, Hicks RA, Smith JL. Yield of Skeletal Surveys in Children ≤18 Months of Age Presenting with Isolated Skull Fractures. *J Pediatr.* 2013; 162(1):86–89

44. Kemp AM, Jaspan T, Griffiths J, et al. Neuroimaging: what neuroradiological features distinguish abusive from non-abusive head trauma? A systematic review. *Archives of disease in childhood.* 2011;96(12):1103–1112

45. Maguire SA, Kemp AM, Lumb RC, Farewell DM. Estimating the probability of abusive head trauma: a pooled analysis. *Pediatrics.* 2011;128(3). Available at: www.pediatrics.org/cgi/content/full/128/3/e550

46. Lindberg DM, Shapiro RA, Blood EA, Steiner RD, Berger RP, Ex Si. Utility of hepatic transaminases in children with concern for abuse. *Pediatrics.* 2013; 131(2):268–275

47. Carpenter RF. The prevalence and distribution of bruising in babies. *Archives of Disease in Childhood.* 1999; 80(4):363–366

48. DeRidder CA, Berkowitz CD, Hicks RA, Laskey AL. Subconjunctival hemorrhages in infants and children: a sign of nonaccidental trauma. *Pediatric Emergency Care.* 2013;29(2):222–226

American Academy
of Pediatrics

DEDICATED TO THE HEALTH OF ALL CHILDREN™

CLINICAL REPORT

Evaluating Children With Fractures for Child Physical Abuse

Emalee G. Flaherty, MD, Jeannette M. Perez-Rossello, MD,
Michael A. Levine, MD, William L. Hennrikus, MD, and the
AMERICAN ACADEMY OF PEDIATRICS COMMITTEE ON CHILD
ABUSE AND NEGLECT, SECTION ON RADIOLOGY, SECTION ON
ENDOCRINOLOGY, and SECTION ON ORTHOPAEDICS, and the
SOCIETY FOR PEDIATRIC RADIOLOGY

KEY WORD
fractures

ABBREVIATIONS
CML—classic metaphyseal lesions
CPR—cardiopulmonary resuscitation
CT—computed tomography
OI—osteogenesis imperfect

www.pediatrics.org/cgi/doi/10.1542/peds.2013-3793

doi:10.1542/peds.2013-3793

All clinical reports from the American Academy of Pediatrics
automatically expire 5 years after publication unless reaffirmed,
revised, or retired at or before that time.

PEDIATRICS (ISSN Numbers: Print, 0031-4005; Online, 1098-4275).

abstract

Fractures are common injuries caused by child abuse. Although the
consequences of failing to diagnose an abusive injury in a child
can be grave, incorrectly diagnosing child abuse in a child whose fractures have another etiology can be distressing for a family. The aim of
this report is to review recent advances in the understanding of fracture specificity, the mechanism of fractures, and other medical diseases that predispose to fractures in infants and children. This
clinical report will aid physicians in developing an evidence-based differential diagnosis and performing the appropriate evaluation when
assessing a child with fractures. *Pediatrics* 2014;133:e477–e489

INTRODUCTION

Fractures are the second most common injury caused by child physical
abuse; bruises are the most common injury.[1] Failure to identify an
injury caused by child abuse and to intervene appropriately may
place a child at risk for further abuse, with potentially permanent
consequences for the child.[2–4] Physical abuse may not be considered
in the physician's differential diagnosis of childhood injury because
the caregiver may have intentionally altered the history to conceal the
abuse.[5] As a result, when fractures are initially evaluated, a diagnosis
of child abuse may be missed.[3] In children younger than 3 years, as
many as 20% of fractures caused by abuse may be misdiagnosed
initially as noninflicted or as attributable to other causes.[3] In addition,
fractures may be missed because radiography is performed before
changes are obvious or the radiographic images are misread or
misinterpreted.[2] However, incorrectly diagnosing physical abuse in a child
with noninflicted fractures has serious consequences for the child and
family. To identify child abuse as the cause of fractures, the physician
must take into consideration the history, the age of the child, the location
and type of fracture, the mechanism that causes the particular type of
fracture, and the presence of other injuries while also considering other
possible causes.

DIFFERENTIAL DIAGNOSIS OF FRACTURES

Trauma: Child Abuse Versus Noninflicted Injuries

Fractures are a common childhood injury and account for between 8%
and 12% of all pediatric injuries.[6–8] In infants and toddlers, physical

abuse is the cause of 12% to 20% of fractures.[9] Although unintentional fractures are much more common than fractures caused by child abuse, the physician needs to remain aware of the possibility of inflicted injury. Although some fracture types are highly suggestive of physical abuse, no pattern can exclude child abuse.[10,11] Specifically, it is important to recognize that any fracture, even fractures that are commonly noninflicted injuries, can be caused by child abuse. Certain details that can help the physician determine whether a fracture was caused by abuse rather than unintentional injury include the history, the child's age and developmental stage, the type and location of the fracture, the age of the fracture, and an understanding of the mechanism that causes the particular type of fracture. The presence of multiple fractures, fractures of different ages or stages of healing, delay in obtaining medical treatment, and the presence of other injuries suspicious for abuse (eg, coexisting injuries to the skin, internal organs, or central nervous system) should alert the physician to possible child abuse.

Child's Age and Development

The physician should consider the child's age and level of development. Approximately 80% of all fractures caused by child abuse occur in children younger than 18 months,[12] and approximately one-quarter of fractures in children younger than 1 year are caused by child abuse.[1,9,13–15] Physical abuse is more likely to be the cause of femoral fractures and humeral fractures in children who are not yet walking compared with children who are ambulatory,[15–18] and the percentage of fractures caused by abuse declines sharply after the child begins to walk.[9,19,20]

Fracture Specificity for Abuse

Fractures With High Specificity for Abuse

As shown in Table 1, certain fractures have high specificity for or strong association with child abuse, particularly in infants, whereas others may have less specificity.[21] Rib fractures in infants, especially those situated posteromedially, and the classic metaphyseal lesions of long bones, have high specificity for child abuse. Fractures of the scapula, spinous process, and sternum also have high specificity for abuse but are uncommon.

Rib fractures are highly suggestive of child abuse. Most abusive rib fractures result from anterior-posterior compression of the chest. For this reason, rib fractures are frequently found in infants who are held around the chest, squeezed, and shaken. Rib fractures have high probability of being caused by abuse.[15,17,21] The positive predictive value of rib fractures for child abuse in children younger than 3 years was 95% in one retrospective study.[22] Other less common causes of rib fractures in infants include significant trauma sustained during childbirth or a motor vehicle crash as well as minor trauma

TABLE 1 Specificity of radiologic findings in infants and toddlers[19]

High specificity[a]
CMLs
Rib fractures, especially posteromedial
Scapular fractures
Spinous process fractures
Sternal fractures
Moderate specificity
Multiple fractures, especially bilateral
Fractures of different ages
Epiphyseal separations
Vertebral body fractures and subluxations
Digital fractures
Complex skull fractures
Common, but low specificity
Subperiosteal new bone formation
Clavicular fractures
Long-bone shaft fractures
Linear skull fractures

[a] Highest specificity applies in infants.

in infants who have increased bone fragility.[23–25]

Cardiopulmonary resuscitation (CPR) has been proposed as a cause of rib fractures, but conventional CPR with 2 fingers of 1 hand rarely causes fractures in children.[26,27] Recent recommendations that CPR be performed using 2 hands encircling the rib cage have raised concerns that this technique might cause rib fractures. An analysis of infants who were discovered during autopsy to have rib fractures and had received 2-handed chest compressions antemortem suggested that 2-handed CPR is associated with anterior-lateral rib fractures of the third to sixth ribs.[28] In this small study, no posterior rib fractures were observed. The fractures in these infants were always multiple, uniformly involved the fourth rib, and were sometimes bilateral. Additional research is needed to examine the relationship between the 2-handed CPR technique and rib fractures.

Classic metaphyseal lesions (CMLs) also have high specificity for child abuse when they occur during the first year of life.[21,29] CMLs are the most common long bone fracture found in infants who die with evidence of inflicted injury.[30] CMLs are planar fractures through the primary spongiosa of the metaphysis. These fractures are caused when torsional and tractional shearing strains are applied across the metaphysis, as may occur with vigorous pulling or twisting of an infant's extremity.[31] Fractures resembling CMLs radiographically have been reported after breech delivery[32] and as a result of treatment of clubfoot.[33]

Depending on the projection of the radiograph, CMLs can have the appearance of a corner or a bucket-handle fracture. Acute injuries can be difficult to visualize radiographically. CMLs commonly heal without subperiosteal new bone formation or marginal sclerosis. They can heal quickly and be undetectable on plain radiographs in 4 to 8 weeks.[31]

Fractures With Moderate Specificity for Abuse

Although many children who have been abused will have only a single fracture,[34] the presence of multiple fractures, fractures of different ages and/or stages of healing, and complex skull fractures have moderate specificity for physical abuse. In addition, epiphyseal separations, vertebral body fractures, and digital fractures have moderate specificity for abuse. The presence of multiple fractures or fractures of different ages can be signs of bone fragility but should also evoke consideration of child abuse. Besides the predictive value of the particular pattern of fractures, many other factors, such as the history and the child's age, must be considered when determining whether the injury was inflicted.

Common Fractures With Low Specificity for Child Abuse

Long bone fractures (other than CMLs), linear skull fractures, clavicle fractures, and isolated findings of subperiosteal new bone formation have low specificity for child abuse. In contrast, the single long bone diaphyseal fracture is the most common fracture pattern identified in abused children.[1,13,34]

An understanding of the extent and type of load that is necessary to cause a particular long bone fracture can help to determine whether a specific fracture is consistent with the injury described by the caregiver.[35,36] Transverse fractures of the long bones are caused by the application of a bending load in a direction that is perpendicular to the bone, whereas spiral fractures are caused by torsion or twisting of a long bone along its long axis. Oblique fractures are caused by a combination of bending and torsion loads.[37] Torus or buckle fractures are the result of compression from axial loading along the length of the bone. Although earlier studies suggested that spiral fractures should always raise suspicion for child abuse,[12] more recent studies do not show that any particular fracture pattern can distinguish between abuse and nonabuse with absolute certainty.[16,38]

Falls are common in childhood.[39] Short falls can cause fractures, but they rarely result in additional significant injury (eg, neurologic injury).[11,40–42] In a retrospective study of short falls, parents reported that 40% of the children before 2 years of age had suffered at least 1 fall from a height of between 6 inches and 4 feet. Approximately one-quarter of these children suffered an injury; bruises were the most common injury observed.[43]

The femur, humerus, and tibia are the most common long bones to be injured by child abuse.[1,34] Femoral fractures in the nonambulatory child are more likely caused by child abuse, whereas these fractures in ambulatory children are most commonly noninflicted.[10,16,43–45]

Certain femur fractures may occur as a result of a noninflicted injury in young children. Several studies have demonstrated that a short fall to the knee may produce a torus or impacted transverse fracture of the distal femoral metadiaphysis.[46,47] Oblique distal femur metaphyseal fractures have been reported in children playing in a stationary activity center, such as an Exersaucer (Evenflo, Picqua, OH).[48]

In both ambulatory and nonambulatory children, under some circumstances, falls on a stairway can cause a spiral femoral fracture. For example, a fall down several steps and landing with 1 leg folded or twisted underneath a child can lead to excessive torsional loading of the femur and a spiral fracture.[46] In ambulatory children, noninflicted femoral fractures have been described in children who fell while running or who fell and landed in a split-leg position.[43]

A fracture of the humeral shaft in a child younger than 18 months has a high likelihood of having been caused by abuse.[15,49,50] In contrast, supracondylar fractures in ambulatory children are usually noninflicted injuries resulting from short falls.[15]

Physicians should also be aware of a particular mechanism reported to produce a noninflicted spiral-oblique fracture of the humerus in 1 case report.[51] When the young infant was rolled from the prone position to the supine while the child's arm is extended, the torsion and stress placed on the extended arm appeared to cause a spiral-oblique fracture of the midshaft of the humerus.

Linear skull fractures of the parietal bone are the most common skull fracture among young children, usually children younger than 1 year.[13] A short fall from several feet onto a hard surface can cause a linear, nondiastatic skull fracture.[19,52] The majority of linear skull fractures are not inflicted.[53] By contrast, complex or bilateral skull fractures are typical of nonaccidental trauma.

Syndromes, Metabolic Disorders, Systemic Disease

Preexisting medical conditions and bone disease may make a child's bones more vulnerable to fracture. Some conditions may manifest skeletal changes, such as metaphyseal irregularity and subperiosteal new bone formation. These entities should be considered in the differential diagnosis of childhood fractures.

Osteogenesis Imperfecta

Osteogenesis imperfecta (OI) is a heterogeneous family of diseases, usually caused by heterozygous mutations of the genes COL1A1 and COL1A2,[54] but mutations in these and other genes can cause autosomal recessive forms of OI. The COL1A1 and COL1A2 genes encode the chains of type I collagen, which forms the structural framework of bone. Although it is a genetic disorder, many children have de novo mutations or autosomal-recessive disease and no family history of bone fragility. In addition, the presentation of the disease within affected members of the same family can be quite variable. Phenotypic expression of the disease depends on the nature of the mutation, its relative abundance attributable to mosaicism, and its expression in target tissues.[55] Some types of OI involve reduced production of collagen, and the symptoms resolve or lessen after puberty.[56] Table 2 lists the various signs and symptoms that can be present in a case of OI.

The diagnosis of OI is often suggested by a family history of fractures, short stature, blue sclera, poor dentition, and radiographic evidence of low bone density or osteopenia. The fractures are most commonly transverse in nature, occurring in the shafts of the

TABLE 2 Characteristics of Osteogenesis Imperfecta

Fragile bones with few, some, or many of the following findings:
- Poor linear growth
- Macrocephaly
- Triangular-shaped face
- Blue sclerae
- Hearing impairment as a result of otosclerosis
- Hypoplastic, translucent, carious, late-erupting, or discolored teeth
- Easy bruisability
- Inguinal and/or umbilical hernias
- Limb deformities
- Hyperextensible joints
- Scoliosis and/or kyphosis
- Wormian bones of the skull
- Demineralized bones

long bones. It is unusual to have multiple long bone fractures or rib fractures, particularly in infancy, without other clinical and radiographic evidence of OI.[57,58]

OI has been misdiagnosed as child abuse.[59] On the other hand, OI is often suggested as the cause of fractures in children who have been abused. If fractures continue to occur when a child is placed in a protective environment, a more thorough evaluation for an underlying bone disease is needed. Child abuse is more common than OI,[60] and children with OI and other metabolic or genetic conditions may also be abused.[61,62]

Preterm Birth

Preterm infants have decreased bone mineralization at birth, but after the first year of life, bone density normalizes.[63,64] Osteopenia of prematurity has been well described as a complication in low birth weight infants.[65] Infants born at less than 28 weeks' gestation or who weigh less than 1500 g at birth are particularly vulnerable. Osteopenia of prematurity is multifactorial. Infants are also at risk if they receive prolonged (for 4 or more weeks) total parenteral nutrition, have bronchopulmonary dysplasia, and/or have received a prolonged course of diuretics or steroids.[66] Osteopenia commonly presents between 6 and 12 weeks of life. Osteopenia of prematurity can be ameliorated if infants are monitored closely and receive the nutritional and mineral supplementation initiated in the NICU.

Fractures associated with osteopenia of prematurity usually occur in the first year of life.[67] Rib fractures are typically encountered incidentally, whereas long bone fractures commonly present with swelling of the extremity. Osteopenia of prematurity can be associated with rickets, and in such cases, metaphyseal irregularities may be present.

Although osteopenia of prematurity may make the infant more vulnerable to fracture, preterm infants are also at an increased risk of abuse.[68]

Vitamin D Deficiency Rickets

Suboptimal vitamin D concentrations and rickets have been proposed as causes of fractures in infants.[69] Vitamin D insufficiency in otherwise healthy infants and toddlers is common. Approximately 40% of infants and toddlers aged 8 to 24 months in an urban clinic had laboratory evidence of vitamin D insufficiency (serum concentrations of 25-hydroxyvitamin D of ≤30 ng/mL).[70] Prolonged breastfeeding without vitamin D supplementation was a critical factor that placed these infants at risk, although increased skin pigmentation and/or lack of sunlight exposure may also have contributed. Rickets is characterized by demineralization, loss of the zone of provisional calcification, widening and irregularity of the physis, and fraying and cupping of the metaphysis.[71] Despite the high prevalence of vitamin D insufficiency in infants and toddlers, rickets is uncommon.[72]

The claim that vitamin D deficiency or insufficiency causes skeletal lesions that lead to the incorrect diagnosis of child abuse in infants is not supported in the literature. A systematic clinical, laboratory, and radiologic assessment should exclude that possibility.[73–75] Schilling et al found no difference in serum concentrations of 25-hydroxyvitamin D in young children with fractures suspicious for abuse and noninflicted fractures.[76] Vitamin D insufficiency was not associated with multiple fractures, in particular rib fractures or CMLs, the high specificity indicators of abuse. Perez-Rossello et al studied radiographs of 40 healthy older infants and toddlers with vitamin D insufficiency and deficiency and concluded that radiographic rachitic changes were uncommon and very mild. In this population, the reported fracture prevalence was zero.[72]

In a study of 45 young children with radiographic evidence of rickets, investigators found that fractures occurred only in those infants and toddlers who were mobile.[77] Fractures were seen in 17.5% of the children, and these children were 8 to 19 months of age. The fractures involved long bones, anterior-lateral and lateral ribs, and metatarsal and metaphyseal regions. The metaphyseal fractures occurred closer to the diaphysis in the background of florid metaphyseal rachitic changes and did not resemble the juxtaphyseal corner or bucket handle pattern of the CML. In infant fatalities in which abuse is suspected, rachitic changes appear to be rare histologically.[78]

Osteomyelitis

Osteomyelitis in infants can present as multiple metaphyseal irregularities potentially resembling CMLs.[79] Typically, the lesions become progressively lytic and sclerotic with substantial subperiosteal new bone formation. Other signs of infection are often present, such as fever, increased erythrocyte sedimentation rate, elevated C-reactive protein concentration, and elevated white blood cell count.

Fractures Secondary to Demineralization From Disuse

Any child with a severe disability that limits or prevents ambulation can be at risk for fractures secondary to disuse demineralization, even with normal handling.[80,81] The fractures are usually diaphyseal rather than CMLs. Often, these fractures occur during physical therapy and range-of-motion exercises. It can be difficult to distinguish between inflicted and noninflicted fractures occurring in these children. At the same time, children with disabilities are at an increased risk of being maltreated.[82–84] When multiple or recurrent fractures occur in a disabled child, a trial change in caregivers may be indicated to determine whether the fractures can be prevented. This is an extreme intervention and should be reserved for unusual circumstances.[63]

Scurvy

Scurvy is caused by insufficient intake of vitamin C, which is important for the synthesis of collagen. Although rare today because formula, human milk, fruits, and vegetables contain vitamin C, scurvy may develop in older infants and children given exclusively cow milk without vitamin supplementation and in children who eat no foods containing vitamin C.[85–87] Although scurvy can result in metaphyseal changes similar to those seen with child abuse, other characteristic bone changes, including osteopenia, increased sclerosis of the zones of provisional calcification, dense epiphyseal rings, and extensive calcification of subperiosteal and soft tissue hemorrhages, will point to the diagnosis of scurvy.

Copper Deficiency

Copper plays a role in cartilage formation. Copper deficiency is a rare condition that may be complicated by bone fractures. Preterm infants are born with lower stores of copper than term infants, because copper is accumulated at a faster rate during the last trimester.[88] Copper insufficiency may be observed in children with severe nutritional disorders, for example, liver failure or short gut syndrome.[89] This deficiency is not likely to be observed in full-term children younger than 6 months of age or preterm infants younger than 2.5 months of age, because fetal copper stores are sufficient for this length of time. In addition, human milk and formula contain sufficient copper to prevent deficiency. Psychomotor retardation, hypotonia, hypopigmentation, pallor, and a sideroblastic anemia are some of the characteristic findings of copper deficiency in infants. Radiologic changes that should lead to further evaluation for possible deficiency include cupping and fraying of the metaphyses, sickle-shaped metaphyseal spurs, significant demineralization, and subperiosteal new bone formation.

Menkes Disease

Menkes disease, also known as Menkes kinky hair syndrome, is a rare congenital defect of copper metabolism.[90] Menkes disease is an X-linked recessive condition and occurs only in boys. Although it has many of the features of dietary copper deficiency, anemia is not associated with Menkes disease. Metaphyseal fragmentation and subperiosteal new bone formation may be observed on radiographs, and the findings may be difficult to distinguish from fractures caused by abuse.[91] Other signs of Menkes disease include sparse, kinky hair, calvarial wormian bones, anterior rib flaring, failure to thrive, and developmental delay. A characteristic finding is tortuous cerebral vessels. Intracranial hemorrhage can occur in Menkes disease but has not been reported in infants with copper deficiency.

Systemic Disease

Chronic renal disease affects bone metabolism because children with chronic renal disease may develop a metabolic acidosis that interferes with vitamin D metabolism. Chronic renal disease can cause renal osteodystrophy resulting in the same radiographic changes as nutritional rickets. Because chronic liver disease (eg, biliary atresia) interferes with vitamin D metabolism, such children may be at an increased risk of fractures. Fanconi syndrome, hypophosphatasia, hypophosphatemic (vitamin D resistant) rickets, hyperparathyroidism, and renal tubular acidosis also cause clinical variants of rickets.

Temporary Brittle Bone Disease Hypothesis

Physicians should be aware of alternative diagnoses that are unsupported by research but are sometimes suggested when an infant has unexplained fractures. In 1993, Paterson proposed that some infants may be born with bones that are temporarily more fragile or vulnerable to fracture in the context of normal handling, which he called "temporary brittle bone disease."[92] Paterson suggested that some trace element deficiency, such as copper or a transient collagen immaturity, caused the disease but provided no scientific data that confirmed his hypotheses and offered no specific test that confirmed temporary brittle bone disease.[61] Subsequent studies did not support his hypotheses, and his case analysis has been refuted.[57,93–95]

Miller hypothesized that temporary brittle bone disease is a result of fetal immobilization or intrauterine confinement that leads to transient bone loss or osteopenia.[96,97] In support of his hypothesis, he reported that 95% of 21 infants with multiple unexplained fractures had decreased fetal movements, according to their mothers.[97,98] Although he used bone densitometry in each patient as a basis for his conclusions, none of the patients had had bone densitometry performed at the time of the fracture. The testing was performed 8 to 21 weeks later, and no infants were tested before 5 months of age. In addition, bone densitometry standards have not been established for infants. He relied on the mother's history of decreased fetal movements and provided no independent measurements of those movements. Palacios and Rodriguez found no evidence that oligohydramnios affects bone mass of the fetus, probably because fetal movement is only restricted in the last trimester of pregnancy by oligohydramnios and because the mechanical loading on the bones stimulating bone formation is conserved.[99]

Medical Evaluation

History of Present Illness

It is essential to obtain a detailed history to determine how an injury occurred. If an injury in a nonverbal child was witnessed, the caregiver should be able to provide details about the child's activity and position before an injury and the child's final position and location after the injury occurred.[46] Verbal children with concerning fractures should be interviewed apart from caregivers and ideally by a professional who is skilled in forensic interviewing.

A comparison of the histories provided by caregivers of children with noninflicted femoral fractures and by caregivers of children whose injuries were caused by abuse is instructive. When an injury was caused by abuse, the caregiver provided either no history of an injury or related a history of a low-energy event. By contrast, 29% of the caregivers of children with noninflicted injuries provided some high-energy explanation, such as a motor vehicle collision or that the child fell from a height.[16] Most of the low-energy mechanisms provided for the noninflicted injuries involved falls including stair falls and siblings landing on the femur during play.[16,46]

The child's response to the event may also provide important clues about the etiology. The majority of children with long bone fractures will have some swelling, pain, or other signs, such as decreased use of the extremity, suggesting a fracture.[100,101] Some children, however, will have minimal external signs of injury.[102] The absence of any history of injury, a vague description of the event, a delay in seeking care, the absence of an explanation for an injury particularly in a nonambulatory child, or an inconsistent explanation should increase the physician's concern that an injury was caused by child abuse (see Table 3).[13,16]

Past Medical History

The past medical history is important and should include details about the mother's pregnancy. If the child was born preterm, the infant's bone mineral content may be reduced, and the infant may be at risk for fracture. A history of total parental nutrition, hepatobiliary disease, diuretic therapy, hypercalciuria, or corticosteroids may make the bones of a low birth weight infant even more vulnerable to fracture. In addition, chronic diseases, such as renal insufficiency or metabolic acidosis, malabsorption, cerebral palsy or other neuromuscular disorders, genetic diseases that affect skeletal development, or any illness that limits mobility, may affect bone strength. A thorough dietary history and history of medications that can

TABLE 3 When Is a Fracture Suspicious for Child Abuse?

- No history of injury
- History of injury not plausible—mechanism described not consistent with the type of fracture, the energy load needed to cause the fracture, or the severity of the injury
- Inconsistent histories or changing histories provided by caregiver
- Fracture in a nonambulatory child
- Fracture of high specificity for child abuse (eg, rib fractures)
- Multiple fractures
- Fractures of different ages
- Other injuries suspicious for child abuse
- Delay in seeking care for an injury

predispose to fractures are important. The physician should inquire about previous injuries including bruises and determine the child's developmental abilities, because children who are not yet mobile are much more likely to have fractures caused by abuse.

Family History

A family history of multiple fractures, early-onset hearing loss, abnormally developed dentition, blue sclera, and short stature should suggest the possibility of OI.

Social History

The physician should obtain a complete psychosocial history, including asking who lives in the home and who has provided care for the child. The history should inquire about intimate partner violence, substance abuse including drugs and alcohol, mental illness, and previous involvement with child protective services and/or law enforcement.

Physical Examination

The child should have a comprehensive physical examination, and the growth chart should be carefully reviewed. Abnormal weight may suggest neglect or endocrine or metabolic disorders. Any signs or symptoms of fractures, such as swelling, limitation of motion, and point tenderness should be documented. The physician should do a complete skin examination to look for bruises and other skin findings because bruises are the most common injury caused by child abuse. The majority of children with fractures do not have bruising associated with the fracture; the presence or absence of such bruising does not help to determine which fractures are caused by child abuse.[103,104] Bruising in a child who is not yet cruising or bruising in unusual locations, such as the ears,

neck, or trunk should raise suspicion for child abuse.[105,106] The child should be examined for other injuries caused by child abuse, in addition to signs of other medical conditions associated with bone fragility. Blue sclerae are seen in certain types of OI. Sparse, kinky hair is associated with Menkes disease. Dentinogenesis imperfecta is occasionally identified in older children with OI.

Laboratory Evaluation

The clinical evaluation should guide the laboratory evaluation. In children with fractures suspicious for abuse, serum calcium, phosphorus, and alkaline phosphatase should be reviewed, although alkaline phosphatase may be elevated with healing fractures. The physician should consider checking serum concentrations of parathyroid hormone and 25-hydroxyvitamin D, as well as urinary calcium excretion (eg, random urinary calcium/creatinine ratio) in all young children with fractures concerning for abuse, but these levels should certainly be assessed if there is radiographic evidence of osteopenia or metabolic bone disease. Screening for abdominal trauma with liver function studies as well as amylase and lipase concentration should be performed when severe or multiple injuries are identified. A urinalysis should be performed to screen for occult blood. Serum copper, vitamin C, and ceruloplasmin concentrations should be considered if the child is at risk for scurvy or copper deficiency and has radiographic findings that include metaphyseal abnormalities.

If OI is suspected, sequence analysis of the *COL1A1* and *COL1A2* genes that are associated with 90% of cases of OI as well as other genes associated with less common autosomal-recessive forms of OI may be more sensitive than biochemical tests of

type I collagen and may identify the mutation to guide testing of other family members.[107] Some of the less common forms of OI are OI types IIB and VII, *CRTAP*; OI type VI, *FKBP10*; OI type VIII, *LEPRE1*; OI type IX, *PPIB*; OI type X, *SERPINH1*; OI type XI, *SP7*; OI type XII, *SERPINF1*; and OI type *XIII*, *BMP1*. DNA sequencing can be performed using genomic DNA isolated from peripheral blood mononuclear cells or even saliva, whereas the biochemical analysis of type I collagen requires a skin biopsy. Doing both DNA analysis and skin biopsy is not indicated in most cases. Consultation with a pediatric geneticist may be helpful in deciding which children to test and which test to order.[108]

Imaging Approach

Children younger than 2 years with fractures suspicious for child abuse should have a radiographic skeletal survey to look for other bone injuries or osseous abnormalities.[109] Additional fractures are identified in approximately 10% of skeletal surveys, with higher yields in infants.[110] Skeletal surveys may be appropriate in some children between ages 2 and 5 years, depending on the clinical suspicion of abuse. If specific clinical findings indicate an injury at a particular site, imaging of that area should be obtained regardless of the child's age.

The American College of Radiology has developed specific practice guidelines for skeletal surveys in children.[111] Twenty-one images are obtained, including frontal images of the appendicular skeleton, frontal and lateral views of the axial skeleton, and oblique views of the chest. Oblique views of the chest have been shown to increase the sensitivity, specificity, and accuracy of the identification of rib fractures.[112] A full 4 skull series should be obtained if there are concerns of head injury. Computed tomography (CT) 3-dimensional models are valuable adjuncts to the radiographs and have the potential to replace the skull series.[113] This has not been studied systematically in this context, however. Because lateral views of the extremities increase yield, some authors suggest that these views be included in the imaging protocol.[114] Fractures may be missed if the guidelines are not followed or if the images are of poor quality.[115] A repeat skeletal survey should be performed approximately 2 to 3 weeks after the initial skeletal survey if child abuse is strongly suspected.[109,116] The follow-up examination may identify fractures not seen on the initial skeletal survey, can clarify uncertain findings identified by the initial skeletal survey, and improves both sensitivity and specificity of the skeletal survey.[116,117] In one study, 13 of 19 fractures found on the follow-up examination were not seen on the initial series.[116] The number of images on the follow-up examination may be limited to 15 views by omitting the views of the skull, pelvis, and lateral spine.[118]

Radiography may assist in assessing the approximate time when an injury occurred because long bone fractures heal following a particular sequence.[119] If the healing pattern is not consistent with the explanation provided, the accuracy of the explanation should be questioned.

Bone scintigraphy may be used to complement the skeletal survey but should not be the sole method of identifying fractures in infants. Although it has high overall sensitivity, it lacks specificity for fracture detection and may fail to identify CMLs and skull fractures.[109,119,120] Scintigraphy does have high sensitivity for identifying rib fractures, which can be difficult to detect before healing. In toddlers and older children, the use of bone scintigraphy or skeletal survey depends on the specific clinical indicators of abuse.[109]

Because brain injuries are often occult, head imaging should be considered for any child younger than 1 year with a fracture suspicious for abuse.[121] Imaging studies may help clarify whether the child has been abused, provide further support for a diagnosis of child abuse, and identify other injuries that require treatment. Additional imaging may be needed if the child has signs or symptoms of chest, abdominal, or neck injury.

Chest CT can identify rib fractures that are not seen on chest radiographs.[122] CT is particularly useful in detecting anterior rib fractures and rib fractures at all stages of healing—early subacute, subacute, and old fractures. Although CT may be more sensitive in identifying these injuries, a chest CT exposes the child to significantly more radiation than chest radiography. Every effort should be made to reduce children's exposure to radiation while at the same time considering the risk to the child if abuse is not identified.[123] Therefore, selective application of this technique in certain clinical settings is appropriate.

Other modalities may become available in the future that will provide more accurate identification of skeletal injuries. Whole-body short tau inverse recovery imaging, a magnetic resonance imaging (MRI) technique, may identify rib fractures not recognized on the radiographic skeletal survey.[124] In a study of 21 infants with suspected abuse, whole-body MRI at 1.5-Tesla was insensitive in the detection of CMLs and rib fractures. In some cases, whole-body MRI identified soft tissue edema and joint effusions that led to the identification of skeletal injuries with additional radiographs.[125] Bone scintigraphy with ^{18}F-sodium fluoride positron emission tomography (^{18}F-NaF PET) bone scan may be useful in cases of equivocal or negative skeletal surveys when there is high clinical suspicion of abuse. If available, a ^{18}F-NaF positron emission tomography bone scan has better contrast and spatial resolution than ^{99m}Tc-labeled methylene diphosphonate.[120]

Although bone densitometry by dual-energy x-ray absorptiometry is useful to predict bone fragility and fracture risk in older adults, interpretation of bone densitometry in children and adolescents is more problematic.[126] In adults, bone densitometry is interpreted using T scores, which describe the number of SDs above or below the average peak bone mass for a gender- and race-adjusted reference group of normal subjects. Because peak bone mass is not achieved until approximately 30 years of age, in children, z scores must be used to express bone density, because z scores express the child's bone mineral density as a function of SDs above or below the average for an age- and gender-matched norm control population.[127] In addition, because bone size influences dual-energy x-ray absorptiometry, z scores must also be adjusted for height z scores.[128] The International Society for Clinical Densitometry recommends that the diagnosis of osteoporosis in childhood should not be made on the basis of low bone mass alone but should also include a clinically significant history of low-impact fracture. The recommendations currently apply to children 5 years and older, although reference data are available for children as young as 3 years.[129,130] Unfortunately, there are limited reference data for the young, nonverbal child who is most at risk for suffering fractures caused by child abuse.

Evaluation of Siblings

Siblings, especially twins, and other young household members of children who have been physically abused should be evaluated for maltreatment.[131] In a study of 795 siblings in 400 households of a child who had been abused or neglected, all siblings in 37% of households and some siblings in 20% of households had suffered some form of maltreatment.[132] In this study, which included all manifestations of maltreatment, siblings were found to be more at risk for maltreatment if the index child suffered moderate or severe maltreatment. In addition to a careful evaluation, imaging should be considered for any siblings younger than 2 years, especially if there are signs of abuse.

DIAGNOSIS

When evaluating a child with a fracture, physicians must take a careful history of any injury event and then determine whether the mechanism described and the severity and timing are consistent with the injury identified (see Table 3).[133] They must consider and evaluate for possible diagnoses in addition to other signs or symptoms of child abuse. A careful evaluation for other injuries is important because the presence of additional injuries that are associated with child abuse increases the likelihood that a particular fracture was inflicted.[16,43] It is important to remember that even if a child has an underlying disorder or disability that could increase the likelihood of a fracture, the child may also have been abused because children with disabilities and other special health care needs are at increased risk of child abuse.[83,84] Physicians should keep an open mind to the possibility of abuse and remember that child abuse occurs in all socioeconomic

groups and across all racial and ethnic groups. Many of these diagnoses are complex. If a physician is uncertain about how to evaluate an injury or if they should suspect a fracture was caused by child abuse, they should consult a child abuse pediatrician or multidisciplinary child abuse team to assist in the evaluation, particularly if the child is nonambulatory or younger than 1 year of age.[134] In certain circumstances, the physician will need to consult an orthopedist, endocrinologist, geneticist, or other subspecialists.

All US states, commonwealths, and territories have mandatory reporting requirements for physicians and other health care providers when child abuse is suspected. Physicians should be aware of and comply with the reporting requirements of their state. Typically, the standard for making a report is when the reporter "suspects" or "has reason to believe" that a child has been abused or neglected. Sometimes determining whether that "reasonable belief" or "reasonable suspicion" standard has been met can be nuanced and complex. The physician should keep in mind that incontrovertible proof of abuse or neglect is not required by state statutes, and there may be cases in which it is reasonable to consult with a child abuse pediatrician about whether a report should be made.

LEAD AUTHOR

Emalee G. Flaherty, MD, FAAP

COMMITTEE ON CHILD ABUSE AND NEGLECT, 2012–2013

Cindy W. Christian, MD, FAAP, Chairperson
James E. Crawford-Jakubiak, MD, FAAP
Emalee G. Flaherty, MD, FAAP
John M. Leventhal, MD, FAAP
James L. Lukefahr, MD, FAAP
Robert D. Sege MD, PhD, FAAP

LIAISONS

Harriet MacMillan, MD – *American Academy of Child and Adolescent Psychiatry*
Catherine M. Nolan, MSW, ACSW – *Administration for Children, Youth, and Families*
Linda Anne Valley, PhD – *Centers for Disease Control and Prevention*

STAFF

Tammy Piazza Hurley

SECTION ON RADIOLOGY EXECUTIVE COMMITTEE, 2012–2013

Christopher I. Cassady, MD, FAAP, Chairperson
Dorothy I. Bulas, MD, FAAP
John A. Cassese, MD, FAAP
Amy R. Mehollin-Ray, MD, FAAP
Maria-Gisela Mercado-Deane, MD, FAAP
Sarah Sarvis Milla, MD, FAAP

STAFF

Vivian Thorne

SECTION ON ENDOCRINOLOGY EXECUTIVE COMMITTEE, 2012–2103

Irene N. Sills, MD, FAAP, Chairperson
Clifford A. Bloch, MD, FAAP
Samuel J. Casella, MD, MSc, FAAP
Joyce M. Lee, MD, FAAP
Jane Lockwood Lynch, MD, FAAP
Kupper A. Wintergerst, MD, FAAP

STAFF

Laura Laskosz, MPH

SECTION ON ORTHOPEDICS EXECUTIVE COMMITTEE, 2012–2013

Richard M. Schwend, MD, FAAP, Chairperson
J. Eric Gordon, MD, FAAP
Norman Y. Otsuka, MD, FAAP
Ellen M. Raney, MD, FAAP
Brian A. Shaw, MD, FAAP
Brian G. Smith, MD, FAAP
Lawrence Wells, MD, FAAP
Paul W. Esposito, MD, USBJD Liaison

STAFF

Niccole Alexander, MPP

REFERENCES

1. Loder RT, Feinberg JR. Orthopaedic injuries in children with nonaccidental trauma: demographics and incidence from the 2000 kids' inpatient database [published correction appears in *J Pediatr Orthop*. 2008;28(6):699]. *J Pediatr Orthop*. 2007;27(4):421–426

2. Jenny C, Hymel KP, Ritzen A, Reinert SE, Hay TC. Analysis of missed cases of abusive head trauma [see comment; published correction appears in *JAMA*. 1999; 282(1):29]. *JAMA*. 1999;281(7):621–626

3. Ravichandiran N, Schuh S, Bejuk M, et al. Delayed identification of pediatric abuse-related fractures. *Pediatrics*. 2010;125(1):60–66

4. Skellern C, Donald T. Suspicious childhood injury: formulation of forensic opinion. *J Paediatr Child Health*. 2011;47(11):771–775

5. O'Neill JA, Jr, Meacham WF, Griffin JP, Sawyers JL. Patterns of injury in the battered child syndrome. *J Trauma*. 1973;13(4):332–339

6. Gallagher SS, Finison K, Guyer B, Goodenough S. The incidence of injuries among 87,000 Massachusetts children and adolescents: results of the 1980–81 Statewide Childhood Injury Prevention Program Surveillance System. *Am J Public Health*. 1984;74(12):1340–1347

7. Spady DW, Saunders DL, Schopflocher DP, Svenson LW. Patterns of injury in children: a population-based approach. *Pediatrics*. 2004;113(3 pt 1):522–529

8. Rennie L, Court-Brown CM, Mok JYQ, Beattie TF. The epidemiology of fractures in children. *Injury*. 2007;38(8):913–922

9. Leventhal JM, Martin KD, Asnes AG. Incidence of fractures attributable to abuse in young hospitalized children: results from analysis of a United States database. *Pediatrics*. 2008;122(3):599–604

10. Schwend RM, Werth C, Johnston A. Femur shaft fractures in toddlers and young children: rarely from child abuse. *J Pediatr Orthop*. 2000;20(4):475–481

11. Hennrikus WL, Shaw BA, Gerardi JA. Injuries when children reportedly fall from a bed or couch. *Clin Orthop Relat Res*. 2003; (407):148–151

12. Worlock P, Stower M, Barbor P. Patterns of fractures in accidental and non-accidental injury in children: a comparative study. *Br Med J (Clin Res Ed)*. 1986;293(6539):100–102

13. Leventhal JM, Thomas SA, Rosenfield NS, Markowitz RI. Fractures in young children. Distinguishing child abuse from unintentional injuries. *Am J Dis Child*. 1993;147(1):87–92

14. Leventhal JM, Larson IA, Abdoo D, et al. Are abusive fractures in young children becoming less common? Changes over 24 years. *Child Abuse Negl*. 2007;31(3):311–322

15. Kemp AM, Dunstan F, Harrison S, et al. Patterns of skeletal fractures in child abuse: systematic review [review]. *BMJ*. 2008;337:a1518

16. Hui C, Joughin E, Goldstein S, et al. Femoral fractures in children younger than three years: the role of nonaccidental injury. *J Pediatr Orthop*. 2008;28(3):297–302

17. Pandya NK, Baldwin K, Wolfgruber H, Christian CW, Drummond DS, Hosalkar HS. Child abuse and orthopaedic injury patterns: analysis at a level I pediatric trauma center. *J Pediatr Orthop*. 2009;29(6):618–625

18. Coffey C, Haley K, Hayes J, Groner JI. The risk of child abuse in infants and toddlers with lower extremity injuries. *J Pediatr Surg*. 2005;40(1):120–123

19. Kleinman PK. The spectrum of non-accidental injuries (child abuse) and its imitators. In: Hodler J, Zollikofer CL, Schulthess GK, eds. Musculoskeletal Diseases 2009–2012. Milan, Italy: Springer Italia; 2009:227–233

20. Clarke NMP, Shelton FRM, Taylor CC, Khan T, Needhirajan S. The incidence of fractures in children under the age of 24 months—in relation to non-accidental injury. *Injury*. 201243(6):762–765

21. Kleinman PK. *Diagnostic Imaging of Child Abuse*. 2nd ed. St. Louis, MO: Mosby; 1998

22. Barsness KA, Cha E-S, Bensard DD, et al. The positive predictive value of rib fractures as an indicator of nonaccidental trauma in children [see comment]. *J Trauma*. 2003;54(6):1107–1110

23. Bulloch B, Schubert CJ, Brophy PD, Johnson N, Reed MH, Shapiro RA. Cause and clinical characteristics of rib fractures in infants. *Pediatrics*. 2000;105(4). Available at: www.pediatrics.org/cgi/content/full/105/4/E48

24. Kleinman PK, Schlesinger AE. Mechanical factors associated with posterior rib fractures: laboratory and case studies. *Pediatr Radiol*. 1997;27(1):87–91

25. Bixby SD, Abo A, Kleinman PK. High-impact trauma causing multiple posteromedial rib fractures in a child. *Pediatr Emerg Care*. 2011;27(3):218–219

26. Feldman KW, Brewer DK. Child abuse, cardiopulmonary resuscitation, and rib fractures. *Pediatrics*. 1984;73(3):339–342

27. Spevak MR, Kleinman PK, Belanger PL, Primack C, Richmond JM. Cardiopulmonary resuscitation and rib fractures in infants. A postmortem radiologic-pathologic study. *JAMA*. 1994;272(8):617–618

28. Matshes EW, Lew EO. Two-handed cardiopulmonary resuscitation can cause rib fractures in infants. *Am J Forensic Med Pathol*. 2010;31(4):303–307

29. Kleinman PK, Perez-Rossello JM, Newton AW, Feldman HA, Kleinman PL. Prevalence of the classic metaphyseal lesion in infants at low versus high risk for abuse. *AJR Am J Roentgenol*. 2011;197(4):1005–1008

30. Kleinman PK, Marks SC, Jr, Richmond JM, Blackbourne BD. Inflicted skeletal injury: a postmortem radiologic-histopathologic study in 31 infants. *AJR Am J Roentgenol*. 1995;165(3):647–650

31. Kleinman PK. Problems in the diagnosis of metaphyseal fractures. *Pediatr Radiol*. 2008;38(suppl 3):S388–S394

32. O'Connell A, Donoghue VB. Can classic metaphyseal lesions follow uncomplicated caesarean section? *Pediatr Radiol*. 2007;37(5):488–491

33. Grayev AM, Boal DK, Wallach DM, Segal LS. Metaphyseal fractures mimicking abuse during treatment for clubfoot [see comment]. *Pediatr Radiol*. 2001;31(8):559–563

34. King J, Diefendorf D, Apthorp J, Negrete VF, Carlson M. Analysis of 429 fractures in 189 battered children. *J Pediatr Orthop*. 1988;8(5):585–589

35. Pierce MC, Bertocci G. Injury biomechanics and child abuse. *Annu Rev Biomed Eng*. 2008;10:85–106

36. Pierce MC, Bertocci GE, Vogeley E, Moreland MS. Evaluating long bone fractures in children: a biomechanical approach with illustrative cases. *Child Abuse Negl*. 2004;28(5):505–524

37. Pierce MC, Bertocci G. Fractures resulting from inflicted trauma: assessing injury and history compatibility. *Clin Pediatr Emerg Med*. 2006;7(3):143–148

38. Rex C, Kay PR. Features of femoral fractures in nonaccidental injury. *J Pediatr Orthop*. 2000;20(3):411–413

39. Haney SB, Starling SP, Heisler KW, Okwara L. Characteristics of falls and risk of injury in children younger than 2 years. *Pediatr Emerg Care*. 2010;26(12):914–918

40. Nimityongskul P, Anderson LD. The likelihood of injuries when children fall out of bed. *J Pediatr Orthop*. 1987;7(2):184–186

41. Lyons TJ, Oates RK. Falling out of bed: a relatively benign occurrence. *Pediatrics.* 1993;92(1):125–127

42. Hansoti B, Beattie T. Can the height of fall predict long bone fracture in children under 24 months? *Eur J Emerg Med.* 2005;12(6):285–286

43. Thomas SA, Rosenfield NS, Leventhal JM, Markowitz RI. Long-bone fractures in young children: distinguishing accidental injuries from child abuse. *Pediatrics.* 1991;88(3):471–476

44. Loder RT, O'Donnell PW, Feinberg JR. Epidemiology and mechanisms of femur fractures in children. *J Pediatr Orthop.* 2006;26(5):561–566

45. Baldwin K, Pandya NK, Wolfgruber H, Drummond DS, Hosalkar HS. Femur fractures in the pediatric population: abuse or accidental trauma? *Clin Orthop Relat Res.* 2011;469(3):798–804

46. Pierce MC, Bertocci GE, Janosky JE, et al. Femur fractures resulting from stair falls among children: an injury plausibility model. *Pediatrics.* 2005;115(6):1712–1722

47. Haney SB, Boos SC, Kutz TJ, Starling SP. Transverse fracture of the distal femoral metadiaphysis: a plausible accidental mechanism. *Pediatr Emerg Care.* 2009;25(12):841–844

48. Grant P, Mata MB, Tidwell M. Femur fracture in infants: a possible accidental etiology. *Pediatrics.* 2001;108(4):1009–1011

49. Pandya NK, Baldwin KD, Wolfgruber H, Drummond DS, Hosalkar HS. Humerus fractures in the pediatric population: an algorithm to identify abuse. *J Pediatr Orthop B.* 2010;19(6):535–541

50. Strait RT, Siegel RM, Shapiro RA. Humeral fractures without obvious etiologies in children less than 3 years of age: when is it abuse? *Pediatrics.* 1995;96(4 pt 1):667–671

51. Hymel KP, Jenny C. Abusive spiral fractures of the humerus: a videotaped exception. *Arch Pediatr Adolesc Med.* 1996;150(2):226–227

52. Laskey AL, Stump TE, Hicks RA, Smith JL. Yield of skeletal surveys in children ≤18 months of age presenting with isolated skull fractures. *J Pediatr.* 2013;162(1):86–89

53. Wood JN, Christian CW, Adams CM, Rubin DM. Skeletal surveys in infants with isolated skull fractures. *Pediatrics.* 2009;123(2). Available at: www.pediatrics.org/cgi/content/full/123/2/e247–e252

54. Byers PH, Steiner RD. Osteogenesis imperfecta. *Annu Rev Med.* 1992;43:269–282

55. Wallis GA, Starman BJ, Zinn AB, Byers PH. Variable expression of osteogenesis imperfecta in a nuclear family is explained by somatic mosaicism for a lethal point mutation in the alpha 1(I) gene (COL1A1) of type I collagen in a parent. *Am J Hum Genet.* 1990;46(6):1034–1040

56. Barsh GS, Byers PH. Reduced secretion of structurally abnormal type I procollagen in a form of osteogenesis imperfecta. *Proc Natl Acad Sci USA.* 1981;78(8):5142–5146

57. Sprigg A. Temporary brittle bone disease versus suspected non-accidental skeletal injury. *Arch Dis Child.* 2011;96(5):411–413

58. Greeley CS, Donaruma-Kwoh M, Vettimattam M, Lobo C, Williard C, Mazur L. Fractures at diagnosis in infants and children with osteogenesis imperfecta. *J Pediatr Orthop.* 2013;33(1):32–36 doi:10.1097/BPO.1090-b1013e318279c318255d

59. Singh Kocher M, Dichtel L. Osteogenesis imperfecta misdiagnosed as child abuse. *J Pediatr Orthop B.* 2011;20(6):440–443

60. Gahagan S, Rimsza ME. Child abuse or osteogenesis imperfecta: how can we tell? *Pediatrics.* 1991;88(5):987–992

61. Ablin DS, Sane SM. Non-accidental injury: confusion with temporary brittle bone disease and mild osteogenesis imperfecta. *Pediatr Radiol.* 1997;27(2):111–113

62. Knight DJ, Bennet GC. Nonaccidental injury in osteogenesis imperfecta: a case report. *J Pediatr Orthop.* 1990;10(4):542–544

63. Jenny C; Committee on Child Abuse and Neglect. Evaluating infants and young children with multiple fractures. *Pediatrics.* 2006;118(3):1299–1303

64. Backström MC, Kuusela A-L, Mäki R. Metabolic bone disease of prematurity. *Ann Med.* 1996;28(4):275–282

65. Naylor KE, Eastell R, Shattuck KE, Alfrey AC, Klein GL. Bone turnover in preterm infants. *Pediatr Res.* 1999;45(3):363–366

66. Harrison CM, Johnson K, McKechnie E. Osteopenia of prematurity: a national survey and review of practice. *Acta Paediatr.* 2008;97(4):407–413

67. Amir J, Katz K, Grunebaum M, Yosipovich Z, Wielunsky E, Reisner SH. Fractures in premature infants. *J Pediatr Orthop.* 1988;8(1):41–44

68. Bugental DB, Happaney K. Predicting infant maltreatment in low-income families: the interactive effects of maternal attributions and child status at birth. *Dev Psychol.* 2004;40(2):234–243

69. Keller KA, Barnes PD. Rickets vs. abuse: a national and international epidemic. *Pediatr Radiol.* 2008;38(11):1210–1216

70. Gordon CM, Feldman HA, Sinclair L, et al. Prevalence of vitamin D deficiency among healthy infants and toddlers. *Arch Pediatr Adolesc Med.* 2008;162(6):505–512

71. Greenspan A. *Orthopedic Imaging: A Practical Approach.* 4th ed. Philadelphia, PA: Lippincott Williams & Wilkins; 2004

72. Perez-Rossello JM, Feldman HA, Kleinman PK, et al. Rachitic changes, demineralization, and fracture risk in healthy infants and toddlers with vitamin D deficiency. *Radiology.* 2012;262(1):234–241

73. Slovis TL, Chapman S. Vitamin D insufficiency/deficiency—a conundrum. *Pediatr Radiol.* 2008;38(11):1153

74. Slovis TL, Chapman S. Evaluating the data concerning vitamin D insufficiency/deficiency and child abuse. *Pediatr Radiol.* 2008;38(11):1221–1224

75. Jenny C. Rickets or abuse? *Pediatr Radiol.* 2008;38(11):1219–1220

76. Schilling S, Wood JN, Levine MA, Langdon D, Christian CW. Vitamin D status in abused and nonabused children younger than 2 years old with fractures. *Pediatrics.* 2011;127(5):835–841

77. Chapman T, Sugar N, Done S, Marasigan J, Wambold N, Feldman K. Fractures in infants and toddlers with rickets. *Pediatr Radiol.* 2010;40(7):1184–1189

78. Perez-Rossello JM, McDonald AG, Rosenberg AE, Ivey SL, Richmond JM, Kleinman PK. Prevalence of rachitic changes in deceased infants: a radiologic and pathologic study. *Pediatr Radiol.* 2011;41(suppl 1):S57

79. Ogden JA. Pediatric osteomyelitis and septic arthritis: the pathology of neonatal disease. *Yale J Biol Med.* 1979;52(5):423–448

80. Whedon GD. Disuse osteoporosis: physiological aspects. *Calcif Tissue Int.* 1984;36(suppl 1):S146–S150

81. Presedo A, Dabney KW, Miller F. Fractures in patients with cerebral palsy. *J Pediatr Orthop.* 2007;27(2):147–153

82. Westcott H. The abuse of disabled children: a review of the literature. *Child Care Health Dev.* 1991;17(4):243–258

83. Sullivan PM, Knutson JF. The association between child maltreatment and disabilities in a hospital-based epidemiological study. *Child Abuse Negl.* 1998;22(4):271–288

84. Sullivan PM, Knutson JF. Maltreatment and disabilities: a population-based epidemiological study. *Child Abuse Negl.* 2000;24(10):1257–1273

85. Olmedo JM, Yiannias JA, Windgassen EB, Gornet MK. Scurvy: a disease almost forgotten. *Int J Dermatol.* 2006;45(8):909–913

86. Larralde M, Santos Muñoz A, Boggio P, Di Gruccio V, Weis I, Schygiel A. Scurvy in a 10-month-old boy. *Int J Dermatol.* 2007;46(2):194–198

87. Nishio H, Matsui K, Tsuji H, Tamura A, Suzuki K. Immunohistochemical study of tyrosine phosphorylation signaling in the involuted thymus. *Forensic Sci Int.* 2000;110(3):189–198

88. Shaw JC. Copper deficiency and non-accidental injury. *Arch Dis Child.* 1988;63(4):448–455

89. Marquardt ML, Done SL, Sandrock M, Berdon WE, Feldman KW. Copper deficiency presenting as metabolic bone disease in extremely low birth weight, short-gut infants. *Pediatrics.* 2012;130(3). Available at: www.pediatrics.org/cgi/content/full/130/3/e695–e698

90. Tümer Z, Møller LB. Menkes disease. *Eur J Hum Genet.* 2010;18(5):511–518

91. Bacopoulou F, Henderson L, Philip SG. Menkes disease mimicking non-accidental injury [published correction appears in *Arch Dis Child.* 2009;94(1):77]. *Arch Dis Child.* 2006;91(11):919

92. Paterson CR, Burns J, McAllion SJ. Osteogenesis imperfecta: the distinction from child abuse and the recognition of a variant form [see comment]. *Am J Med Genet.* 1993;45(2):187–192

93. Chapman S, Hall CM. Non-accidental injury or brittle bones. *Pediatr Radiol.* 1997;27(2):106–110

94. Paterson CR. Temporary brittle bone disease: fractures in medical care. *Acta Paediatr.* 2009;98(12):1935–1938

95. Paterson CR. Temporary brittle bone disease: the current position. *Arch Dis Child.* 2011;96(9):901–902

96. Miller ME. The lesson of temporary brittle bone disease: all bones are not created equal. *Bone.* 2003;33(4):466–474

97. Miller ME. Temporary brittle bone disease: a true entity? *Semin Perinatol.* 1999;23(2):174–182

98. Miller ME, Hangartner TN. Temporary brittle bone disease: association with decreased fetal movement and osteopenia. *Calcif Tissue Int.* 1999;64(2):137–143

99. Palacios J, Rodriguez JI. Extrinsic fetal akinesia and skeletal development: a study in oligohydramnios sequence. *Teratology.* 1990;42(1):1–5

100. Rivara FP, Parish RA, Mueller BA. Extremity injuries in children: predictive value of clinical findings. *Pediatrics.* 1986;78(5):803–807

101. Taitz J, Moran K, O'Meara M. Long bone fractures in children under 3 years of age: is abuse being missed in emergency department presentations? *J Paediatr Child Health.* 2004;40(4):170–174

102. Farrell C, Rubin DM, Downes K, Dormans J, Christian CW. Symptoms and time to medical care in children with accidental extremity fractures. *Pediatrics.* 2012;129(1). Available at: www.pediatrics.org/cgi/content/full/129/1/ e128–133

103. Peters ML, Starling SP, Barnes-Eley ML, Heisler KW. The presence of bruising associated with fractures. *Arch Pediatr Adolesc Med.* 2008;162(9):877–881

104. Valvano TJ, Binns HJ, Flaherty EG, Leonhardt DE. Does bruising help determine which fractures are caused by abuse? *Child Maltreat.* 2009;14(4):376–381

105. Sugar NF, Taylor JA, Feldman KW; Puget Sound Pediatric Research Network. Bruises in infants and toddlers: those who don't cruise rarely bruise. *Arch Pediatr Adolesc Med.* 1999;153(4):399–403

106. Pierce MC, Kaczor K, Aldridge S, O'Flynn J, Lorenz DJ. Bruising characteristics discriminating physical child abuse from accidental trauma. *Pediatrics.* 2010;125(1):67–74

107. Shapiro JR, Sponsellor PD. Osteogenesis imperfecta: questions and answers. *Curr Opin Pediatr.* 2009;21(6):709–716

108. Marlowe A, Pepin MG, Byers PH. Testing for osteogenesis imperfecta in cases of suspected non-accidental injury. *J Med Genet.* 2002;39(6):382–386

109. American Academy of Pediatrics; Section on Radiology; American Academy of Pediatrics. Diagnostic imaging of child abuse. *Pediatrics.* 2009;123(5):1430–1435

110. Duffy SO, Squires J, Fromkin JB, Berger RP. Use of skeletal surveys to evaluate for physical abuse: analysis of 703 consecutive skeletal surveys. *Pediatrics.* 2011;127(1). Available at: www.pediatrics.org/cgi/content/full/127/1/e47–e52

111. American College of Radiology. *ACR Practice Guidelines for Skeletal Surveys in Children.* 2011. Available at: www.acr.org/~/media/ACR/Documents/PGTS/guidelines/Skeletal_Surveys.pdf. Accessed May 5, 2013

112. Ingram JD, Connell J, Hay TC, Strain JD, MacKenzie T. Oblique radiographs of the chest in nonaccidental trauma. *Emerg Radiol.* 2000;7(1):42–46

113. Prabhu SP, Newton AW, Perez-Rossello JM, Kleinman PK. Three-dimensional skull models as a problem-solving tool in suspected child abuse. *Pediatr Radiol.* 2013;43(5):575–581

114. Karmazyn B, Duhn RD, Jennings SG, et al. Long bone fracture detection in suspected child abuse: contribution of lateral views [published online ahead of print October 6, 2011]. *Pediatr Radiol.* doi: 10.1007/s00247-011-2248-3

115. van Rijn RR. How should we image skeletal injuries in child abuse? *Pediatr Radiol.* 2009;39(suppl 2):S226–S229

116. Kleinman PK, Nimkin K, Spevak MR, et al. Follow-up skeletal surveys in suspected child abuse. *AJR Am J Roentgenol.* 1996;167(4):893–896

117. Bennett BL, Chua MS, Care M, Kachelmeyer A, Mahabee-Gittens M. Retrospective review to determine the utility of follow-up skeletal surveys in child abuse evaluations when the initial skeletal survey is normal. *BMC Res Notes.* 2011;4(1):354

118. Harlan SR, Nixon GW, Campbell KA, Hansen K, Prince JS. Follow-up skeletal surveys for nonaccidental trauma: can a more limited survey be performed? *Pediatr Radiol.* 2009;39(9):962–968

119. Mandelstam SA, Cook D, Fitzgerald M, Ditchfield MR. Complementary use of radiological skeletal survey and bone scintigraphy in detection of bony injuries in suspected child abuse. *Arch Dis Child.* 2003;88(5):387–390, discussion 387–390

120. Drubach LA, Johnston PR, Newton AW, Perez-Rossello JM, Grant FD, Kleinman PK. Skeletal trauma in child abuse: detection with 18F-NaF PET. *Radiology.* 2010;255(1):173–181

121. Rubin DM, Christian CW, Bilaniuk LT, Zazyczny KA, Durbin DR. Occult head injury in high-risk abused children. *Pediatrics.* 2003;111(6 pt 1):1382–1386

122. Wootton-Gorges SL, Stein-Wexler R, Walton JW, Rosas AJ, Coulter KP, Rogers KK. Comparison of computed tomography and chest radiography in the detection of rib fractures in abused infants. *Child Abuse Negl.* 2008;32(6):659–663

123. Brody AS, Frush DP, Huda W, Brent RL; American Academy of Pediatrics Section on Radiology. Radiation risk to children from computed tomography. *Pediatrics.* 2007;120(3):677–682

124. Stranzinger E, Kellenberger CJ, Braunschweig S, Hopper R, Huisman TAGM. Whole-body STIR MR imaging in suspected child abuse: an alternative to skeletal survey radiography? *Eur J Radiol Extra.* 2007;63(1):43–47

125. Perez-Rossello JM, Connolly SA, Newton AW, Zou KH, Kleinman PK. Whole-body MRI

in suspected infant abuse. *AJR Am J Roentgenol.* 2010;195(3):744–750

126. Bachrach LK, Sills IN; Section on Endocrinology. Clinical report—bone densitometry in children and adolescents. *Pediatrics.* 2011;127(1):189–194

127. Khoury DJ, Szalay EA. Bone mineral density correlation with fractures in nonambulatory pediatric patients. *J Pediatr Orthop.* 2007;27(5):562–566

128. Zemel BS, Kalkwarf HJ, Gilsanz V, et al. Revised reference curves for bone mineral content and areal bone mineral density according to age and sex for black and non-black children: results of the bone mineral density in childhood study. *J*

Clin Endocrinol Metab. 2011;96(10):3160–3169

129. Gordon CM, Baim S, Bianchi M-L, et al; International Society for Clinical Densitometry. Special report on the 2007 Pediatric Position Development Conference of the International Society for Clinical Densitometry. *South Med J.* 2008;101(7):740–743

130. Henderson RC, Lark RK, Newman JE, et al. Pediatric reference data for dual x-ray absorptiometric measures of normal bone density in the distal femur. *AJR Am J Roentgenol.* 2002;178(2):439–443

131. Lindberg DM, Shapiro RA, Laskey AL, Pallin DJ, Blood EA, Berger RP; ExSTRA Inves-

tigators. Prevalence of abusive injuries in siblings and household contacts of physically abused children. *Pediatrics.* 2012; 130(2):193–201

132. Hamilton-Giachritsis CE, Browne KD. A retrospective study of risk to siblings in abusing families. *J Fam Psychol.* 2005;19 (4):619–624

133. Asnes AG, Leventhal JM. Managing child abuse: general principles. *Pediatr Rev.* 2010;31(2):47–55

134. Banaszkiewicz PA, Scotland TR, Myerscough EJ. Fractures in children younger than age 1 year: importance of collaboration with child protection services. *J Pediatr Orthop.* 2002;22(6):740–744

RESEARCH ARTICLE

Potential Opportunities for Prevention or Earlier Diagnosis of Child Physical Abuse in the Inpatient Setting

Henry T. Puls, MD,[a] James D. Anderst, MD, MSCI,[b] Jessica L. Bettenhausen, MD,[a] Abbey Masonbrink, MD, MPH,[a] Jessica L. Markham, MD,[a] Laura Plencner, MD,[a] Molly Krager, MD,[a] Matthew B. Johnson, MD,[a] Jacqueline M. Walker, MD,[a] Christopher S. Greeley, MD,[c] Matthew Hall, PhD[a,d]

ABSTRACT

OBJECTIVES: To compare rates of previous inpatient visits among children hospitalized with child physical abuse (CPA) with controls as well as between individual abuse types.

METHODS: In this study, we used the Pediatric Health Information System administrative database of 44 children's hospitals. Children <6 years of age hospitalized with CPA between January 1, 2011, and September 30, 2015, were identified by discharge codes and propensity matched to accidental injury controls. Rates for previous visit types were calculated per 10 000 months of life. χ^2 and Poisson regression were used to compare proportions and rates.

RESULTS: There were 5425 children hospitalized for CPA. Of abuse and accident cases, 13.1% and 13.2% had a previous inpatient visit, respectively. At previous visits, abused children had higher rates of fractures (rate ratio [RR] = 3.0 times; $P = .018$), head injuries (RR = 3.5 times; $P = .005$), symptoms concerning for occult abusive head trauma (AHT) (eg, isolated vomiting, seizures, brief resolved unexplained events) (RR = 1.4 times; $P = .054$), and perinatal conditions (eg, prematurity) (RR = 1.3 times; $P = .014$) compared with controls. Head injuries and symptoms concerning for occult AHT also more frequently preceded cases of AHT compared with other types of abuse (both $P < .001$).

CONCLUSIONS: Infants hospitalized with perinatal-related conditions, symptoms concerning for occult AHT, and injuries are inpatient populations who may benefit from abuse prevention efforts and/or risk assessments. Head injuries and symptoms concerning for occult AHT (eg, isolated vomiting, seizures, and brief resolved unexplained events) may represent missed opportunities to diagnose AHT in the inpatient setting; however, this requires further study.

[a]Divisions of Hospital Medicine and [b]Child Abuse and Neglect, Department of Pediatrics, Children's Mercy Hospital, School of Medicine, University of Missouri–Kansas City, Kansas City, Missouri; [c]Division of Child Abuse and Neglect, Department of Pediatrics, Baylor College of Medicine, Houston, Texas; and [d]Children's Hospital Association, Lenexa, Kansas

www.hospitalpediatrics.org

DOI:https://doi.org/10.1542/hpeds.2017-0109

Copyright © 2018 by the American Academy of Pediatrics

Address correspondence to Henry T. Puls, MD, Division of Hospital Medicine, Department of Pediatrics, Children's Mercy Hospital, 2401 Gillham Rd, Kansas City, MO 64108. E-mail: htpuls@cmh.edu

HOSPITAL PEDIATRICS (ISSN Numbers: Print, 2154-1663; Online, 2154-1671).

FINANCIAL DISCLOSURE: The authors have indicated they have no financial relationships relevant to this article to disclose.

FUNDING: No external funding.

POTENTIAL CONFLICT OF INTEREST: The authors have indicated they have no potential conflicts of interest to disclose.

Dr Puls participated in the study design, analysis and interpretation of data, and was the primary author of the manuscript; Drs Anderst, Bettenhausen, Masonbrink, Markham, Plencner, Krager, Johnson, Walker, and Greeley participated in the study design and analysis and interpretation of data; Dr Hall participated in the study design, acquisition of data, and analysis and interpretation of data; and all authors provided critical revision of the manuscript and approved the final manuscript as submitted.

Child physical abuse (CPA) remains a prevalent problem with the rates of abuse-related hospitalizations, abusive head trauma (AHT), and fatalities remaining stable or increasing in recent years.[1–4] Primary prevention is directed toward the general population and attempts to stop maltreatment from occurring.[5] Hospital-based primary prevention efforts have principally targeted newborns during their birth hospitalizations. Unfortunately, these efforts have not clearly led to reductions in abuse.[6,7]

Secondary prevention efforts are focused on subpopulations at higher risk for abuse.[5] Children with psychosocial risk factors for abuse have been shown to have higher hospitalization rates.[8,9] Additionally, hospitalization in early infancy has been associated with future maltreatment in general,[10] as well as CPA, specifically.[11] These data suggest that some hospitalized children may be at higher risk for abuse and may also benefit from secondary prevention.

The early diagnosis of CPA can be difficult, and it is frequently missed at ambulatory or emergency department encounters[12–16] in part because it accounts for a minority of clinical presentations.[2,17–19] In addition to prevention opportunities, inpatient visits preceding abuse may also represent opportunities for earlier diagnosis of CPA. However, the incidence of hospitalizations and the various diagnoses preceding abuse, as well as how often abuse may be missed in the inpatient setting, remain largely unknown.

Our primary objective with this study was to compare children hospitalized for abuse with children hospitalized with accidental injuries (ie, matched controls) on their rates of having any previous inpatient visits as well as their specific previous visit type (eg, injuries, nonspecific symptoms concerning for occult abuse, and noninjuries). Our secondary objective was to compare the rates of previous visit types between types of abuse.

METHODS
Data Source

In this study, we used the Pediatric Health Information System (PHIS) administrative database managed by the Children's Hospital Association (Lenexa, KS). The PHIS contains deidentified *International Classification of Diseases, Ninth Revision, Clinical Modification* (ICD-9-CM) discharge codes and administrative and financial data for all observation and inpatient visits at 44 children's hospitals in the United States. An encrypted patient identifier permits longitudinal tracking of patients between encounters within the same PHIS hospital.

Study Population

Our study population included children <6 years of age with a first-time CPA hospitalization at a PHIS hospital from January 1, 2011, to September 30, 2015. We used a previously published coding scheme using validated abuse codes to identify children hospitalized for CPA.[2,20,21] In short, this scheme requires that 1 of the following 4 criteria be met: (1) ICD-9-CM codes for an injury (800–959) and abuse (995.50, 995.54, 995.55, 995.59, or E967), (2) ICD-9-CM codes for an injury and assault (E960, E966, E968), (3) ICD-9-CM codes for retinal hemorrhages (362.81) or anoxic brain injury (348.1) and abuse, or (4) any ICD-9-CM code for shaken infant syndrome (995.55). Exclusion criteria included late-onset injury effects, e-codes indicating that the injury occurred at a location not typical for abuse (eg, farms), or an abuse code at any previous encounter.[2] We classified abuse hospitalizations by injury type: fracture, AHT, abusive abdominal trauma, burns, skin, other (eg, lung contusion), and multiple.[2] AHT included but was not limited to isolated skull fractures, subdural hemorrhages, retinal hemorrhages, and/or anoxic brain injury. Patient characteristics included age, sex, race and/or ethnicity, payer, zip code–based median household income, ICU use, median ICU days, hospital length of stay, median total costs (based on standardized cost-to-charge ratios),[22] and in-hospital mortality. Each child hospitalized with CPA was propensity matched by using a greedy algorithm with up to 2 children hospitalized with an accidental injury similar to previous work (E880–E888, E916–E921, E923–E928, and E810–E829) on the basis of age, race and/or ethnicity, sex, and insurance type.[15,23–25]

Previous Inpatient Visits

We identified which children had any lifetime inpatient visit preceding their CPA or accidental injury hospitalizations. Normal birth hospitalizations were not counted as previous inpatient visits. Only visits closest to the abuse hospitalization and their primary discharge diagnoses were used to strengthen their conceptual association (ie, only 1 previous inpatient visit per case and control were investigated). All previous visits were categorized into 3 broad categories: (1) injuries, (2) nonspecific symptoms concerning for occult abuse, and (3) noninjuries.

First, we identified children diagnosed with an injury at a previous inpatient visit. We categorized previous injury visits as fractures, head injuries, and skin injuries with the same ICD-9-CM codes used to identify their respective abusive injury types. Next, we identified previous visits during which symptoms concerning for occult injury were diagnosed. Informed by previous literature describing misdiagnoses commonly made in cases of missed abuse,[12–14,16] all authors (blinded to the frequencies of ICD-9-CM codes) reached consensus as to which noninjury ICD-9-CM codes from previous visits could conceptually represent occult AHT on a physiologic basis (Supplemental Table 3). These diagnoses were broken into 2 groups: (1) symptoms specifically concerning for occult AHT (ie, vomiting alone, gastroesophageal reflux [GERD], seizures, neurologic abnormalities, or abnormal breathing including apnea or brief resolved unexplained events [BRUEs; formerly apparent life-threatening events]) or (2) fussiness and/or feeding difficulties. Finally, all remaining diagnoses were designated as noninjury visits and organized by Clinical Classifications Software (CCS).[26] The CCS is a categorization scheme that groups the thousands of ICD-9-CM diagnoses into a smaller number of clinically meaningful categories. We included the 3 most common CCS categories, and all remaining noninjury encounters were collapsed into noninjury, other.

Statistical Analysis

We summarized patient characteristics with frequencies and percentages and used χ^2 tests to determine statistical differences between abuse cases and the accidental injury controls as well as between individual abuse types. Because children varied in their exposure for having previous visits simply because of differences in age, the rates of different previous inpatient visit types were reported as per 10 000 months of life with 95% confidence intervals (CIs). The median number of days and interquartile range (IQR) between previous inpatient visits and the abuse hospitalizations quantified their temporal relationships. We used χ^2 and Poisson regression, controlling for hospital clustering with random intercepts for each hospital, to calculate associations of categorical and continuous variables with abuse type. All statistical analyses were performed by using SAS version 9.4 (SAS Institute, Inc, Cary, NC). P values <.05 were considered statistically significant. This study was deemed nonhuman subjects research by the Institutional Review Board at Children's Mercy Hospital.

RESULTS
Characteristics of Abuse Cases and Controls

There were 5425 children hospitalized with CPA. Abused children most often had multiple abusive injuries (39.3%) (Table 1). The most common combinations of multiple abusive injuries were AHT and skin, fracture and skin, and AHT and other injuries, which respectively accounted for 30.8%, 24.0%, and 5.1% of those with multiple abusive injuries. Figure 1 shows the distribution of abusive injuries.

Abused children were most commonly <6 months of age, boys, non-Hispanic white, with public insurance, and from the lowest quartile of median household income, but ~14% were from the highest income quartile. The overall median cost per hospitalization was ~$11 000 and highest for AHT and abusive abdominal trauma, both of which cost over $22 000. The overall mortality rate was 6.2% and was highest for abusive abdominal trauma (10.8%) and AHT (10.4%).

There were 10 836 children hospitalized with accidental injuries who were matched to the CPA hospitalizations. There were no significant differences in demographics between CPA cases and accidental injury

controls, but CPA cases had longer lengths of stay, greater ICU use, more ICU days, and higher mortality (all P < .001) (Supplemental Table 4).

Frequencies of Previous Inpatient Visits

There were 711 (13.1%) abused and 1433 (13.2%) accidental injury children who had a previous inpatient visit at the same children's hospital where they were later hospitalized for physical abuse or accidental injuries. Children with abusive abdominal trauma, burns, and other abusive injuries occurred in small numbers and had such low (none in some cases) rates of previous inpatient visits that we excluded them from the analysis of previous visits. The frequencies of each previous visit type or diagnosis for abused children are shown in Fig 2.

Abuse Cases Compared With Controls

CPA cases (107.5 per 10 000 months of life [95% CI: 99.6–115.5]) were not significantly different from accidental injury controls (102.5 [95% CI: 97.2–107.8]) in their rates of having any lifetime previous inpatient visit (P = .29). However, CPA cases were more often diagnosed with injuries (rate ratio [RR] = 3.2 times; P < .001) and nonspecific symptoms concerning for occult abuse (RR = 1.4 times; P = .03) at previous inpatient visits compared with accidental injury controls (Table 2). Specifically, fractures (RR = 3 times; P = .02), head injuries (RR = 3.5 times; P = .005), and symptoms concerning for occult AHT (RR = 1.4 times; P = .05) more often preceded CPA compared with accidental injuries. Although CPA cases and controls had similar rates of previous noninjury inpatient visits overall, perinatal conditions (predominately diagnoses of prematurity or low birth weight) were diagnosed at a rate 1.3 times higher among CPA cases compared with controls (P = .01).

Comparisons Between Abuse Types
Previous Injury Inpatient Visits

Head injuries were the most frequent injury diagnosed at previous inpatient visits among abused children (2.1 [95% CI: 1.0–3.2]) (Supplemental Table 5) and preceded AHT at a rate 10.3 to 14.7 times higher than other types of abuse (P < .001;

Fig 3). The rates of previous fractures (1.8 [95% CI: 0.8–2.8]) and skin injuries (0.8 [95% CI: 0.1–1.4]) did not significantly differ between the individual types of abuse.

Previous Inpatient Visits for Nonspecific Symptoms Concerning for Occult Abuse

Nonspecific symptoms concerning for occult abuse were most often specifically concerning for occult AHT (10.4 [95% CI: 8.0–12.9]) and their rates were 2.4 to 4.2 times higher for children subsequently diagnosed with AHT compared with other abusive injuries (P < .001). They preceded AHT by the shortest time, a median of 52 days (IQR 16–90), which was significantly shorter than 67 days (IQR 32–230) for all abused children and 199 days (IQR 67–1201) for abusive skin injuries (P = .04). Fussiness and/or feeding difficulties were less common (2.3 [95% CI: 1.1–3.4]) and did not vary in their rates between types of abuse or median times between encounters.

Inpatient Visits Concerning for Missed Cases of AHT

Of all cases of AHT (n = 2423), both isolated and those with other concurrent abusive injuries, 2.2% had a previous inpatient visit during which either head injuries (n =11) or symptoms concerning for occult AHT (n = 42) were diagnosed. However, by using only those children with AHT who had a previous inpatient visit as the denominator (n = 271), we found that 19.6% received 1 of these diagnoses concerning for possible missed AHT.

Previous Noninjury Inpatient Visits

Diseases of the respiratory system (21.8 [95% CI: 18.2–25.3]) was the most common category of noninjury diagnoses among abused children and were predominantly cases of bronchiolitis, asthma, or pneumonia. Second and third most common were conditions originating in the perinatal period (19.1 [95% CI: 15.7–22.4]) and congenital anomalies (10.3 [95% CI: 7.8–12.7]), which were most often diagnoses of prematurity or low birth weight and congenital heart disease, respectively. The median number of days between previous noninjury inpatient visits and abuse hospitalizations were 125.5 days (IQR 47–425.5) for respiratory

TABLE 1 Demographics of Children Hospitalized for Physical Abuse

Characteristic	Overall	Type of Abusive Injury						
		Fracture	AHT	Abdomen	Burn	Skin	Other	Multiple
No. patients, n (%)	5425 (100)	959 (17.7)	1368 (25.2)	37 (0.7)	141 (2.6)	693 (12.8)	96 (1.8)	2131 (39.3)
Age, y, n (%)								
<0.5	2717 (50.1)	606 (63.2)	899 (65.7)	4 (10.8)	17 (12.1)	215 (31)	39 (40.6)	937 (44)
0.5–1	998 (18.4)	205 (21.4)	283 (20.7)	3 (8.1)	25 (17.7)	99 (14.3)	16 (16.7)	367 (17.2)
1–3	1472 (27.1)	127 (13.2)	163 (11.9)	25 (67.6)	85 (60.3)	303 (43.7)	32 (33.3)	737 (34.6)
3–5	238 (4.4)	21 (2.2)	23 (1.7)	5 (13.5)	14 (9.9)	76 (11)	9 (9.4)	90 (4.2)
Sex[a], n (%)								
Male	3174 (58.6)	551 (57.5)	829 (60.6)	25 (67.6)	85 (60.3)	406 (58.7)	49 (51.6)	1229 (57.8)
Race and/or ethnicity, n (%)								
Non-Hispanic white	2642 (48.7)	446 (46.5)	655 (47.9)	9 (24.3)	39 (27.7)	366 (52.8)	45 (46.9)	1082 (50.8)
Non-Hispanic African American	1290 (23.8)	253 (26.4)	276 (20.2)	15 (40.5)	83 (58.9)	157 (22.7)	30 (31.3)	476 (22.3)
Hispanic	851 (15.7)	152 (15.8)	236 (17.3)	4 (10.8)	7 (5)	101 (14.6)	15 (15.6)	336 (15.8)
Other	642 (11.8)	108 (11.3)	201 (14.7)	9 (24.3)	12 (8.5)	69 (10)	6 (6.3)	237 (11.1)
Payor, n (%)								
Public	4579 (84.4)	800 (83.4)	1109 (81.1)	35 (94.6)	126 (89.4)	592 (85.4)	79 (82.3)	1838 (86.3)
Private	715 (13.2)	141 (14.7)	225 (16.4)	2 (5.4)	10 (7.1)	79 (11.4)	15 (15.6)	243 (11.4)
Other	131 (2.4)	18 (1.9)	34 (2.5)	0 (0.0)	5 (3.5)	22 (3.2)	2 (2.1)	50 (2.3)
Median household income quartile[a], n (%)								
Lowest	1914 (36.2)	343 (36.7)	450 (33.8)	14 (37.8)	58 (41.4)	239 (35.2)	35 (36.8)	775 (37.4)
Less than average	1405 (26.6)	236 (25.2)	358 (26.9)	11 (29.7)	39 (27.9)	171 (25.2)	24 (25.3)	566 (27.3)
Greater than average	1208 (22.8)	215 (23)	321 (24.1)	8 (21.6)	26 (18.6)	155 (22.8)	23 (24.2)	460 (22.2)
Highest	763 (14.4)	141 (15.1)	203 (15.2)	4 (10.8)	17 (12.1)	114 (16.8)	13 (13.7)	271 (13.1)
ICU use, n (%)	2009 (37)	65 (6.8)	861 (62.9)	22 (59.5)	37 (26.2)	50 (7.2)	27 (28.1)	947 (44.4)
ICU length of stay, d, median (IQR)	4 (2–8)	2 (1–4)	4 (2–8)	3 (2–7)	5 (2–13)	2 (1–4)	5 (2–10)	3 (2–8)
Length of stay, d, median (IQR)	3 (2–8)	2 (1–3)	6 (3–14)	8 (4–21)	4 (2–10)	1 (1–3)	2 (1–7.5)	4 (2–10)
Total cost, dollars, median (IQR)	11 020 (53 149–29 003)	5891 (3748–9403)	22 700 (11 373–50 751)	25 816 (14 851–66 761)	8846 (3571–25 625)	4988 (3050–7812)	7477 (3441–22 310)	14 636 (6969–37 460)
In-hospital mortality, n (%)	338 (6.2)	6 (0.6)	142 (10.4)	4 (10.8)	1 (0.7)	6 (0.9)	5 (5.2)	174 (8.2)

P values obtained from χ^2 tests. All P values ≤ .001 except otherwise noted.
[a] P values not significant.

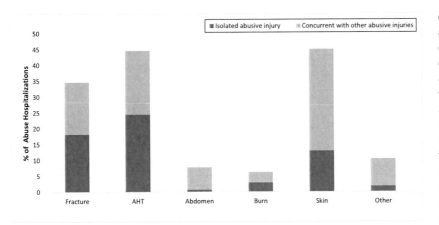

FIGURE 1 The distribution of abusive injury types. The 2131 (39.3%) children with multiple abusive injuries have been distributed to the mutually exclusive abusive injury categories (lighter bars).

diseases, 102.5 days (IQR 57–244) for perinatal-related discharges, and 237 days (IQR 60.5–704) for congenital-related discharges.

DISCUSSION

At previous inpatient visits, abused children had higher rates of injuries (fractures and head injuries), symptoms concerning for

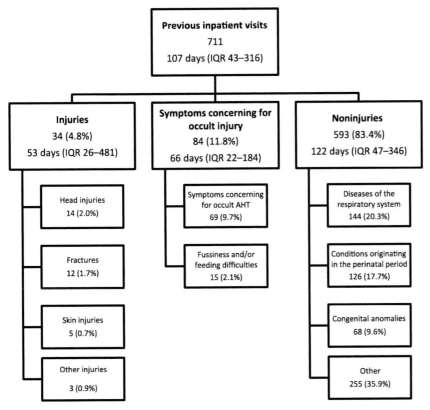

FIGURE 2 Frequencies of diagnoses (% of all previous inpatient visits) of inpatient visits before abuse hospitalizations. Median number of days (IQR) between hospitalizations are listed for all previous inpatient visits as well as the 3 broad categories of previous visit types (injuries, symptoms concerning for injuries, and noninjuries).

occult AHT (eg, isolated vomiting, BRUEs), and prematurity-related conditions compared with controls. Given their commonality and higher rates among abused children, infants hospitalized with prematurity or low birth weight appear to be inpatient populations who may benefit from primary and/or secondary prevention efforts. We found that head injuries and symptoms concerning for occult AHT more frequently preceded abuse in general compared with controls as well as specifically AHT compared with other types of abusive injuries, suggesting that some of these previous visits may represent missed opportunities to diagnose AHT. Overall, these possible missed events appear to be rare, but of the AHT cases with a previous inpatient visit, ~1 in 5 had 1 of these diagnoses concerning for missed abuse. Despite these important differences, abused children did not significantly differ from matched accidental injury controls in their having any previous inpatient visit at the same children's hospital (each ~13%).

Abused children had higher rates of perinatal-related (eg, prematurity) diagnoses compared with controls, and perinatal-related conditions accounted for ~1 in 6 previous inpatient visits among abused children. Our results are in agreement with previous findings that prematurity and low birth weight are associated with increased risk for physical abuse[10,27–30] but that congenital anomalies (eg, spina bifida) may not be.[28] Our results support NICUs as areas at children's hospitals that may particularly benefit from abuse prevention efforts. It is disappointing that primary abuse prevention efforts (The Period of PURPLE Crying and the Pennsylvania Shaken Baby Syndrome Prevention Program) employed during newborn hospitalizations have not clearly lead to reductions in AHT.[6,7] How frequently these programs are used in NICUs or if they are more effective for this unique patient population, however, is unclear. Further study should better identify which abuse prevention strategies may be most efficacious for NICU populations.

TABLE 2 Rates per 10 000 Months of Life (95% CIs) of Primary Discharge Diagnoses for Previous Inpatient Visits of Abused Children Compared With Accidental Injury Controls

	Overall	Abuse	Accident	P^a
No. patients	16 261	5425	10 836	—
Exposure months	205 976	66 111	139 865	—
Inpatient visits	104.1 (99.7–108.5)	107.5 (99.6–115.5)	102.5 (97.2–107.8)	.29
Injury	2.7 (2–3.4)	5.1 (3.4–6.9)	1.6 (0.9–2.2)	<.001
Head injuries	1.1 (0.7–1.6)	2.1 (1–3.2)	0.6 (0.2–1.1)	.005
Fractures	1(0.6–1.5)	1.8 (0.8–2.8)	0.6 (0.2–1.1)	.02
Skin injuries	0.4 (0.1–0.7)	0.8 (0.1–1.4)	0.2 (0–0.5)	.08
Symptoms concerning for occult injury[b]	10.4 (9–11.8)	12.7 (10–15.4)	9.4 (7.8–11)	.03
Symptoms concerning for occult AHT[b]	8.6 (7.3–9.9)	10.4 (8–12.9)	7.7 (6.3–9.2)	.05
Fussiness and/or feeding difficulties[b]	1.8 (1.3–2.4)	2.3 (1.1–3.4)	1.6 (1–2.3)	.34
Noninjury[c]	90.9 (86.8–95.1)	89.7 (82.5–96.9)	91.5 (86.5–96.5)	.69
Diseases of the respiratory system	22.7 (20.7–24.8)	21.8 (18.2–25.3)	23.2 (20.6–25.7)	.54
Certain conditions originating in the perinatal period	15.9 (14.2–17.6)	19.1 (15.7–22.4)	14.4 (12.4–16.4)	.01
Congenital anomalies	10.3 (8.9–11.7)	10.3 (7.8–12.7)	10.3 (8.6–12)	.99
Other	42 (39.2–44.8)	38.6 (33.8–43.3)	43.7 (40.2–47.1)	.09

—, not applicable.

[a] P values obtained from Poisson regression comparing median times between previous visits and the abuse hospitalizations across abusive injury types.

[b] Based on previous researchers' reporting of symptoms common among missed cases of abuse.[12–14,16]

[c] ICD-9-CM codes categorized by CCS level 1 groups.

We found that head injuries and symptoms concerning for occult AHT more frequently preceded abuse cases compared with controls as well as AHT compared with other abusive injuries and within a shorter median time. These results appear to validate previous case series' findings that isolated vomiting, GERD, seizures, neurologic abnormalities, apnea, and BRUEs are misdiagnoses commonly made in cases of missed AHT.[12–16,31] Although our methods do not allow definite relationships to be made between encounters or allow for precise estimates of missed AHT, our findings raise concern that some of these previous visits represent missed opportunities to diagnose AHT and provide a base to improve occult injury detection in the inpatient setting.

Early identification of physical abuse remains critical given that it tends to be recurrent, often with increasing severity and mortality.[15,32–34] Unfortunately, an estimated 20% to 36% of abused children have emergency department or outpatient encounters during which their abuse was missed.[12–16] Our findings suggest that inpatient encounters are a minimal contributor to the overall prevalence of missed AHT. However, they also suggest that an upper limit estimate of the proportion of children who may have their AHT missed by inpatient providers may be as high as that seen in outpatient and emergency department settings. Abused children were more likely to have previous injury-related hospitalizations compared with controls in our study, which supports previous findings that abuse is more likely to be substantiated with a greater number of past injuries.[35] These data support a heightened attention to medical histories in assessing children's risk for abuse, something that may have informed the ultimate abuse diagnoses in our study. A majority of the possible missed cases of AHT in this study, however, were in children for whom only concerning symptoms were diagnosed and not discrete injuries. Among these concerning symptoms were BRUEs. An estimated 1% to 2% of children presenting for BRUEs have an abusive etiology,[18,19] but only half may be appropriately identified on their first admission.[19] BRUEs due to AHT more often have a 911 call before presentation, vomiting, or irritability.[18] Similar factors to differentiate abused from nonabused children presenting with isolated vomiting or GERD are unknown, making the detection of abuse difficult given the high prevalence of these symptoms in inpatient settings.

Overall, our study identified a number of conditions (ie, prematurity, symptoms concerning for occult AHT, and injuries) in the inpatient setting that represent either precursors to abuse (ie, risk) or cases in which abuse may have already occurred but had gone undetected. Perhaps screening infants hospitalized with these conditions (or all infants given their risk for sustaining the most severe abusive injuries) for unmet social needs and adverse social determinants of health may improve the prevention and/or detection of abuse. There are screening tools effective at identifying and leading to referrals to address social needs.[36,37] The impacts of these interventions in the inpatient setting on preventing abuse remain to be determined, but their preliminary success in the outpatient setting is encouraging.[38,39]

This study has several limitations. First, identification of CPA with a hospitalized cohort at children's hospitals will underestimate abuse.[40,41] Although identification of abuse with ICD-9-CM codes in the inpatient setting has high specificity (>90%), its sensitivity (73.5%) varies between institutions and can be limited by coding inaccuracies, reluctance to formally diagnose abuse, or some abuse diagnoses may have been assigned after discharge once further investigations were completed.[20,21] Second, we likely underestimate the incidence of previous visits and chronic health conditions (eg, prematurity) because medical encounters occurring outside the hospital during which the abuse or accidental injury hospitalizations occurred would not have

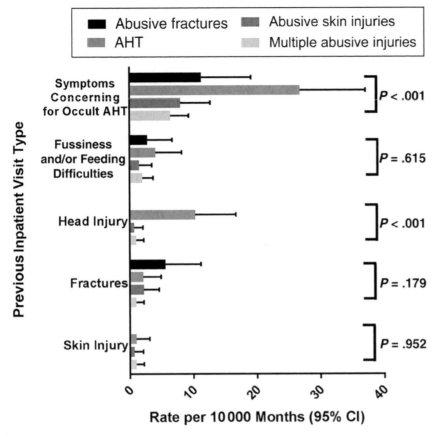

FIGURE 3 The age-adjusted rates of previous inpatient visits among each subsequent type of abusive injury in the 711 abused children who had a previous inpatient visit.

been captured, only primary discharge diagnoses were investigated, and only the visits most recent to the abuse were used. Third, rates of previous visits among the accidental injury controls may not reflect the total population of hospitalized children. However, use of nonabusive injury controls is common,[15,23–25] and lower sensitivity for abuse coding would suggest that some of the controls were in fact cases of abuse, pushing our results toward the null. Lastly, owing to this study's design, definite relationships between previous inpatient visits and later abuse hospitalizations cannot be made. Some previous visits may have been identified as abuse but not coded as such, or some may have truly been unrelated to later abuse. Regardless, we provide an estimation and characterization of the possible missed opportunities to diagnose AHT as well as allowing for a clearer characterization of prevention opportunities within children's hospitals. In

addition, we identify key areas for future investigations and/or interventions that can improve the prevention or early detection of abuse.

CONCLUSIONS

Infants hospitalized with prematurity, low birth weight, symptoms concerning for occult AHT, and injuries are inpatient populations at children's hospitals who may benefit from abuse prevention and/or risk assessments. Diagnoses of head injuries, vomiting, GERD, seizures, neurologic abnormalities, apnea, and BRUEs were more likely to precede AHT specifically and may represent missed opportunities to diagnosis AHT in the inpatient setting. Although missed AHT in the inpatient setting appears rare overall, a similar proportion of AHT may be missed in the inpatient setting (1 in 5) compared with other clinical settings, but further study is needed to confirm these findings.

REFERENCES

1. Farst K, Ambadwar PB, King AJ, Bird TM, Robbins JM. Trends in hospitalization rates and severity of injuries from abuse in young children, 1997-2009. *Pediatrics.* 2013;131(6). Available at: www.pediatrics. org/cgi/content/full/131/6/e1796

2. Leventhal JM, Martin KD, Gaither JR. Using US data to estimate the incidence of serious physical abuse in children. *Pediatrics.* 2012;129(3):458–464

3. Berger RP, Fromkin JB, Stutz H, et al. Abusive head trauma during a time of increased unemployment: a multicenter analysis. *Pediatrics.* 2011;128(4):637–643

4. Wood JN, Medina SP, Feudtner C, et al. Local macroeconomic trends and hospital admissions for child abuse, 2000-2009. *Pediatrics.* 2012;130(2). Available at: www.pediatrics.org/cgi/ content/full/130/2/e358

5. US Department of Health & Human Services, Administration for Children and Families, Children's Bureau. Framework for prevention of child maltreatment. Available at: https://www.childwelfare.gov/ topics/preventing/overview/framework/. Accessed June 8, 2017

6. Dias MS, Rottmund CM, Cappos KM, et al. Association of a postnatal parent education program for abusive head trauma with subsequent pediatric abusive head trauma hospitalization rates. *JAMA Pediatr.* 2017;171(3):223–229

7. Zolotor AJ, Runyan DK, Shanahan M, et al. Effectiveness of a statewide abusive head trauma prevention program in North Carolina. *JAMA Pediatr.* 2015;169(12):1126–1131

8. Leventhal JM, Pew MC, Berg AT, Garber RB. Use of health services by children who were identified during the postpartum period as being at high risk of child abuse or neglect. *Pediatrics.* 1996;97(3):331–335

9. Flores G, Abreu M, Chaisson CE, Sun D. Keeping children out of hospitals: parents' and physicians' perspectives on how pediatric hospitalizations for ambulatory care-sensitive conditions can be avoided. *Pediatrics.* 2003;112(5):1021–1030

10. Sidebotham P, Heron J; ALSPAC Study Team. Child maltreatment in the "children of the nineties:" the role of the child. *Child Abuse Negl.* 2003;27(3):337–352

11. McPhilips H, Gallaher M, Koepsell T. Children hospitalized early and increased risk for future serious injury. *Inj Prev.* 2001;7(2):150–154

12. King WK, Kiesel EL, Simon HK. Child abuse fatalities: are we missing opportunities for intervention? *Pediatr Emerg Care.* 2006;22(4):211–214

13. Jenny C, Hymel KP, Ritzen A, Reinert SE, Hay TC. Analysis of missed cases of abusive head trauma. *JAMA.* 1999;281(7):621–626

14. Letson MM, Cooper JN, Deans KJ, et al. Prior opportunities to identify abuse in children with abusive head trauma. *Child Abuse Negl.* 2016;60:36–45

15. Sheets LK, Leach ME, Koszewski IJ, Lessmeier AM, Nugent M, Simpson P. Sentinel injuries in infants evaluated for child physical abuse. *Pediatrics.* 2013; 131(4):701–707

16. Thorpe EL, Zuckerbraun NS, Wolford JE, Berger RP. Missed opportunities to diagnose child physical abuse. *Pediatr Emerg Care.* 2014;30(11):771–776

17. Lindberg DM, Beaty B, Juarez-Colunga E, Wood JN, Runyan DK. Testing for abuse in children with sentinel injuries. *Pediatrics.* 2015;136(5):831–838

18. Guenther E, Powers A, Srivastava R, Bonkowsky JL. Abusive head trauma in children presenting with an apparent life-threatening event. *J Pediatr.* 2010; 157(5):821–825

19. Bonkowsky JL, Guenther E, Filloux FM, Srivastava R. Death, child abuse, and adverse neurological outcome of infants after an apparent life-threatening event. *Pediatrics.* 2008;122(1):125–131

20. Hooft A, Ronda J, Schaeffer P, Asnes AG, Leventhal JM. Identification of physical abuse cases in hospitalized children: accuracy of International Classification of Diseases codes. *J Pediatr.* 2013;162(1): 80–85

21. Hooft AM, Asnes AG, Livingston N, et al. The accuracy of ICD codes: identifying physical abuse in 4 children's hospitals. *Acad Pediatr.* 2015;15(4):444–450

22. Peltz A, Hall M, Rubin DM, et al. Hospital utilization among children with the highest annual inpatient cost. *Pediatrics.* 2016;137(2):e20151829

23. Wood JN, Feudtner C, Medina SP, Luan X, Localio R, Rubin DM. Variation in occult injury screening for children with suspected abuse in selected US children's hospitals. *Pediatrics.* 2012; 130(5):853–860

24. Friedman LS, Sheppard S, Friedman D. A retrospective cohort study of suspected child maltreatment cases resulting in hospitalization. *Injury.* 2012;43(11):1881–1887

25. Forjuoh SN. Child maltreatment related injuries: incidence, hospital charges, and correlates of hospitalization. *Child Abuse Negl.* 2000;24(8):1019–1025

26. Healthcare Cost and Utilization Project. Clinical Classifications Software (CCS) for ICD-9-CM. Available at: https://www.hcup-us.ahrq.gov/toolssoftware/ccs/ccs.jsp. Accessed February 6, 2017

27. Risch EC, Owora A, Nandyal R, Chaffin M, Bonner BL. Risk for child maltreatment among infants discharged from a neonatal intensive care unit: a sibling comparison. *Child Maltreat.* 2014;19(2):92–100

28. Van Horne BS, Moffitt KB, Canfield MA, et al. Maltreatment of children under age 2 with specific birth defects: a population-based study. *Pediatrics.* 2015; 136(6). Available at: www.pediatrics.org/cgi/content/full/136/6/e1504

29. Wu SS, Ma CX, Carter RL, et al. Risk factors for infant maltreatment: a population-based study. *Child Abuse Negl.* 2004;28(12):1253–1264

30. Kelly P, Thompson JMD, Koh J, et al. Perinatal risk and protective factors for pediatric abusive head trauma: a multicenter case-control study. *J Pediatr.* 2017;187:240–246.e4

31. Selassie AW, Borg K, Busch C, Russell WS. Abusive head trauma in young children: a population-based study. *Pediatr Emerg Care.* 2013;29(3):283–291

32. Deans KJ, Thackeray J, Groner JI, Cooper JN, Minneci PC. Risk factors for recurrent injuries in victims of suspected non-accidental trauma: a retrospective cohort study. *BMC Pediatr.* 2014;14:217

33. Deans KJ, Thackeray J, Askegard-Giesmann JR, Earley E, Groner JI, Minneci PC. Mortality increases with recurrent episodes of nonaccidental trauma in children. *J Trauma Acute Care Surg.* 2013;75(1):161–165

34. Thackeray J, Minneci PC, Cooper JN, Groner JI, Deans KJ. Predictors of increasing injury severity across suspected recurrent episodes of non-accidental trauma: a retrospective cohort study. *BMC Pediatr.* 2016;16:8

35. Spivey MI, Schnitzer PG, Kruse RL, Slusher P, Jaffe DM. Association of injury visits in children and child maltreatment reports. *J Emerg Med.* 2009;36(2):207–214

36. Colvin JD, Bettenhausen JL, Anderson-Carpenter KD, et al. Multiple behavior change intervention to improve detection of unmet social needs and resulting resource referrals. *Acad Pediatr.* 2016;16(2):168–174

37. Gottlieb LM, Hessler D, Long D, et al. Effects of social needs screening and in-person service navigation on child health: a randomized clinical trial. *JAMA Pediatr.* 2016;170(11):e162521

38. Dubowitz H, Feigelman S, Lane W, Kim J. Pediatric primary care to help prevent child maltreatment: the Safe Environment for Every Kid (SEEK) model. *Pediatrics.* 2009;123(3):858–864

39. Dubowitz H, Lane WG, Semiatin JN, Magder LS. The SEEK model of pediatric primary care: can child maltreatment be prevented in a low-risk population? *Acad Pediatr.* 2012;12(4):259–268

40. Allareddy V, Asad R, Lee MK, et al. Hospital based emergency department visits attributed to child physical abuse in United States: predictors of in-hospital mortality. *PLoS One.* 2014;9(2):e100110

41. Trokel M, Waddimba A, Griffith J, Sege R. Variation in the diagnosis of child abuse in severely injured infants [published correction appears in *Pediatrics.* 2006; 118(3):1324]. *Pediatrics.* 2006;117(3): 722–728

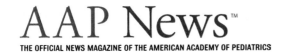

THE OFFICIAL NEWS MAGAZINE OF THE AMERICAN ACADEMY OF PEDIATRICS

:: April-6-2018

How Pediatricians Can Assess for Child Neglect, Support At-Risk Families

Dr. Ryan D. Brown, MD, FAAP

C hild maltreatment is a medical condition that affects hundreds of thousands of children yearly, according to the U.S. Department of Health and Human Services (HHS). In 2012, an estimated 686,000 children were victims of maltreatment, and 1,640 children died.

Child abuse and neglect have been shown to affect males and females of all ages, races and socioeconomic backgrounds.

About 75% of child maltreatment cases are neglect, according to HHS. This is more than all other forms of child abuse combined. Neglect also is the No. 1 killer of children who die as a result of child maltreatment.

Neglect is an omission in care by a parent or caregiver, which can lead to significant harm or risk of significant harm. Neglect can come in multiple forms, including nutritional, medical, educational, supervisory and even dental. In a nutshell, neglect occurs when a child's need for food, clothing, shelter, education, supervision, protection or health care is not met.

The vast majority of neglect cases can be prevented with education, resources and support for the family. Pediatricians may feel overwhelmed by the number of surveys, assessments and tools that are available to evaluate parents and children. However, the following questions can help assess for child neglect when evaluating the family for the first time:

- Was this pregnancy planned?
- Who lives in the house with the child?
- Who will be caring for the child?
- Do you have a car seat for the child?
- Do you have adequate clothing for the child?
- Does your house have running water and electricity?

Lack of a paternal desire for a child has been shown to be associated with physical abuse, whereas from a maternal perspective, neglect and psychological maltreatment can manifest. Also, according to the National Child Abuse and Neglect Data System, children whose single parent had a live-in partner had more than eight times the rate of maltreatment overall, over 10 times the rate of abuse and more than six times the rate of neglect compared to children living with married, biological parents. Therefore, it is optimal for every member of the house to have a sense of ownership of the child's well-being.

Many caregivers who work rely on some form of child care. Nearly half of children under 5 years of age attend out-of-home child care, according to the U.S. Census Bureau. A safe and nurturing child care setting can be beneficial to both the physical and developmental well-being of the child. Information for parents on how to select a child care provider or babysitter can be found at www.aap.org/healthychildcare.

Nutritional neglect in infants and children results from inadequate nutrition to maintain physical growth, development and intelligence. Failure to thrive is the most common consequence of nutritional neglect. However, allowing the ingestion of an abundance of calories that can lead to obesity and other health consequences can be construed as a form of maltreatment.

Pediatricians can reduce nutritional neglect by referring families to local resources and services such as charities, thrift stores and food banks. They also should know the eligibility criteria for and how families can enroll in the Special Supplemental Nutrition Program for Women, Infants, and Children (WIC) and the Supplemental Nutrition Assistance Program (SNAP, formerly known as food stamps). It may be helpful to have applications in the office. AAP guidance on helping families in poverty is available at www.aap.org/poverty.

Communication, education and a trusting partnership between the pediatrician and caregiver can help secure a happy, healthy and safe future for the child.

Dr. Brown is a member of the AAP Council on Child Abuse and Neglect.

Special Needs, Higher Abuse Risks

Dr. Andrew Sirotnak, MD, FAAP, Editor in Chief, *Pediatrics in Review Editorial Board*

C hild maltreatment is a challenging issue to address in the office or hospital setting, and children with special health care needs and disabilities can be at higher risk for maltreatment. Just as importantly, they also are at higher risk for injuries that can happen during routine care, for example, because of immobility and osteopenia, or bleeding abnormalities due to the adverse effects of chronic medications on liver function.

The October issue of Pediatrics in Review includes a wonderful review, "Child Abuse in Children and Youth with Special health Care Needs," by Drs. Brodie, McColgan, Spector and Turchi. (See page 110 of this collection.) It highlights the vital role that the primary care physician plays for special needs children and their families: Providing a trusted medical home, ensuring access to general and subspecialty care, and advocating for access to community-based services and, of course, financial coverage for medical and behavioral services across the life span.

This is an important review that highlights a number of educational gaps and provides a number of resources for the primary care provider. What stands out in this review for our readers and young physicians and trainees? I will highlight two key points here.

First, there are many resources within the American Academy of Pediatrics, including the AAP Council on Child Abuse and Neglect, that can provide continuing education as well as quick office-based resources for making the diagnosis.

For example, there are bruising patterns that may raise concerns for physical abuse. Sentinel injury literature reminds us that bruising over soft tissue surfaces, head, neck, face, and torso must be evaluated carefully for the possibility of inflicted injury, which often can occur in the context of frustration during care or discipline.

A number of years ago, in collaboration with the parent of a child with autism spectrum disorder, I helped create a community-based educational video on self-injurious behavior (SIB). As a child abuse pediatrician, I rarely get consulted on children with disabilities and physical abuse injuries, but from working with this parent I learned firsthand how challenging behaviors may lead to frustration on the part of a caregiver and harm for the child. We often forget these children may be in the care of babysitters, residential treatment facilities, or respite placements—caregivers who may not know the child or be able to cope with the behaviors as well as the child's parents.

Second, making this video reminded me of the important partnership between parents of a special needs child and their medical home pediatrician. Practical office-based suggestions include making sure SIB is on the problem list, with examples of the specific injury patterns; placing photos in the chart to document injury; and developing a short explanatory letter that could be in the record as a flag or "FYI" regarding the need to be aware of SIB as a presentation for injuries.

Advocating for health, welfare and safety for children with disabilities or special health care needs is inherent to our makeup as pediatricians and includes ensuring the child is safe from abuse and/or neglect. As AAP members, we have a wealth of resources for this task. Check out the practice resources and parenting resources from the AAP, listed at the end of the review, as well as the teaching slides that accompany this worthwhile article.

Child Abuse in Children and Youth with Special Health Care Needs

Nicola Brodie, MD,* Maria D. McColgan, MD,[†] Nancy D. Spector, MD,[‡] Renee M. Turchi, MD, MPH[§]

*Department of Pediatrics, [†]Child Protection Program, [‡]Executive Leadership in Academic Medicine Program, and [§]Center for Children and Youth with Special Health Care Needs, Drexel University College of Medicine, St Christopher's Hospital for Children, Philadelphia, PA

Education Gap

As the number of children and youth with special health care needs increases, it is imperative that pediatricians garner the skills to identify patients at increased risk for abuse, to correctly differentiate child abuse and neglect from accidental injury or sequelae of specific disease processes, to appropriately report child abuse, and to integrate prevention strategies into the medical home for our most vulnerable patients.

Objectives   After completing this article, readers should be able to:

1. Detail the definition and epidemiology of children with special health care needs.

2. Describe the epidemiology of child abuse and neglect.

3. Review the prevalence of abuse in children with special health care needs.

4. Determine the psychosocial and environmental risk factors for child abuse and neglect.

5. Differentiate the findings associated with physical abuse from those of accidental injury or illness.

6. List unique barriers to identifying and reporting abuse in children with special health care needs.

7. Identify strategies to prevent child abuse in children with special health care needs.

8. Recognize the importance of a medical home for children and youth with chronic conditions and physical and cognitive limitations.

AUTHOR DISCLOSURE Drs Brodie and Turchi have disclosed no financial relationships relevant to this article. Dr McColgan has disclosed that she is principal investigator for Children's Trust Fund's Family Safe Zone Project, that she provides expert witness testimony and expert opinion in legal cases, and that she owns employee stock in Tenet Health. Dr Spector has disclosed that she is coinvestigator on PCORI CDR-1306-03556, Bringing I-PASS to the Bedside: A Communication Bundle to Improve Patient Safety and Experience; that she mentored implementation of the I-PASS Program as coinvestigator on AHRQ 1R18HS023291; and that she is a member of the Coordinating Council and Scientific Oversight Committees and co-chair of the Educational Executive and Dissemination Committees for both projects. Dr McColgan's current affiliation is The CARES Institute, Rowan University School of Osteopathic Medicine, Stratford, NJ. This commentary does not contain a discussion of an unapproved/investigative use of a commercial product/device.

ABBREVIATION

AAP   American Academy of Pediatrics

CASE

A 14-year-old boy with intellectual disability and moderate spastic cerebral palsy presents to the emergency department with 1 day of fussiness and pain. At examination, he is noted to be nonverbal and thin and has swelling and tenderness of his left thigh. On radiographs, he is noted to have diffuse osteopenia with cortical thinning, as well as a left midshaft femur fracture. When questioned about the injury, his parents report no history of trauma.

INTRODUCTION

Child abuse is defined as "all forms of physical and/or emotional ill treatment, sexual abuse, neglect, or negligent treatment or commercial or other exploitation, resulting in actual or potential harm to the child's health, survival, development or dignity in the context of a relationship of responsibility, trust or power." (1) Child abuse can be thought of in 4 broad categories: physical abuse, sexual abuse, psychological and emotional abuse, and neglect. In 2014, 702,000 children were confirmed victims of child abuse and neglect in the United States, and data collected via telephone survey of caregivers and children suggest that this number may be even higher. (2) Every year, about 4% to 16% of children are physically abused, and 1 in 10 is neglected or psychologically abused. During childhood, 5% to 10% of girls and up to 5% of boys are exposed to penetrative sexual abuse, and up to 3 times this number are exposed to any type of sexual abuse. (3)

While abuse is a pressing public health concern in the general pediatric population, there are specific patient populations who are at even higher risk for abuse and neglect. Risk factors for abuse have been divided into 3 categories: factors related to the child, such as special health care needs or a child who is the product of an unplanned pregnancy; factors related to the parent, such as a personal history of abuse, poor impulse control, or substance abuse; and factors related to the environment, such as poverty and social isolation. (4)

The Centers for Disease Control and Prevention identifies "special needs that may increase caregiver burden," such as intellectual disability or chronic physical illness, as a major risk factor for child abuse. (5) Children with special health care needs are defined as "those who have or are at increased risk for a chronic physical, developmental, behavioral, or emotional condition and who also require health and related services of a type or amount beyond that required by children generally." (6) It is imperative to note that this definition is not based on specific diagnoses or functional status but rather on increased service use or need. Increased risk can be both biological and environmental. On the basis of this definition, the National Survey of Children and Youth with Special Health Care Needs in 2009 to 2010 demonstrated an overall national prevalence of 15.1% of children with special health care needs. Owing

to advances in medical technology for all children and youth, as well as the improved survival of extremely premature infants, this number has increased over time and represents an increase from 12.8% in 2001 and 13.9% in 2005. (2)

The definition of children with special health care needs can encompass a wide range of abilities; however, this article will focus primarily on a subset of this patient population known as *children with medical complexity*, which comprises those with multisystem acquired or congenital disease and children with severe functional impairment secondary to a neurological condition. (7) These patients require an additional level of experience, expertise, and resources to achieve optimal health outcomes and are particularly fragile and vulnerable.

SCOPE OF THE PROBLEM

While it is difficult to estimate the rates of abuse in the general population, it is particularly challenging to enumerate in children with special health care needs. Defining the special needs population presents a challenge, as there are various definitions used for special health care needs and disabilities in the literature. Additionally, the prevalence of maltreatment in the United States is often challenging to calculate, as individual states use different definitions of "child abuse and neglect." (8) Finally, it can be difficult to determine whether the disability is the precipitating agent for abuse or whether abuse caused the disability, and the potential for reverse causation cannot be excluded in population-based studies. Despite the difficulty in calculating rates of abuse in children with special health care needs, several studies indicate that children with special health care needs experience all types of abuse at higher rates than their peers. (9)(10)

A landmark study published in 2000 noted that children with disabilities were nearly 4 times more likely to be physically abused or neglected and more than 3 times more likely to be sexually abused when compared to children without disabilities. (9) Additionally, a study conducted by using forensic interviews showed that increasing levels of impairment were associated with an increased risk of sexual abuse. (11) Finally, in the first review to provide pooled estimates of the prevalence and risk of abuse against children with disabilities, it was estimated that up to one-quarter of children with disabilities will be a victim of child abuse or neglect in their lifetimes. (12)

With clear evidence that children and youth with special health care needs are particularly vulnerable to all types of abuse, it becomes imperative to understand the specific risk factors for abuse and the unique challenges faced by this population, as well as the ways in which pediatricians can appropriately identify and prevent abuse.

SPECIFIC RISK FACTORS

Several studies have sought to identify reasons why children and youth with special health care needs are more vulnerable to abuse than their typically developing peers. Reasons for this disparity include societal stigma, negative traditional beliefs or ignorance within communities, lack of social support for caregivers, and heightened vulnerability as a result of the need for increased care. (12) Children and youth may have behavioral issues that are difficult to manage or may not be able to communicate abuse when it happens, which leads to the inability to report abuse when it occurs. Finally, parents and caregivers often lack adequate support systems, which creates an environment in which abuse is more likely to occur. Thus, risk factors for abuse that are unique to children with special health care needs relate to the child's underlying diagnosis and associated limitations, the increased need for assistance in activities of daily living, and the increased caregiver burden associated with having a child with special health care needs.

Specific special needs have been correlated with increased risk for specific types of abuse. A longitudinal cohort study in two counties in New York demonstrated an increased risk of neglect among children with a low verbal IQ or who were anxious or withdrawn. They also found that children who required special education were at an increased risk of sexual abuse but that low IQ was not an independent risk factor for physical abuse. (13) A retrospective birth cohort study conducted in the United Kingdom provided the odds ratio for abuse on the basis of several different types of disability, including cerebral palsy, conduct disorder, speech or language disorder, learning disability, sensory disorders, and autism. (14) Findings suggest that children with cerebral palsy were at increased risk of physical abuse and neglect; autism and hearing or vision impairments did not predispose children to abuse or neglect in this study. Investigators in another study posit that children with special health care needs who are reliant on others for assistance with self-care may be at increased risk for sexual abuse specifically because they may be used to others touching their bodies and may be less able to recognize inappropriate contact or touch. (15)

Parental stress also plays a major role in increasing the risk for child abuse in children with special health care needs. Parents of children with special health care needs face unique challenges in caring for their children, including the burden of additional parenting tasks, such as arranging and attending frequent medical appointments, developing appropriate behavioral management plans in children who do not have the same level of understanding as their age-matched peers, parenting without clear benchmarks for success, integrating their child's care with both medical and nonmedical needed services, and the feeling of having to parent under public scrutiny. (16)

In a clinical report entitled "Maltreatment of Children with Disabilities," several parental stressors are identified that may contribute to child abuse in children with special health care needs:

1. Parents or caregivers may experience additional stress because children with disabilities may not respond to traditional means of discipline.
2. Children with disabilities place additional physical, economic, emotional, and social demands on their families.
3. Parents and caregivers who have a limited social support system may be at increased risk of maltreating their children with disabilities because they may feel overwhelmed. (8)

IDENTIFICATION OF CHILD ABUSE

The identification of child abuse can be difficult for the pediatrician, as patients do not always present with clear physical examination findings, particularly in the case of childhood sexual abuse. Guidelines exist for the identification of abuse in the general pediatric population, including appropriate diagnostic testing to evaluate for underlying medical conditions; these guidelines are summarized in the clinical report "The Evaluation of Suspected Childhood Physical Abuse," published by the American Academy of Pediatrics (AAP) Committee on Child Abuse and Neglect. (4) However, unique challenges exist in the identification of child abuse in children with special health care needs. These challenges may be related to the patient's medical condition or to factors involved in caring appropriately for these children.

Medical conditions that may mimic abuse in the patient with special health care needs include but are not limited to motor and balance issues, bleeding disorders, osteoporosis or osteopenia, self-injurious behavior, and developmental delay.

Motor and Balance Issues

Patients with motor and balance issues, such as poor coordination or wheelchair dependence, may present with many concerning skin findings for physical abuse. The pediatrician should differentiate between skin findings consistent with an appropriate mechanism of injury and skin findings that raise red flags for abuse. Few rigorous studies have been conducted to examine variations in bruising patterns among patients with limited or restricted mobility when compared to their peers. One study showed a significant decrease in the number of skin markings in patients with no ability to ambulate when compared to patients with some ability to ambulate with assistance. (17) However, no additional differences in skin findings were noted. Goldberg et al (18) found that patients with clinically significant mobility limitations that required maximal assistance with transfers and self-care were more likely to have bruising than their peers but that the location of bruising differed (Table). Specifically, the lower legs were often bruised in children without disabilities but not in children who were wheelchair bound. In contrast, the feet, back and lumbar areas, and pelvis were more frequently bruised in children who were wheelchair dependent, and children with severe mobility restrictions were more likely to sustain bruises at older ages when compared to their peers. These differences were postulated to be secondary to the increasing difficulty in transferring these patients, particularly as they grow in size. (18) However, children with mobility limitations did not have a higher frequency of bruising at other sites, which raise concern for abuse in the general population, such as the neck, ears, chin, anterior chest, or buttocks. (4)(19)

These studies indicate the importance of accounting for specific mobility status in patients when determining whether a skin finding is consistent with the mechanism of injury described. A patient who is unable to ambulate is significantly less likely to have bruising of the lower extremities from a benign etiologic cause than a patient with some ability to ambulate independently. However, patients who are wheelchair dependent may develop lower-extremity bruising related to their equipment, particularly bruises at the site of foot and ankle splints. Therefore, it behooves the pediatrician to examine each case on

an individual basis, and suspicion should be raised if the mechanism of injury does not align with the child's mobility status.

Bleeding Disorders

Patients with bleeding disorders may present with unexplained bruising or bleeding, which raises concerns for physical abuse or abusive head trauma. It is important to consider bleeding disorders in the evaluation of children with suspected nonaccidental trauma, especially at young ages. Platelet number should be assessed, and disorders of platelet function should be considered, especially in the context of medications, which may influence platelet activity. Nonverbal patients with bruising as the only finding concerning for abuse should always be screened for hemophilia and Von Willebrand disease; frequently, other screening for bleeding diatheses is undertaken. (20) In patients with a known bleeding disorder, the specific manifestations of that disorder should be taken into account when assessing the likelihood of nonaccidental trauma. For example, a patient with hemophilia may be particularly prone to bruising, but a finding of patterned bruising is always concerning for child abuse.

Osteoporosis and Osteopenia

Patients who have limited mobility or who do not bear weight are at increased risk for osteoporosis and associated fractures. Specifically, children with spastic cerebral palsy have been studied in depth to assess their risk for long bone fractures, which may be mistaken for physical abuse. These studies showed that children with cerebral palsy are at increased risk for accidental or nontraumatic long bone fractures, at a rate of about 4% per year. (21) Specific risk factors for fractures included limited mobility, feeding difficulties, anticonvulsant use, and history of prior fractures. (22) Children and youth with limited mobility should have preventive measures taken to foster adequate bone health and mineralization in the primary care medical home or in partnership with specialty care when indicated.

TABLE. Bruising Patterns That Raise Concern for Physical Abuse

	POSSIBLY ACCIDENTAL PATTERNS	PATTERNS CONCERNING FOR ABUSE
Children without mobility limitations	Lower extremities	Torso Ears Neck (19)
Children with limited mobility	Feet Lumbar spine Thighs Pelvis Hands and arms (18)	Lower extremities Anterior chest Ears Neck Chin Buttocks

Self-injurious Behavior

Children with special health care needs engage in self-injurious behavior more frequently than their typically developing peers, and this behavior is more persistent as children get older. (23) Risk factors for self-injurious behavior include a diagnosis of autism spectrum disorder, as well as specific genetic syndromes such as Prader-Willi, Lesch-Nyhan, fragile X, Cornelia de Lange, and Smith-Magenis. (24) Studies have demonstrated the usual topography of these injuries to most frequently include head-banging, eye-poking, and hand-mouthing, which can result in serious morbidity. (23) These injuries can be mistaken for physical abuse; thus, vigilance on the part of the primary care provider is important. On the other hand, there is some evidence to suggest that there may be an increase in self-injurious behaviors, particularly in children with autism spectrum disorders, when they are exposed to chronic maltreatment and abuse; (25) thus, increasing intensity of self-injurious behaviors always merits further investigation.

Developmental Delay

It is important to take into account both a patient's developmental age and his or her chronological age when assessing whether an injury may be the result of nonaccidental trauma. This is relevant with regard to motor development milestones but also with regard to cognitive milestones. Patients with intellectual disability may be more prone to accidental toxic or drug ingestion, as their physical ability to access potentially harmful substances in the home may be beyond their ability to understand the consequences of their actions. This is particularly true in patients with severe intellectual disability, cognitive delays, hyperphagia, or other genetic syndromes, such as Prader-Willi.

PREVENTION OF ABUSE

The AAP clinical report "The Pediatrician's Role in Child Maltreatment Prevention" provides guidance on child maltreatment prevention through strengthening families and promoting stable nurturing families. (26) At a minimum, pediatricians of children with special health care needs should consider providing disability-specific injury prevention recommendations to all families as part of their anticipatory guidance to help families minimize their child's risk of injury. For example, the AAP Committee on Injury and Poison Prevention provides clear illustrated guidelines for the safe transportation of patients with technology dependence and specific medical needs to prevent serious injury. (27) Additionally, it behooves the pediatrician to develop

strategies for recognizing overwhelmed parents who are at risk of harming their children. In fact, investigators in 1 study found that the single best way to protect children with special health care needs from abuse is to address the needs of their caretakers. This should include parental training in topics such as child behavior management, stress management skills, and respite care and community supports. (15)

The pediatrician need not work alone in a vacuum to prevent child abuse. Community partners can be extremely helpful in preventing parents from becoming overwhelmed and include, but are not limited to, home nursing agencies, child advocacy agencies, medical child care, school and educational settings, and community programs that provide home visiting and assistance in navigating the health care system to families of children with special health care needs. One national organization is Family Voices (http://www.familyvoices.org/), which provides resources and support to families of children with special health care needs and advocates for family-centered care. Indeed, the role of the medical home, or the provision of care that is "accessible, continuous, comprehensive, family centered, coordinated, compassionate, and culturally effective," cannot be emphasized enough in the prevention of abuse of children and youth with special health care needs. (28)

CASE RESOLUTION

In light of the unexplained fracture, the provider becomes suspicious for potential physical abuse. A thorough physical examination demonstrates a nonverbal, wheelchair-dependent child with spasticity in all 4 extremities. A skin examination shows a small bruise on the lateral aspect of the left thigh, but no other bruises are identified. The provider notes that the patient has several risk factors for abuse, including special health care needs, limited mobility and communication, developmental delay, and multiple caretakers. However, the provider also recognizes that the patient is at increased risk for accidental femur fracture because of his limited mobility, spasticity, and low bone mineral density. As a mandated reporter, the provider reports her suspicion for abuse to child protective services. A thorough investigation of the home and family is undertaken. A more comprehensive interview with the family suggests that the patient's femur fracture was most likely accidental and was sustained during a transfer from wheelchair to bathtub and that the patient's parents feel overwhelmed by their child's extensive needs. A referral is made to the local home-visiting intervention program to assist the family in managing their child's care, and the child remains in the care of his family, without further concerns for nonaccidental trauma.

CONCLUSION

Children and youth with special health care needs are particularly vulnerable to all types of child abuse, including physical abuse, sexual abuse, emotional abuse, and neglect due to their increased medical, emotional, and psychosocial needs for care, as well as stressors on their caregivers. The pediatrician must be trained in differentiating abuse from injuries related to an underlying medical diagnosis. Additionally, pediatricians should work collaboratively within the context of the patient- and family-centered medical home and their available partners, recognizing patients and families with risk factors for abuse, with the goal of preventing child abuse in this particularly vulnerable patient population.

Summary

1. Longitudinal epidemiologic surveillance data indicate that children and youth with special health care needs are a growing population in the United States, secondary to advances in medical technology and improved survival of premature infants. (2)

2. On the basis of strong research evidence, children and youth with special health care needs are at increased risk for child abuse because of increased need for care and additional parental and caregiver stressors. (8)(9)(10)

3. On the basis of some research evidence, as well as consensus, there are unique challenges to the identification of abuse in children with special health care needs, such as the differentiation of abuse from accidental trauma based on risk factors such as osteopenia, spasticity, higher rates of fracture or soft-tissue trauma, and limited mobility that requires transfers by assistive person, as well as recognizing abuse in nonverbal patients. (18)(20)(22)

4. The medical home model provides a framework for preventing abuse in vulnerable children while partnering with the community and families. (26)(28)

To view teaching slides that accompany this article, visit http://pedsinreview.aappublications.org/content/38/10/463.supplemental.

Child Abuse in Children and Youth with Special Healthcare Needs

Nicola Brodie, MD
Maria McColgan, MD
Nancy Spector, MD
Renee Turchi, MD, MPH

Pediatrics in Review

American Academy of Pediatrics
DEDICATED TO THE HEALTH OF ALL CHILDREN®

References for this article are at http://pedsinreview.aappublications.org/content/38/10/463.

Additional Resources for Pediatricians

AAP Textbook of Pediatric Care, 2nd Edition
• Chapter 367: Physical Abuse and Neglect - https://pediatriccare.solutions.aap.org/chapter.aspx?sectionId=124919066&bookId=1626
Point-of-Care Quick Reference
• Physical Abuse and Neglect - https://pediatriccare.solutions.aap.org/content.aspx?gbosid=245973

Parent Resources from the AAP at HealthyChildren.org

• What to Know about Child Abuse: https://www.healthychildren.org/English/safety-prevention/at-home/Pages/What-to-Know-about-Child-Abuse.aspx

• Social & Economic Factors Associated with Developmental Disabilities: https://www.healthychildren.org/English/health-issues/conditions/developmental-disabilities/Pages/Social-Economic-Factors-Associated-with-Developmental-Disabilities.aspx

For a comprehensive library of AAP parent handouts, please go to the *Pediatric Patient Education* site at http://patiented.aap.org.

Childhood Maltreatment and Disability Diagnosis: Sorting Out Causality

Dr. Lydia Furman, MD, Associate Editor, *Pediatrics*

In a recently released issue of Pediatrics, Dr. Miriam McLean and colleagues explore maltreatment risk among children with disabilities in Western Australia 1990-2010 using large population-based registries (10.1542/peds.2016-1817). The authors accessed 4 administrative databases which included a range of disability diagnoses identified or recorded at birth or hospital admission, and through receipt of educational services or mental health care. Diagnoses included intellectual disability, Down syndrome (coded as a separate disorder), birth defect or cerebral palsy, autism, conduct disorder, and other mental health or behavioral disorders. Among all children with disabilities, 15.6% had at least one co-morbidity, and among those with intellectual disability, 62.6% had one or more co-morbidities. Basic demographic information about parents included socioeconomic level based on neighborhood census tract, and any history of hospital contact for mental health, substance abuse or interpersonal violence. Finally, episodes of maltreatment allegation and substantiation were obtained from the Department for Child Protection and Family Support.

Overall, and after controlling for other risk factors, children with a disability diagnosis did have a significantly higher risk of both maltreatment allegation and substantiation than children without disability. While this result makes sense, it is not the whole answer, since risk was not distributed evenly across diagnoses, and not all disabilities appeared to confer added risk. I will note, for example, that children with Down syndrome were not at increased risk. The authors speculate on causes for the uneven distribution of maltreatment risk across the spectrum of disabilities, but clearly more research will be needed since large databases lack many details such as the child's age of diagnosis, the chronicity and severity of the disorder, and data on parental resources, supports and stressors, that might shed light on the question.

What interests me most is the issue of causality, which the authors do address in their Discussion. Children with mild or moderate intellectual disability, mental/behavioral problems and those with conduct disorder had a higher risk of maltreatment, even after accounting for family and neighborhood risk factors. The authors also noted that the disabilities most strongly associated with maltreatment appeared to co-occur with clusters of social risk, such as parental mental health problems, living in poor neighborhoods and having young parents. Is it possible that the mental/behavioral problems, intellectual disability and conduct problems are actually a result of rather than a cause of maltreatment? While risk could be bi-directional (i.e. maltreatment could both cause and result in mental/behavioral health issues), good evidence causally links childhood physical abuse with childhood (and adult) mental health problems.[1-3] Both family stress and lower socioeconomic status, even without physical maltreatment, are causally linked to lowered childhood IQ.[4,5] The public health impact of sorting out the direction of the association (between maltreatment and both childhood mental/behavioral problems and IQ) is not trivial, since presumably preventive programming should be focused on the cause rather than the result of the problem. I believe this study has raised more questions than it has answered, and hopefully more excellent research will follow.

References

1. McCrory E, De Brito SA, Viding E. The link between child abuse and psychopathology: A review of neurobiological and genetic research. Journal of the Royal Society of Medicine. 2012;105: 151-156.

2. Mulvaney MK, Mebert CJ. Parental corporal punishment predicts behavior problems in early childhood. J Fam Psychol. 2007; 21:389-97.

3. Teicher MH, Samson JA. Annual Research Review: Enduring neurobiological effects of childhood abuse and neglect. J Child Psychol Psychiatry. 2016; 57: 241-66.

4. Marcus Jenkins JV, Woolley DP, Hooper SR, De Bellis MD. Direct and Indirect Effects of Brain Volume, Socioeconomic Status and Family Stress on Child IQ. J Child and Adolesc Behav. 2013;1:1000107.

5. Ursache A, Noble KG, Pediatric Imaging, Neurocognition and Genetics Study. Socioeconomic status, white matter, and executive function in children. Brain Behav. 2016 Aug 2;6(10):e00531.

Maltreatment Risk Among Children With Disabilities

Miriam J. Maclean, BPsych(Hons), MSc, PhD, Scott Sims, MBiostat, BSC, Carol Bower, MSC, MB, BS, PhD, FAPHM, Helen Leonard, MBChB, MPH, Fiona J. Stanley, MD, MSC, FFPHM, FAFPHM, Melissa O'Donnell, BPsych(Hons), MPsych, Dip Ed, PhD

BACKGROUND: Children with disabilities are at increased risk of child maltreatment; however, there is a gap in the evidence about whether all disabilities are at equal risk and whether risk factors vary according to the type of disability.

METHODS: A population-based record-linkage study of all children born in Western Australia between 1990 and 2010. Children with disabilities were identified by using population-based registers and risk of maltreatment determined by allegations reported to the Department for Child Protection and Family Support.

RESULTS: Although children with disabilities make up 10.4% of the population, they represent 25.9% of children with a maltreatment allegation and 29.0% of those with a substantiated allegation; however, increased risk of maltreatment was not consistent across all disability types. Children with intellectual disability, mental/behavioral problems, and conduct disorder continued to have increased risk of an allegation and substantiated allegation after adjusting for child, family, and neighborhood risk factors. In contrast, adjusting for these factors resulted in children with autism having a lower risk, and children with Down syndrome and birth defects/cerebral palsy having the same risk as children without disability.

CONCLUSIONS: The prevalence of disabilities in the child protection system suggests a need for awareness of the scope of issues faced by these children and the need for interagency collaboration to ensure children's complex needs are met. Supports are needed for families with children with disabilities to assist in meeting the child's health and developmental needs, but also to support the parents in managing the often more complex parenting environment.

Telethon Kids Institute, University of Western Australia, Perth, Western Australia.

Dr Maclean conceptualized and designed the study, and drafted the initial manuscript; Mr Sims carried out the initial analyses, and reviewed and revised the manuscript; Drs Bower, Leonard, and Stanley contributed to the design of the study, and reviewed and revised the manuscript; Dr O'Donnell contributed to the conceptualization and design of the study, and critically reviewed the manuscript; and all authors approved the final manuscript as submitted.

DOI: 10.1542/peds.2016-1817

Accepted for publication Jan 26, 2017

Address correspondence to Melissa O'Donnell, PhD, Telethon Kids Institute, University of Western Australia, 100 Roberts Rd, Subiaco, Australia, 6008. E-mail: Melissa.O'Donnell@telethonkids.org.au

PEDIATRICS (ISSN Numbers: Print, 0031-4005; Online, 1098-4275).

FINANCIAL DISCLOSURE: The authors have indicated they have no financial relationships relevant to this article to disclose.

WHAT'S KNOWN ON THIS SUBJECT: Children with disabilities experience elevated rates of child abuse and neglect. Only a few population-based studies have been conducted producing mixed evidence regarding maltreatment risk for children with different types of disabilities.

WHAT THIS STUDY ADDS: Children with disabilities account for 1 in 3 substantiated maltreatment allegations; however, maltreatment risk was not consistent across all disabilities. Children with intellectual disability, mental/behavioral problems, and conduct disorder had increased risk, but not autism, Down syndrome, or birth defects.

To cite: Maclean MJ, Sims S, Bower C, et al. Maltreatment Risk Among Children With Disabilities. *Pediatrics.* 2017; 139(4):e20161817

Group	Databases	ICD-9 Codes	ICD-10 Codes
ID	IDEA, HMDS, MHIS	317–319	F70-F79
Down syndrome	IDEA, WARDA, HMDS, MHIS	758.0	Q90
Birth defects/cerebral palsy (all congenital malformations and cerebral palsy)	WARDA[a]		
Autism	IDEA, HMDS, MHIS	299.0	F84.0, F84.1
Conduct disorder	HMDS, MHIS	312, 314.0	F90-F92
Mental and behavioral disorder[b] (all other mental/behavioral disorders apart from autism, conduct disorder, and intellectual disability)	HMDS, MHIS	290–316 (excluding 299.0, 312, 314.0)	F00-F69, F80-F99 (excluding F84.0, F84.1, F90-F92
Any disability	Any of the above	Any of the above	Any of the above

[a] http://kemh.health.wa.gov.au/services/register_developmental_anomalies/diagnostic_codes_birth_defects.htm.
[b] This includes organic disorders, disorders due to psychoactive substance use, schizophrenia-type disorders, mood disorders, behavioral syndromes, stress-related disorders, personality disorders, specific developmental disorders, behavioral and emotional disorders.

An estimated 5.1% of children worldwide have a moderate to severe disability.[1] Research shows that children with disabilities experience elevated rates of child abuse and neglect.[2-6] However, there are critical knowledge gaps, leading US researchers Kendall-Tackett et al[7] to state "there is an appalling gap in the states' ability to protect abused and neglected children with disabilities."

At the most basic level, states/countries need to know the proportion of children within their child protection systems who have disabilities, and their types of disability.[7] Risk of maltreatment is associated with child characteristics, such as age and ethnicity; parent factors, such as young age, mental health problems, and substance abuse; and neighborhood factors, such as socioeconomic disadvantage.[6] Families of children with disabilities more frequently experience risk factors associated with a higher risk of maltreatment.[8] However, the risk for maltreatment among children with disabilities has not been explored taking into account the multiple risk factors that often cooccur in the context of these families.

The few population-based studies conducted have produced mixed evidence regarding maltreatment risk for children with different types of disabilities,[4,9,10] and it remains unclear whether disability types, such as intellectual disability (ID), are associated with increased risk. The aims of this research were to report the prevalence of different disabilities within the child protection system in an Australian state, and to assess risk of maltreatment in various types of disability taking into account child, family, and neighborhood risk factors.

METHODS

Population and Data Sources

We conducted a population-based record-linkage study of all children born in Western Australia (WA) between 1990 and 2010 using de-identified administrative data. Disability information was obtained from 4 sources that had information for the whole study period 1990 to 2010. The first is the WA Register of Developmental Anomalies (WARDA),[11] which includes structural or functional birth defects that are present before birth and diagnosed by age 6, and cerebral palsy. WARDA

receives notifications of birth defects from the Midwives Notification System, the Hospital Morbidity Data System (HMDS), and other services (eg, genetic, pathology, and private practitioners). The second is the population-based Intellectual Disability Exploring Answers (IDEA)[12] database, which provides WA state data on individuals with ID and/or autism, by using information provided by the Disability Services Commission for individuals of any age with ID who are provided with services, and the Department of Education (individuals with ID receiving education support, predominantly aged 5–17 years). The IDEA database also collects information on severity of ID, and for cases obtained through the Disability Services Commission, the probable cause by using diagnostic information reviewed from medical records. Cases could be classified as caused by chromosomal disorders, metabolic disorders, prenatal exposure to alcohol, postnatal injury, cultural-familial (family history of ID/environmental disadvantage), and so forth.[13] The third is HMDS, which contains information on all public and private hospital discharges, including up to 21 diagnostic codes by using the International Classification of Diseases (ICD) codes (ICD-9:1990–June 1999, ICD-10: July 1999–2010, see Table 1). The fourth is the Mental Health Information System (MHIS), containing information on all mental health–related public and private inpatient admissions and public outpatient contacts with diagnoses captured by using ICD codes. This study has ethics approval from the WA Department of Health Human Research Ethics Committee.

Disability for this article was defined as any limitation or impairment that may affect everyday activities ranging from intellectual, physical, and psychological conditions.[14] This broad definition includes psychological conditions, which are often not diagnosed until adolescence, as well as disabilities typically diagnosed at birth or soon after. Children's disabilities were identified through the 4 data sources of WARDA, IDEA, HMDS and MHIS, and disability groups were categorized as shown in Table 1. Disability categories were chosen because they were consistent with our definition, were the main disability groups identified in the sources, and their sample sizes were adequate for analyses. Children could be grouped in >1 category if they had comorbid conditions; however, Down syndrome (DS) was grouped separately because it is both a birth defect and causes ID. Of the 54 532 children who had ID, birth defect/cerebral palsy, autism, conduct disorder, or a mental/behavioral disorder, 15.6% had ≥1 comorbidities. For children with ID, there was a high rate of comorbidity with other conditions (62.6%).

We also included an additional analysis of 2 birth defect categories from the WARDA, spina bifida (n = 192) and cleft lip and/or palate (n = 525), to compare with previous research.[15]

The disability data were linked to records from Births Registrations (1990–2010), the Midwives Notification System (1990–2010), Mortality Database (1990–2010), and the Department of Child Protection and Family Support (CPFS) (1990–2010). Using probabilistic linkage of common identifiers, such as name, address, and birth date, the data were linked by the Department of Health's Data Linkage Branch in which extensive clerical review also was conducted as per their process, with a linkage quality of 97% to 98%.[16,17] The identifiers were separated from the clinical or service information to maximize privacy during the linkage process, with only de-identified information provided to researchers.

The child's sex, Aboriginality, birth weight, and gestational age were obtained from Births Registrations and Midwives Notification System, along with parents' marital status and age at the time of birth. Neighborhood-level socioeconomic status was determined by the Index of Relative Social Disadvantage from the Australian Bureau of Statistics by using the Birth and Midwives data.[18] Five levels of disadvantage were assigned to census collection districts (~200 households) ranging from 1 (most disadvantaged) to 5 (least disadvantaged). Parents' history of hospital discharges and contacts (pre- and post-birth) for mental health, substance-related issues, and assault-related injuries were ascertained from HMDS and the MHIS (1970–2010). The Mortality Register was used to censor observations at date of death.

The CPFS records provided data on children's entire history of maltreatment allegations from birth onward, including age of allegation and type of maltreatment. Allegations consist of reports made to CPFS regarding alleged child abuse and neglect. An allegation is substantiated by CPFS when after investigation there is reasonable cause to believe the child has been, is being, or is likely to be abused, neglected, or otherwise harmed. After a substantiated allegation, children could be removed from their families and enter out-of-home care.

Statistical Analysis

In addition to descriptive analysis, Cox regression was used to estimate the adjusted and unadjusted hazard ratio (HR) and 95% confidence interval (CI) for the time in months from birth to first maltreatment allegation, adjusted for disability types and other risk factors. Results in which the 95% CIs did not include the null value of 1 were considered statistically significant. Records were censored at their date of death and

if there was no child maltreatment allegation by the end of follow-up. The main analyses first assessed the HR for child maltreatment allegations by using a dichotomous disability covariate (disability versus no disability), and second by using 6 dichotomous covariates (6 disability types) in addition to adjusting for child, family, and neighborhood risk factors. In the categorical disability analysis (6 disability groups), children with comorbidities could be categorized in >1 group (except DS) and analyzed accordingly. Further Cox regression analyses investigated time to a substantiated allegation and time to a period of out-of-home care. In our analyses, we assumed the values of these covariates were determined at the point when follow-up began on each child (time = 0; ie, at birth) and that these did not change over the period of observation. As we are not confident when diagnoses began, we did not add a time-varying covariate for disability and have stated this in the limitations. Additional analyses examined risk of allegations related to aspects of ID, including severity, comorbidity, cause, and the specific birth defects of spina bifida and cleft lip and/or palate. Further analyses also were conducted to investigate type of maltreatment allegation (neglect, physical and sexual abuse) for all disability groups and ID severity (Supplemental Information).

RESULTS

Risk of Allegations

Of the 524 534 children in the population cohort, 4.6% had a maltreatment allegation (Table 2). Overall, 25.9% of child maltreatment allegations and 29.0% of substantiated allegations involved a child with a disability. Maltreatment allegations varied by disability type; children with ID comprised 6.7% allegations, similar to birth defects/cerebral palsy (6.6%), and conduct disorder (4.5%), with the largest number of allegations for children with mental/behavioral disorders (15.6%). Only a small proportion of allegations included children with DS (0.1%) or autism (0.7%).

Age at first maltreatment allegation was similar across disability types, with a mean age of 4.8 years, and fairly similar to children without disabilities (4.2 years). Type of maltreatment allegation also was similar across disability groups (neglect ~25%, physical abuse ~24%, sexual abuse ~19%, and emotional abuse ~3.5%). This pattern was generally similar to children without disabilities, except proportions were slightly higher for neglect and physical abuse. The only groups that varied to a large degree were children with ID who had a higher proportion of neglect (33%) and children with conduct disorder who had more physical abuse (31%).

Before adjusting for child, family, and neighborhood characteristics, children with a disability had more than a twofold increased risk of having a maltreatment allegation (HR 2.64, 95% CI 2.56–2.74) and a threefold increased risk of a substantiated allegation (HR 3.09, 95% CI 2.97–3.22) compared with children without a disability (see Table 3). All disability types other than DS were associated with a significantly increased risk for having a maltreatment allegation before adjustment. The highest HRs were for conduct disorder (HR 5.14, 95% CI 4.83–5.47), followed by ID (HR 3.86, 95% CI 3.67–4.06) and mental/behavioral disorders (HR 3.69, 95% CI 3.56–3.82). The risk of substantiated allegation also was higher.

Adjustment for Demographic and Psychosocial Characteristics

As shown in the Supplemental Tables, demographic and psychosocial characteristics vary across disability type. Accounting for child, family, and

neighborhood risk factors partially attenuated the relationship between disabilities and maltreatment, particularly for conduct disorder and mental/behavioral disorders, and changed the relationship for autism from increased to decreased risk (Table 3). After controlling for other risk factors, children with a disability still had an increased risk of maltreatment allegations (HR 1.74, 95% CI 1.68–1.80) and substantiated allegations (HR 1.89, 95% CI 1.80–1.98) compared with children without disabilities.

Risk was highest for children with IDs (HR 2.14, 95% CI 2.00–2.28), followed by conduct disorder and mental/behavioral disorders. There was significantly lower risk of maltreatment allegations for children with autism (HR 0.74, 95% CI 0.63–0.89), and children with DS also had lower risk, although did not reach significance (HR 0.69, 95% CI 0.46–1.02). Risk of maltreatment allegations did not differ between children with birth defects/ cerebral palsy and children with no disabilities (HR 0.99, 95% CI 0.93– 1.05), although they had a slightly elevated risk of a substantiated allegation (HR 1.10, 95% CI 1.01– 1.20) and entering out-of-home care (HR 1.32, 95% CI 1.18–1.49, see Supplemental Information). Analysis by type of maltreatment allegation found relatively consistent results, with the exception of maltreatment involving sexual abuse, in which autism was protective and birth defects/cerebral palsy showed no increased risk. However, caution should be taken when interpreting results due to smaller sample sizes and therefore unreliable estimates (Supplemental Information).

Supplementary multivariate analysis of spina bifida and cleft lip and/ or palate was conducted, finding an increased risk of substantiated allegation in the univariate analysis (HR 1.94, 95% CI 1.01–3.72; HR 1.61, 95% CI 1.01–2.56, respectively), but

after adjustment found no increased risk (HR 0.74, 95% CI 0.33–1.65; HR 0.81, 95% CI 0.42–1.55, respectively). Caution should be taken with this finding due to small sample size.

Aboriginal children had an increased risk of a maltreatment allegation of almost 6.5 times compared with non-Aboriginal children; however, this risk dropped to 1.64 (95% CI 1.57– 1.70) once other factors were taken into account, particularly as they had a higher risk of other family and social risk factors. The proportion of Aboriginal children with disability was 14.2%, compared with 10.1% for non-Aboriginal children. They had a higher proportion of children with ID (3.2% vs 1.5%) and mental/ behavioral disorder (17.5% versus 14.3%), both of which had higher risks of maltreatment allegations.

Severity and Cause of ID

For children with ID, less severe disability was related to increased likelihood of maltreatment allegations (Table 4). After controlling for other risk factors, children with borderline-mild ID had an almost threefold increased likelihood of maltreatment allegations (HR 2.73, 95% CI 2.45–3.04), and children with mild-moderate ID were at twofold increased likelihood of allegations (HR 2.01, 95% CI 1.85–2.17). The risk associated with severe ID did not differ significantly from children without ID (HR 1.30, 95% CI 0.95– 1.79). When broken down by type of maltreatment allegation, the findings were relatively consistent except that for children with severe ID, they were at increased risk of neglect (Supplemental Information).

Among children with ID, a supplementary analysis found an increased maltreatment risk for children for whom the recorded cause of disability was postnatal injury (HR 5.14, 95% CI 2.99–8.83), prenatal exposure to alcohol (HR 2.01, 95% CI 1.30–3.11), other birth

TABLE 2 Characteristics of Study Population and Level of Child Protection Involvement

Characteristic	Total	No Allegation		Any Allegation		Any Substantiated Allegation		Entered Out-of-Home Care	
	n	n	%	n	%	n	%	n	%
Number	524 534	500 518		24 016		11 560		5596	
Sex									
Male	268 651	257 108	51.4	11 543	48.1	5472	47.3	2810	50.2
Female	255 831	243 362	48.6	12 469	51.9	6088	52.6	2786	49.8
Aboriginality									
Non-Aboriginal	492 740	475 379	95.0	17 361	72.3	7771	67.2	3506	62.7
Aboriginal	31 612	24 975	5.0	6637	27.6	3779	32.7	2085	37.3
Missing	182	164	0.03	18	0.1	10	0.1	5	0.09
Socioeconomic status									
1 (most disadvantaged)	120 565	37 560	7.5	11 506	47.9	5811	50.3	2903	51.9
2	120 126	81 247	16.2	5805	24.2	2749	23.4	1335	23.9
3	99 811	66 313	13.5	3344	13.9	1550	13.4	726	13.0
4	94 009	136 417	27.3	2097	8.7	923	8.0	420	7.5
5 (least disadvantaged)	87 330	177 067	35.4	1120	4.7	445	3.8	173	3.1
Missing	2693	1914	0.4	144	0.6	82	0.7	39	0.7
Disability type									
ID	8551	6952	1.4	1599	6.7	905	7.8	527	9.4
Down syndrome	552	521	0.1	31	0.1	15	0.1	8	0.1
Birth defect/cerebral palsy	30 090	28 501	5.7	1589	6.6	860	7.4	498	8.9
Autism	2253	2078	0.4	175	0.7	89	0.8	56	1.0
Conduct disorder	3924	2846	0.6	1078	4.5	573	5.0	318	5.7
Mental and behavioral disorder	19 813	16 062	3.2	3751	15.6	2073	17.9	1004	17.9
Any disability	54 535	48 324	9.7	6211	25.9	3352	29.0	1709	30.5
Maternal age, y									
<20	30 019	25 194	5.0	4825	20.1	2406	20.8	1162	20.8
20–29	252 817	239 044	47.8	13 773	57.3	6638	57.4	3162	56.5
30+	241 642	236 228	47.2	5414	22.5	2516	21.8	1272	22.7
Missing	56	52	0.01	4	0.02	0	0.0	0	0.0
Paternal age, y									
<20	9522	8107	1.6	1415	5.9	687	5.9	327	5.8
20–29	175 262	165 343	33.0	9919	41.3	4649	40.2	2074	37.1
30+	314 549	307 078	61.4	7471	31.1	3257	28.2	1518	27.1
Missing	25 201	19 990	4.0	5211	21.7	2967	25.7	1677	30.0
Gestational age, wk									
<37	38 702	35 767	7.1	2935	12.2	1606	13.9	945	16.9
37+	485 157	464 117	92.7	21 040	87.6	9933	85.9	4642	83.0
Birth weight for gestational age									
<10th percentile	52 489	48 271	9.6	4218	17.6	2182	18.9	1164	20.8
>10th percentile	471 322	451 566	90.2	19 756	82.3	9357	80.9	4423	79.0
Marital status									
Single	51 697	44 091	8.8	7606	31.7	4000	34.6	2223	39.7
Married/defacto	470 751	454 529	90.8	16 222	67.5	7436	64.3	3302	59.0
Missing	2086	1898	0.4	188	0.8	124	1.1	71	1.3
Maternal mental health–related admission									
Yes	86 956	75 459	15.1	11 497	47.9	6153	53.2	3573	63.8
No	437 578	425 059	84.9	12 519	52.1	5407	46.8	2023	36.2
Maternal substance-related admission									
Yes	41 150	31 278	6.3	9872	41.1	5756	49.8	3597	64.3
No	483 384	469 240	93.7	14 144	58.9	5804	50.2	1999	26.9
Paternal mental health–related admission									
Yes	46 689	41 323	8.3	5366	22.3	2756	23.8	1506	26.9
No	477 845	459 195	91.7	18 650	77.6	8804	76.2	4090	73.1
Paternal substance-related admission									
Yes	43 431	37 212	7.4	6219	25.9	3371	29.2	1932	34.5
No	481 103	463 306	92.6	17 797	74.1	8189	70.8	3664	65.5

TABLE 3 Risk of Maltreatment Allegation and Substantiated Maltreatment Allegation by Disability

Characteristic	Risk of Maltreatment Allegation			Risk of Substantiated Maltreatment Allegation		
	Crude HR (95% CI)	Adjusted HR (Disability Yes Versus No)[a]	Adjusted HR (6-Disability Category)[b]	Crude HR (95% CI)	Adjusted HR (Disability Yes Versus No)[a]	Adjusted HR (6-Disability Category)[b]
Sex						
Male	Ref	Ref	Ref	Ref	Ref	Ref
Female	1.14 (1.12–1.17)	1.19 (1.15–1.22)	1.21 (1.17–1.24)	1.18 (1.14–1.22)	1.28 (1.22–1.33)	1.30 (1.25–1.36)
Aboriginality						
Non-Aboriginal	Ref	Ref	Ref	Ref	Ref	Ref
Aboriginal	6.47 (6.29–6.66)	1.64 (1.57–1.71)	1.64 (1.57–1.70)	7.90 (7.60–8.22)	1.78 (1.68–1.89)	1.78 (1.68–1.88)
Socioeconomic status						
1 (most disadvantaged)	7.04 (6.62–7.49)	2.65 (2.47–2.84)	2.62 (2.44–2.80)	8.83 (8.02–9.73)	2.81 (2.52–3.14)	2.78 (2.48–3.10)
2	3.54 (3.32–3.78)	2.08 (1.94–2.23)	2.07 (1.93–2.22)	4.21 (3.81–4.65)	2.34 (2.09–2.62)	2.32 (2.07–2.59)
3	2.47 (2.31–2.64)	1.70 (1.58–1.83)	1.70 (1.57–1.83)	2.89 (2.60–3.21)	1.88 (1.67–2.12)	1.88 (1.67–2.12)
4	1.72 (1.59–1.85)	1.40 (1.29–1.51)	1.40 (1.30–1.52)	1.90 (1.70–2.13)	1.47 (1.29–1.67)	1.47 (1.30–1.67)
5 (least disadvantaged)	Ref	Ref	Ref	Ref	Ref	Ref
Maternal age						
<20	7.18 (6.90–7.46)	2.02 (1.91–2.15)	2.00 (1.88–2.12)	7.43 (7.02–7.86)	1.80 (1.65–1.96)	1.78 (1.63–1.94)
20–29	2.26 (2.19–2.33)	1.40 (1.35–1.46)	1.39 (1.34–1.45)	2.35 (2.24–2.46)	1.38 (1.30–1.47)	1.36 (1.28–1.45)
≥30	Ref	Ref	Ref	Ref	Ref	Ref
Paternal age						
<20	6.60 (6.23–6.99)	1.18 (1.10–1.27)	1.20 (1.11–1.28)	7.04 (6.48–7.64)	1.20 (1.08–1.33)	1.22 (1.10–1.35)
20–29	2.25 (2.18–2.32)	1.14 (1.10–1.18)	1.14 (1.10–1.18)	2.41 (2.30–2.52)	1.16 (1.10–1.23)	1.16 (1.10–1.23)
≥30	Ref	Ref	Ref	Ref	Ref	Ref
Marital status						
Single	4.48 (4.36–4.60)	1.56 (1.51–1.62)	1.55 (1.49–1.61)	4.97 (4.79–5.17)	1.57 (1.49–1.66)	1.56 (1.48–1.65)
Married/defacto	Ref	Ref	Ref	Ref	Ref	Ref
Estimated gestation						
<37 wk	1.86 (1.79–1.94)	1.25 (1.20–1.31)	1.29 (1.23–1.35)	2.13 (2.02–2.24)	1.33 (1.25–1.42)	1.35 (1.27–1.44)
Birth weight for gestational age						
<10th percentile	1.90 (1.84–1.96)	1.23 (1.18–1.28)	1.23 (1.18–1.28)	2.06 (1.96–2.15)	1.26 (1.19–1.33)	1.25 (1.18–1.33)
Maternal mental health–related admission						
Yes	4.77 (4.65–4.90)	2.32 (2.24–2.39)	2.28 (2.21–2.36)	5.76 (5.57–5.98)	2.47 (2.35–2.59)	2.43 (2.31–2.55)
Maternal substance-related admission						
Yes	8.61 (8.39–8.84)	2.82 (2.72–2.92)	2.78 (2.69–2.89)	11.68 (11.26–12.12)	3.36 (3.19–3.54)	3.33 (3.16–3.50)
Paternal mental health–related admission						
Yes	2.92 (2.83–3.01)	1.68 (1.62–1.74)	1.65 (1.59–1.71)	3.12 (2.99–3.26)	1.69 (1.61–1.78)	1.66 (1.58–1.75)
Paternal substance-related admission						
Yes	3.85 (3.74–3.97)	1.86 (1.79–1.93)	1.85 (1.78–1.91)	4.45 (4.28–4.64)	2.10 (1.99–2.21)	2.09 (1.98–2.20)
Any disability						
Yes	2.64 (2.56–2.72)	1.74 (1.68–1.80)		3.09 (2.97–3.22)	1.89 (1.80–1.98)	
ID						
Yes	3.86 (3.67–4.06)		2.14 (2.00–2.28)	4.51 (4.21–4.83)		2.15 (1.96–2.35)
Down syndrome						
Yes	1.15 (0.80–1.66)		0.69 (0.46–1.02)	1.08 (0.63–1.86)		0.48 (0.25–0.93)

TABLE 3 Continued

Characteristic	Risk of Maltreatment Allegation			Risk of Substantiated Maltreatment Allegation		
	Crude HR (95% CI)	Adjusted HR (Disability Yes Versus No)[a]	Adjusted HR (6-Disability Category)[b]	Crude HR (95% CI)	Adjusted HR (Disability Yes Versus No)[a]	Adjusted HR (6-Disability Category)[b]
Birth defect/cerebral palsy						
Yes	1.12 (1.06–1.18)		0.99 (0.93–1.05)	1.27 (1.19–1.37)		1.10 (1.01–1.20)
Autism						
Yes	1.53 (1.32–1.78)		0.74 (0.63–0.89)	1.65 (1.34–2.03)		0.87 (0.68–1.11)
Conduct disorder						
Yes	5.14 (4.83–5.47)		1.84 (1.70–1.98)	5.57 (5.12–6.06)		1.74 (1.56–1.93)
Mental and behavioral disorder						
Yes	3.69 (3.56–3.82)		1.62 (1.55–1.69)	4.37 (4.17–4.59)		1.74 (1.64–1.85)

Ref, reference category.
[a] Adjusted by sex, Aboriginality, socioeconomic status, maternal age, paternal age, marital status, estimated gestation, birth weight for gestational age, parental mental health–related admissions, parental substance-related admissions and whether they had a disability.
[b] Adjusted by sex, Aboriginality, socioeconomic status, maternal age, paternal age, marital status, estimated gestation, birth weight for gestational age, parental mental health–related admissions, parental substance-related admissions and disability groups.

defects (HR 9.49, 95% CI 2.20–41.06), and cultural-familial (HR 4.13, 95% CI 3.01–5.66).

Comorbidity

Comorbidity was common. Of the 8551 children with ID, 5350 (62.6%) also have at least 1 of the following: birth defect/cerebral palsy, autism, conduct disorder, or a mental/behavioral diagnosis. The presence of comorbid ID significantly increased the likelihood of having a maltreatment allegation for children with birth defect/cerebral palsy, autism, or mental health and behavioral disorders (Table 5). Children with autism but no ID showed a nonsignificant increased risk, probably due to volatility of estimates due to small numbers.

DISCUSSION

Children with disabilities make up 10.4% of the WA population; however, they account for 1 in 4 maltreatment allegations and 1 in 3 substantiated allegations. This disproportionate representation of children with disabilities in maltreatment allegations are consistent with international findings.[9] Importantly, the increased risk of maltreatment allegations was not consistent across all disability types. Overrepresented groups included children with ID, conduct disorder, and mental/behavioral disorders.

Previous studies have included various disability types, but there is no consistent method for defining and grouping disability types, which reduces comparability. Also, different countries may have different thresholds and processes around child maltreatment allegations, which reduces comparability. Nevertheless, comparisons with previous studies shed light on some consistent findings. Unadjusted results show significantly elevated risk of allegations for all disability types except DS, with a more than threefold increased risk of allegations for mental/behavioral disorders, conduct disorder, and ID. After adjusting for risk factors, children with ID, mental/behavioral problems, and conduct disorder continued to have increased risk of allegations and substantiated allegations, consistent with previous research.[4,9,10] Likewise, children with ID continued to have increased risk of allegations, consistent with some but not all previous population studies.[4,9]

In contrast, after adjustment, children with autism, DS, and birth defects/cerebral palsy showed no increased risk for an allegation; however, for substantiated maltreatment, children with birth defects/cerebral palsy had a slightly increased risk, which just reached significance. Our results of no increased risk for autism and DS are consistent with previous research despite different lengths of follow-up.[4,9] However, our finding of no increased risk for spina bifida or cleft lip and/or palate after adjustment was the opposite of previous findings.[15]

Possible explanations for the lower risk for children with DS and autism include that these disabilities are comparatively well recognized, understood, and supported. Parents tended to be older, better off socioeconomically, and for DS, the ready availability of prenatal screening in WA means most parents have had the opportunity for prenatal diagnosis and the choice to continue with the pregnancy.[19]

We cannot specifically address the directionality of maltreatment and disability in our study. However, the stronger relationship between disability types that could be caused by or share a pathway with maltreatment is consistent with studies that found the relationship with maltreatment was stronger (eg, Sullivan and Knutson[9]) or present (eg, Spencer et al[4]) only for disabilities such as conduct disorder,

TABLE 4 Risk of Maltreatment Allegation by Severity of ID

Severity of ID	Number	Multivariate HR[a]
Borderline-mild	2775	2.73 (2.45–3.04)
Mild-moderate	4077	2.01 (1.85–2.17)
Severe	552	1.30 (0.95–1.79)
Unknown	1147	1.57 (1.22–2.03)
No ID	515 983	Ref

Ref, reference category.
[a] Adjusted by sex, Aboriginality, socioeconomic status, maternal age, paternal age, marital status, estimated gestation, birth weight for gestational age, parental mental health–related admissions, and parental substance-related admissions.

TABLE 5 Risk of Maltreatment Allegation by Comorbidity With IDs

Disability Group (With and Without ID)[a]	Number	Multivariate HR[b]
Down syndrome	552	0.77 (0.51–1.17)
Birth defect/cerebral palsy with ID	2606	1.78 (1.54–2.04)
Birth defect/cerebral palsy no ID	27 484	0.96 (0.90–1.02)
Autism with ID	2120	1.21 (1.02–1.45)
Autism no ID	133	1.71 (0.92–3.19)
Conduct with ID	485	1.83 (1.51–2.23)
Conduct no ID	3439	1.92 (1.78–2.08)
Mental disorders with ID	1587	2.13 (1.86–2.43)
Mental disorders no ID	18 226	1.63 (1.55–1.70)

[a] Reference group is children not in that disability group.
[b] Adjusted by sex, Aboriginality, socioeconomic status, maternal age, paternal age, marital status, estimated gestation, birth weight for gestational age, parental mental health–related admissions, and parental substance-related admissions.

mental/behavioral problems, and ID. Together with our examination of the recorded cause of ID, finding increased risk for postnatal injury, prenatal exposure to alcohol, and cultural-familial causes lends further support to this. As an example of potential complexities, the case of maternal alcohol use during pregnancy (causing ID) and continuing after birth may affect parenting a child with complex needs resulting in child protection involvement. This should be examined in future research.

Regardless of causality, the disability types most strongly associated with maltreatment often cooccurred with a constellation of other risk factors, such as parents who are young or who have been hospitalized for mental health or substance use, and living in more disadvantaged neighborhoods. These families already face additional stressors and have fewer resources to access services for their children's special needs.

The inverse relationship between severity of ID and risk

of maltreatment is consistent with other research.[3] It has been suggested that where children's disabilities are more profound, parents may have more realistic expectations, or children may be less able to function in ways that are provocative (eg, talking back). Furthermore, clustering of mild ID within families is relatively common, and linked to socioeconomic disadvantage.[20] In combination with our finding that ID with cultural-familial causes was associated with increased maltreatment, it may be that a number of children with mild ID are more likely to experience maltreatment because they have a higher-risk family profile. It is important that qualitative research investigates further factors that may increase risk and identify support strategies and interventions that may assist families.

The relationship between disability and child maltreatment was partially attenuated after adjusting for demographic and psychosocial risk factors. These findings indicate that disability is an important risk factor for maltreatment, but not all disabled children should be considered at increased risk, and that other risk factors at the child, family, and neighborhood levels also play an important role. From our analyses, socioeconomic disadvantage, teenage parents, maternal mental health, and substance use admissions were strong risk factors for maltreatment. Factors at these different levels need to be considered when assessing the needs of families to ameliorate risks.

Although the use of administrative data allows complete case ascertainment of children with maltreatment allegations from birth onward in WA, it does have limitations. Obviously, maltreatment will be included only if it is reported. Although we have comprehensively ascertained disability from a number of population-level data sources, not all children with disabilities will be identified. Comorbidities also will be underascertained, as the MHIS captures only 1 diagnosis. During the study period, it is expected that there would be changes in the prevalence of diagnoses over time, which would have affected the prevalence of ICD codes. For example, previous research found a rise in the prevalence of autism diagnoses in 1994 with the introduction of the *Diagnostic and Statistical Manual of Mental Disorders, Fourth Edition*, and in 1997 with the formalization of assessment procedures.[21] In addition, a number of important variables could not be obtained using our data, including the child's level of functioning, age of diagnosis, type and amount of support services families are receiving, family functioning, and parents' own disability status. The other issue is

the timing of the onset of disability/condition in relation to maltreatment to provide further evidence of directionality, whether maltreatment may be a cause for some conditions (eg, conduct disorder) or contributes as a risk factor to maltreatment. We also cannot rule out that children with disabilities are likely to have increased service use; therefore, higher scrutiny and increased likelihood to be reported for maltreatment, which should be considered in future research.

The prevalence of disabilities in the child protection population suggests the need for awareness by agencies of the scope of issues faced by children in the system and interagency collaboration to ensure children's complex needs are met. In addition, supports are needed for families of children with disabilities not only to assist in meeting the child's health and developmental needs, but also to support parents in managing the often more complex parenting environment, including dealing with challenging behavior. Research indicates that family-centered care with coordination of services, continuity of care, and respite care are important factors in reducing child protection risk.[22, 23] As signatories to the United Nations Conventions on the Rights of the Child and Rights of Persons with Disabilities, governments have committed to assist parents in the performance of their child-rearing responsibilities, and that persons with disabilities and their family members should receive the necessary assistance to enable families to contribute toward the full and equal enjoyment of the rights of persons with disabilities.

This highlights the important role governments and society have in ensuring that children with disabilities and their families have the appropriate services and support structures in place to enable them to achieve their full potential and ensure their well-being.

ACKNOWLEDGMENTS

The authors acknowledge the partnership of the WA Government Departments of Health, Child Protection, Education, Disability Services, and Corrective Services and the Attorney General who provided support as well as data for this project. This article does not necessarily reflect the views of the government departments involved in this research. We also thank the WA Data Linkage Branch for linking the data.

ABBREVIATIONS

CI: confidence interval
CPFS: Department of Child Protection and Family Support
DS: Down syndrome
HMDS: Hospital Morbidity Data System
HR: hazard ratio
ICD: *International Classification of Diseases*
ID: intellectual disability
IDEA: Intellectual Disability Exploring Answers
MHIS: Mental Health Information System
WA: Western Australia
WARDA: Western Australian Register of Developmental Anomalies

FUNDING: This work was supported by an Australian Research Council Linkage Project Grant (LP100200507) and an Australian Research Council Discovery Grant (DP110100967). Dr O'Donnell is supported by a National Health and Medical Research Council Early Career Fellowship (1012439).

POTENTIAL CONFLICT OF INTEREST: The authors have indicated they have no potential conflicts of interest to disclose.

REFERENCES

1. World Health Organisation. *World Report on Disability*. Geneva, Switzerland: World Health Organisation; 2011

2. Sullivan PM, Knutson JF. The association between child maltreatment and disabilities in a hospital-based epidemiological study. *Child Abuse Negl*. 1998;22(4):271–288

3. Verdugo MA, Bermejo BG, Fuertes J. The maltreatment of intellectually handicapped children and adolescents. *Child Abuse Negl*. 1995;19(2):205–215

4. Spencer N, Devereux E, Wallace A, et al. Disabling conditions and registration for child abuse and neglect: a population-based study. *Pediatrics*. 2005;116(3):609–613

5. Westcott HL, Jones DPH. The abuse of disabled children. *J Child Psychol Psychiatry*. 1999;40(4):497–506

6. O'Donnell M, Nassar N, Leonard H, et al. Characteristics of non-Aboriginal and Aboriginal children and families with substantiated child maltreatment: a population-based study. *Int J Epidemiol*. 2010;39(3):921–928

7. Kendall-Tackett K, Lyon T, Taliaferro G, Little L. Why child maltreatment researchers should include children's disability status in their maltreatment studies. *Child Abuse Negl*. 2005;29(2):147–151

8. Fisher M, Hodapp R, Dykens E. Child abuse among children with disabilities: What we know and what we need to know. *Int Rev Res Ment Retard*. 2008;35:251–289

9. Sullivan PM, Knutson JF. Maltreatment and disabilities: a population-based epidemiological study. *Child Abuse Negl*. 2000;24(10):1257–1273

10. Jaudes PK, Mackey-Bilaver L. Do chronic conditions increase young children's risk of being maltreated? *Child Abuse Negl*. 2008;32(7):671–681

11. Bower C, Baynam G, Rudy E, et al. *Report of the Western Australian Register of Developmental Anomalies 1980–2014*. Perth, Australia: King Edward Memorial Hospital; 2015

12. Petterson B, Leonard H, Bourke J, et al. IDEA (Intellectual Disability Exploring Answers): a population-based database for intellectual disability in Western Australia. *Ann Hum Biol*. 2005;32(2):237–243

13. Bourke J, De Klerk N, Smith T, Leonard H. Population-based prevalence of intellectual disability and autism spectrum disorder in Western Australia: a comparison with previous estimates. *Medicine (Baltimore)*. 2016;95(21):e3737

14. Australian Bureau of Statistics. Children with a disability. *Australian Social Trends, Jun 2012*. Canberra, Australia: Australian Bureau of Statistics; 2012

15. Van Horne BS, Moffitt KB, Canfield MA, et al. Maltreatment of children under age 2 with specific birth defects: a population-based study. *Pediatrics*. 2015;136(6). Available at: www.pediatrics.org/cgi/content/full/136/6/e1504

16. Kelman CW, Bass AJ, Holman CD. Research use of linked health data— a best practice protocol. *Aust N Z J Public Health*. 2002;26(3):251–255

17. Department of Health. Data linkage— making the right connections. 2016. Available at: www.datalinkage-wa. org.au/sites/default/files/Data%20 Linkage%20Branch%20-%20 Linkage%20Quality.pdf. Accessed December 14, 2016

18. Australian Bureau of Statistics. *Socio-Economic Indexes for Areas (SEIFA) - Technical Paper*. Canberra, Australia: Australian Bureau of Statistics; 2008

19. Collins VR, Muggli EE, Riley M, Palma S, Halliday JL. Is Down syndrome a disappearing birth defect? *J Pediatr*. 2008;152(1):20–24, 24.e1

20. Bower C, Leonard H, Petterson B. Intellectual disability in Western Australia. *J Paediatr Child Health*. 2000;36(3):213–215

21. Nassar N, Dixon G, Bourke J, et al. Autism spectrum disorders in young children: effect of changes in diagnostic practices. *Int J Epidemiol*. 2009;38(5):1245–1254

22. O'Brien J, O'Brien J. Planned respite care: hope for families under pressure. *Aust J Soc Issues*. 2001;36(1):51–65

23. Hodgetts S, Nicholas D, Zwaigenbaum L, McConnell D. Parents' and professionals' perceptions of family-centered care for children with autism spectrum disorder across service sectors. *Soc Sci Med*. 2013;96:138–146

Community Poverty and Child Abuse: Sadly a Potentially Lethal Combination

Dr. Lewis First, MD, MS, Editor in Chief, *Pediatrics*

The role of poverty as a contributor to disparities in the health and well being of children and adults has become a major area of concern for all of us dedicated to improving the health of children. While we know that poverty is associated with adverse childhood experiences such as infant and child maltreatment, the magnitude of just how concerning this association can be, in terms of child mortality, has not been well documented until this week, when we release a study that warrants all of our attention. Farrell et al. (10.1542/peds.2016-1616) have compiled a serial cross-sectional analysis of child abuse fatalities in the US in children 0-4 years of age over a 15 year period (1999-2014) using Centers for Disease Control mortality files, and linked this information to data on population and poverty from the US Census. Although the data on both child abuse fatalities and poverty are devastating to read about, when the two are put together, the results become even more tragic. For example, counties with the highest rates of poverty in terms of population density had three times the rate of child abuse fatalities. This information is extremely disheartening. We view this study as a call to arms for us to work to develop strategies to overcome the effect of poverty through strategies that can provide the protective resiliencies needed to these low income communities.

To help us better understand what we can do and provide further insight on the import of this study, we have invited Dr. Robert (Bob) Block, former AAP President and Medical Director of the AAP's Center on Healthy Resilient Children (10.1542/peds.2017-0357) to offer an accompanying commentary. (See page 128 of this collection.) Both this study and commentary remind us of why we do what we do as child health care professionals—and perhaps will be just what it takes to have us advocate even harder for the interventions and resources needed to overcome poverty and in doing so reduce child mortality in this country and around the world.

No Surprise: The Rate of Fatal Child Abuse and Neglect Fatalities Is Related to Poverty

Robert W. Block, MD, FAAP

In this issue of *Pediatrics*, Farrell et al[1] describe research linking poverty with child maltreatment fatalities. The American Academy of Pediatrics has addressed the overall issue of the effects of poverty in a recent policy statement.[2] An increasing number of reports linking ecology with outcomes for both adults and children have been published describing risk factors for overall health, brain health, and lifetime health trajectories.[3,4] Given the sociologic, economic, medical, and myriad other challenges related to poverty, it is not surprising that the authors report a significant increase in fatal child maltreatment related specifically to socioeconomic status. What may be surprising is that although this fact is both intuitive and now statistically proven, given the significant percentage of children living in poverty, the United States has yet to develop a comprehensive plan to address the issue.

Toxic stress, allostatic load, and childhood adversities have all been explored during the last 15 to 20 years, usually concluding that childhood brain development, as well as childhood skill acquisition, social competence, hope, and empathy, are negatively affected by the challenges encountered by families living in poverty. Usually impoverished families live among other families grouped together in impoverished neighborhoods within geographical portions of a larger community. Consequently, the pediatrician in practice cannot address a single family's economic issues without involvement of other programs aimed at reducing poverty in a community. Acknowledging a high rate of poverty, and educating community leaders to work together to address both the economic and child health and development challenges of poverty, could lead to a reduction in frustrations, drug use, family violence, and other negative factors influenced by the toxic stress of poverty.

It is important to note that although poverty is often a reflection of generations of impoverished parents and their children, poverty is sometimes the result of changes in the overall economies of the country, thrusting previously lower to middle-class families into an era of new challenges. Either way, the stresses related to poverty (eg, food insecurity, poor education, unsafe neighborhoods often involving gun violence, access to jobs) can create a frustration level for parents that results in fatal maltreatment of their children. "That's how I was raised," has been heard nationally after high-profile child maltreatment cases reached the press. Finding a way to provide parenting education to folks who are increasingly worried about rent payments, food, finding a job, recovering from addictions, suffering from a low level of education, and other challenges is a daunting task. Developing health plans, including contraception, and addressing the social determinates of health are more than a health system

Department of Pediatrics, University of Oklahoma/Tulsa University School of Community Medicine, Tulsa, Oklahoma

Opinions expressed in these commentaries are those of the author and not necessarily those of the American Academy of Pediatrics or its Committees.

DOI: 10.1542/peds.2017-0357

Accepted for publication Feb 14, 2017

Address correspondence to Robert W. Block, MD, FAAP, Department of Pediatrics, University of Oklahoma/Tulsa University School of Community Medicine, 4502 E. 41st St, Tulsa, OK 74114. E-mail: rblock@aap.net

PEDIATRICS (ISSN Numbers: Print, 0031-4005; Online, 1098-4275).

FINANCIAL DISCLOSURE: The author has indicated he has no financial relationships relevant to this article to disclose.

FUNDING: No external funding.

POTENTIAL CONFLICT OF INTEREST: The author has indicated he has no potential conflicts of interest to disclose.

COMPANION PAPER: A companion to this article can be found online at www.pediatrics.org/cgi/doi/10.1542/peds.2016-1616.

To cite: Block RW. No Surprise: The Rate of Fatal Child Abuse and Neglect Fatalities Is Related to Poverty. *Pediatrics.* 2017;139(5):e20170357

or individual physician responsibility. Unless the United States begins to emphasize the prevention of new poverty, and finds ways to create resiliency among both parents and children, our current situation will not change. Although we may find ways to significantly reduce poverty, the article by Farrell et al[1] is an important reminder of the significant consequences thrust upon an overrepresented portion of our children.

REFERENCES

1. Farrell CA, Fleegler EW, Monuteaux MC, Wilson CR, Christian CW, Lee LK. Community poverty and the risk of child abuse fatalities in the United States. *Pediatrics*. 2017;139(5):e20161616

2. Gitterman BA, Flanagan PJ, Cotton WH, et al; Council on Community Pediatrics. Poverty and child health in the United States. *Pediatrics*. 2016;137(4): e20160339

3. Felitti VJ, Anda RF, Nordenberg D, et al. Relationship of childhood abuse and household dysfunction to many of the leading causes of death in adults. The Adverse Childhood Experiences (ACE) study. *Am J Prev Med*. 1998;14(4): 245–258

4. Block RW. All adults once were children. *J Pediatr Surg*. 2016;51(1):23–27

Community Poverty and Child Abuse Fatalities in the United States

Caitlin A. Farrell, MD,[a,b] Eric W. Fleegler, MD, MPH,[a,b] Michael C. Monuteaux, ScD,[a,b] Celeste R. Wilson, MD,[b,c] Cindy W. Christian, MD,[d,e] Lois K. Lee, MD, MPH[a,b]

BACKGROUND AND OBJECTIVE: Child maltreatment remains a problem in the United States, and individual poverty is a recognized risk factor for abuse. Children in impoverished communities are at risk for negative health outcomes, but the relationship of community poverty to child abuse fatalities is not known. Our objective was to evaluate the association between county poverty concentration and rates of fatal child abuse.

METHODS: This was a retrospective, cross-sectional analysis of child abuse fatalities in US children 0 to 4 years of age from 1999 to 2014 by using the Centers for Disease Control and Prevention Compressed Mortality Files. Population and poverty statistics were obtained from US Census data. National child abuse fatality rates were calculated for each category of community poverty concentration. Multivariate negative binomial regression modeling assessed the relationship between county poverty concentration and child abuse fatalities.

RESULTS: From 1999 to 2014, 11 149 children 0 to 4 years old died of child abuse; 45% (5053) were <1 year old, 56% (6283) were boys, and 58% (6480) were white. The overall rate of fatal child abuse was 3.5 per 100 000 children 0 to 4 years old. In the multivariate model, counties with the highest poverty concentration had >3 times the rate of child abuse fatalities compared with counties with the lowest poverty concentration (adjusted incidence rate ratio, 3.03; 95% confidence interval, 2.4–3.79).

CONCLUSIONS: Higher county poverty concentration is associated with increased rates of child abuse fatalities. This finding should inform public health officials in targeting high-risk areas for interventions and resources.

abstract

Divisions of [a]Emergency Medicine and [c]General Pediatrics, Boston Children's Hospital, Boston, Massachusetts; [b]Department of Pediatrics, Harvard Medical School, Boston, Massachusetts; [d]Division of General Pediatrics, Children's Hospital of Philadelphia, Philadelphia, Pennsylvania; and [e]Department of Pediatrics, Perelman School of Medicine, University of Pennsylvania, Philadelphia, Pennsylvania

Dr Farrell conceptualized and designed the study, completed the statistical analyses, and drafted the initial manuscript; Dr Fleegler contributed to the conceptualization and design of the study and reviewed and revised the manuscript; Dr Monuteaux assisted with the statistical analyses and critically reviewed the manuscript; Drs Wilson and Christian contributed to the design of the study and reviewed and revised the manuscript; Dr Lee contributed to the conceptualization and design of the study, supervised the statistical analyses and initial drafting of the manuscript, and reviewed and revised the manuscript; and all authors approved the final manuscript as submitted and agree to be accountable for all aspects of the work.

This work was presented at the annual meeting of the Eastern Society for Pediatric Research; March 21, 2015; Philadelphia, PA; and at the annual meeting of the Pediatric Academic Societies; April 28, 2015; San Diego, CA.

DOI: 10.1542/peds.2016-1616

Accepted for publication Feb 14, 2017

WHAT'S KNOWN ON THIS SUBJECT: Fatal child abuse remains a substantial problem for young children in this country. Although individual poverty is a well-recognized risk factor for child abuse, the role of community poverty on child abuse fatalities is not well described.

WHAT THIS STUDY ADDS: Using national death certificate data, we noted higher rates of child abuse fatalities in counties with higher concentrations of poverty over 15 years of study. This study can inform public health officials targeting at-risk groups for interventions and resources.

To cite: Farrell CA, Fleegler EW, Monuteaux MC, et al. Community Poverty and Child Abuse Fatalities in the United States. *Pediatrics.* 2017;139(5):e20161616

ARTICLE

Despite widespread reforms in child welfare practices over recent decades, child maltreatment, including physical, sexual, or emotional abuse and neglect, remains a substantial problem in the United States. In 2014, an estimated 702 000 children <18 years old were abused or neglected.[1,2] Fatal cases of abuse, although less common, disproportionally affect the youngest children, with 71% of fatalities occurring in those <3 years old.[1] In their 2016 report to Congress, the Commission to Eliminate Child Abuse and Neglect Fatalities presented recommendations, including targeting resources to high-risk populations and calling for improved collection of data for child abuse fatalities.[3]

Individual poverty is a well-known risk factor for child maltreatment, and the role of community-level poverty on nonfatal child maltreatment is becoming better understood.[4–11] For decades, developmental psychologists have recognized that a child's community and surrounding economic conditions are part of the macrosystem that affect a child's growth and development.[12] In 2016, the American Academy of Pediatrics published a policy statement on poverty and child health in the United States and stated that poverty contributes to many child health disparities, including infant mortality, language development, and injury.[13–15]

Despite the increasing understanding about the role of poverty in child health, including child maltreatment, the relationship between community poverty concentration and fatal child abuse on a national scale is not as well described.[16] As government and child protective agencies strive to target high-risk communities for preventive interventions and resources, understanding community poverty concentration as a risk factor for fatal abuse is

critical.[17] Our objective was to analyze the association between community poverty concentration and child abuse fatality rates, and we hypothesized a positive association between county-level poverty concentration and rates of fatal abuse.

METHODS

Study Design and Data Sources

This is a retrospective, cross-sectional analysis of child abuse fatalities in US children 0 to 4 years old from 1999 to 2014 using mortality data from the Centers for Disease Control and Prevention (CDC) Compressed Mortality Files (CMF), an administrative database maintained by the National Center for Health Statistics (NCHS).[18] The CMF is comprised of death certificate data from 50 states and the District of Columbia. The NCHS calculates mortality statistics for each county. In accordance with World Health Organization regulations, NCHS classifies cause of death according to the *International Classification of Diseases, Tenth Revision* (ICD-10) and reports deaths annually.[18] Population statistics and poverty data, reported as the percent of the population living below the federally defined poverty threshold, were obtained from the US Census Bureau.[19] Because the study included only fatalities, it did not meet the definition of human subjects research and was deemed exempt from institutional review board approval.

Study Measures

The primary study outcome was child abuse fatality rates. A secondary outcome was child abuse fatality rates over time. Deaths due to child abuse were identified within the CMF by external cause of injury codes. The use of the International Classification of Diseases, Ninth Edition (ICD-9), Clinical Modification codes to identify cases of child abuse

in administrative data sets has been previously described.[7,20] Beginning in 1999, the CMF used ICD-10 codes to classify cause of death. The external cause-of-injury mortality matrix, first developed for ICD-9 and modified for ICD-10, reports both mechanism of death and intent (eg, assault/homicide).[21,22] Therefore, fatalities were identified in the CMF by using the ICD-10 codes for assault, consistent with the previous work to identify child abuse (ICD-10 codes X85–X92, X96–Y09, and Y87.1, which correspond to ICD-9 codes E960–E969).[20] To target the population most at risk for fatal abusive injuries and to avoid including victims of peer violence, the study population was limited to children 0 to 4 years old. National and state fatality rates were calculated as deaths per 100 000 children 0 to 4 years old.[19]

Because our study question explores the association between community poverty and child abuse fatalities, the primary predictor variables were county poverty concentration and year. County poverty concentration, defined as percent of the population living below the federally defined poverty threshold, was categorized into discrete subgroups (0%–4.9%, 5%–9.9%, 10%–14.9%, 15%–19.9%, and ≥20%) based on previously published studies.[20,23,24] The federal poverty threshold for a family of 4 was $17 029 in 1999 and was $24 250 in 2014. Fatality rates for each subgroup of counties were calculated as deaths per 100 000 children 0 to 4 years old.

Previous researchers have noted the role of community racial demographics when studying socioeconomic factors and health outcomes. Therefore, racial composition of the county (defined as percent of the county population that is African American) was included a priori in our analysis.[15,25–28] Children of non-white and non–African American races (including Asian or Pacific Islander, American Indian, or

TABLE 1 Demographics of US Children and Child Abuse Fatalities, 1999 to 2014

Demographics	US Population, N (%)	Child Abuse Deaths, N (%)	Child Abuse Fatality Rates (per 100 000)	Child Abuse Fatality IRR	95% CI
Total	317 004 331	11 149 (100)	3.5	—	—
Age, y					
<1	63 638 859 (20)	5053 (45)	7.9	3.3	3.2–3.4
1–4	253 365 472 (80)	6096 (55)	2.4	Reference	—
Sex					
Boy	162 002 938 (51)	6283 (56)	3.9	1.2	1.2–1.3
Girl	155 001 393 (49)	4866 (44)	3.1	Reference	—
Race					
White	242 603 344 (77)	6480 (58)	2.7	Reference	—
African American	52 066 751 (16)	4174 (37)	8.0	3.0	2.9–3.1
Other	22 334 236 (7)	495 (5)	2.2	0.8	0.8–0.9

US population includes total population of each demographic subcategory (ie, age <1 y, girls) during the 1999–2014 study period. Fatality rates are calculated as deaths per 100 000 children 0 to 4 y old. For each demographic subcategory, fatality rates are calculated as deaths per 100 000 children in that category (ie, age <1 y, girls). —, reference populations.

Alaskan Native) comprised only 7% of the population and were included together as "other" races. The CMF began including a variable for Hispanic ethnicity in 1999; however, misclassification for this ethnic group on death certificates has been noted. As a result, this component of race/ethnicity was not included in our analysis.[29,30]

In addition to the county-level primary predictor variables, we calculated child abuse fatality rates across strata of individual demographic variables (age, race, and sex). When reporting demographics, the race of the individual child (not the racial composition of the county) is reported. The CMF does not include the poverty level of the individual child's family, thus, individual socioeconomic status is not included in the descriptive demographic results.

Statistical Analysis

We determined frequencies of child abuse deaths among US children 0 to 4 years old and calculated annual rates of child abuse fatalities by individual demographic variable (age, sex, and race) and by community poverty concentration. We performed a multivariate negative binomial regression with fatality rate as the outcome and county poverty

concentration as the independent variable, controlling for county racial composition and year. In this model, poverty concentration was modeled with indicator variables by using the categorized subgroups described above, with the lowest poverty concentration category set as the referent. Adjusted incidence rate ratios (aIRR) for each subsequent subgroup of poverty concentration were calculated. Because our goal was to study the association of community-level poverty concentration, our multivariate analysis was focused on community-level variables. Collinearity diagnostics were performed among the variables.

As a secondary analysis, we estimated another negative binomial model with year as a piecewise linear function, with knots placed at 2007 and 2009. This model facilitated comparisons of the slope of child abuse fatality rates for the years before (1999–2007), during (2008–2009), and after (2010–2014) the recent economic recession. All analyses were performed by using Stata 13 (Stata Corp, College Station, TX).

RESULTS

From 1999 to 2014, 11 149 children 0 to 4 years old died of abuse. Infants

<12 months old comprise 20% of US children 0 to 4 years old, but represent 45% (5053) of the child abuse deaths (Table 1). African American children 0 to 4 years old, who represent 16% of US children 0 to 4 years old, were disproportionally represented among the fatalities, accounting for 37% (4174) in the child abuse fatality group (Table 1).

The national child abuse fatality rate for the study period was 3.5 deaths per 100 000 children 0 to 4 years old. The fatality rate for children <12 months old was higher at 7.9 deaths per 100 000, compared with the fatality rate for children 1 to 4 years old (2.4/100 000; incidence rate ratio [IRR], 3.3; 95% confidence interval [CI], 3.2–3.4) (Table 1). Boys had a higher fatality rate (3.9/100 000 boys) compared with girls (3.1/100 000 girls; IRR, 1.2; 95% CI, 1.2–1.3). White children had a fatality rate of 2.7 deaths per 100 000 white children. In contrast, for African American children, the child abuse fatality rate was 8.0 deaths per 100 000 African American children (IRR, 3.0; 95% CI, 2.9–3.1).

In counties with the lowest poverty concentration (0%–4.9%), the fatality rate was lowest at 1.3 deaths per 100 000 children. The fatality rate increased with each poverty concentration level. Fatality rates by age, sex, and race of the individual child within each subgroup of community poverty concentration are reported in Table 2. Infants in counties with ≥20% poverty concentration were at highest risk of fatal abuse with a fatality rate of 9.6 deaths per 100 000 infants (Table 2). The fatality rate for African American children in the counties with the lowest poverty concentration (5.1/100 000 African American children 0–4 years old) is higher than the fatality rate for white children in areas of highest poverty concentration (3.2/100 000 white children 0–4 years old).

TABLE 2 Child Abuse Fatality Rates Across Multilevel Variables: Individual Demographic Variables of Age, Sex, and Race and Community Variable of Poverty Concentration, 1999 to 2014

	US Population, N (%)	Child Abuse Deaths N (%)	Child Abuse Fatality Rates (per 100 000)							
			Overall	<1 y	1–4 y	Boys	Girls	White	African American	Other
Total	317 004 331	11 149	3.5	7.9	2.4	3.9	3.1	2.7	8.0	2.2
Poverty concentration[a]										
0%–4.9%	6 866 054 (2)	90 (1)	1.3	4.0	0.7	1.3	1.3	1.1	5.1	0.8
5%–9.9%	74 843 354 (24)	1768 (16)	2.4	5.6	1.6	2.5	2.2	2.0	5.6	1.8
10%–14.9%	110 465 460 (35)	4037 (36)	3.7	8.3	2.5	4.1	3.2	2.9	8.5	2.3
15%–19.9%	88 261 271 (28)	3608 (32)	4.1	9.0	2.8	4.5	3.6	3.0	8.9	1.9
≥20%	36 563 073 (11)	1646 (15)	4.5	9.6	3.2	5.0	4.0	3.2	7.7	4.1

Fatality rates are calculated as deaths per 100 000 children 0 to 4 y old. For each subcategory, fatality rates are calculated as deaths per 100 000 children living in that subcategory (ie, 0%–4.9% poverty concentration).

[a] Percent of the county living below the federal poverty level.

County-level poverty concentration across the United States in 2010 as well as the state cumulative child abuse fatality rates from 1999 to 2014 are displayed in Fig 1. Larger areas of high-poverty concentration are noted throughout the Southeast and Southwest. Higher child abuse fatality rates are generally noted in states with higher poverty concentration (Fig 2).

In the multivariate negative binomial regression model, counties with a higher poverty concentration were associated with increased aIRR for fatal child abuse when compared with counties with the lowest poverty concentration level of 0% to 4.9%. Counties with poverty concentration levels of 5% to 9.9% had an aIRR of 1.80 (95% CI, 1.45–2.23) compared with the lowest poverty category. Counties with >10% poverty concentration had more than twice the incidence rate compared with the lowest poverty category: 10% to 14.9% poverty concentration: aIRR, 2.68 (95% CI, 2.16–3.32); 15% to 19.9% poverty concentration: aIRR, 3.03 (95% CI, 2.44–3.77); and ≥20% poverty concentration: aIRR, 3.03 (95% CI, 2.43–3.79). In this model, counties were noted to have a slight increase in child abuse fatality rate for every percent increase in the African American population (aIRR, 1.01; 95% CI, 1.01–1.01). Diagnostics

did not demonstrate collinearity between the variables.

In our subanalysis excluding children who were victims of assault with a firearm, we had similar results. When compared with counties in the lowest poverty category, we had the following results: county poverty concentration, 5% to 9.9%: aIRR, 1.78 (95% CI, 1.42–2.22); 10% to 14.9% poverty concentration: aIRR, 2.68 (95% CI, 2.14–3.33); 15% to 19.9% poverty concentration: aIRR, 2.95 (95% CI, 2.36–3.68); and ≥20% poverty concentration: aIRR, 2.96 (95% CI, 2.36–3.72).

Annual child abuse fatality rates for each poverty concentration over time are presented in Fig 3, with higher fatality rates noted in counties with higher poverty concentration. Child abuse fatality rates demonstrated a small, but statistically significant decrease over time (aIRR, 0.98; 95% CI, 0.97–0.98). There was no statistically significant difference in the slopes of child abuse fatality rates when comparing the prerecession, recession, and postrecession time periods.

DISCUSSION

This study demonstrates increased rates of child abuse fatalities for young children in communities of higher poverty concentration compared with those living in less

impoverished areas. The greatest difference is observed when comparing counties with a poverty concentration <5% to counties with a >10% poverty concentration, where the incidence rate of child abuse fatalities is >2.5 times higher. There were also racial differences, with higher child abuse fatality rates for African American children compared with white children across all poverty concentrations.

The effects of poverty on children are wide-reaching. Health disparities exist for children in poverty, ranging from increased lead levels, increased revisit rates after tonsillectomy, structural differences in brain development, as well as fatalities from unintentional injuries.[9,31-33] Poor health outcomes, including increased rates of nonfatal child abuse have been reported when comparing areas of high poverty (>20% or >40% of population living in poverty) to areas of low poverty concentration (with substantiated abuse rates 4 times higher in areas of >40% poverty).[28,32]

Although the individual poverty of a child's family has been recognized as a risk factor for abuse[4,34,35] and for hospitalization from abuse,[7,10] the relationship of community poverty on fatal child abuse is less well understood.[14,36,37] Local studies have noted increased rates of child abuse in impoverished communities.[28,38,39]

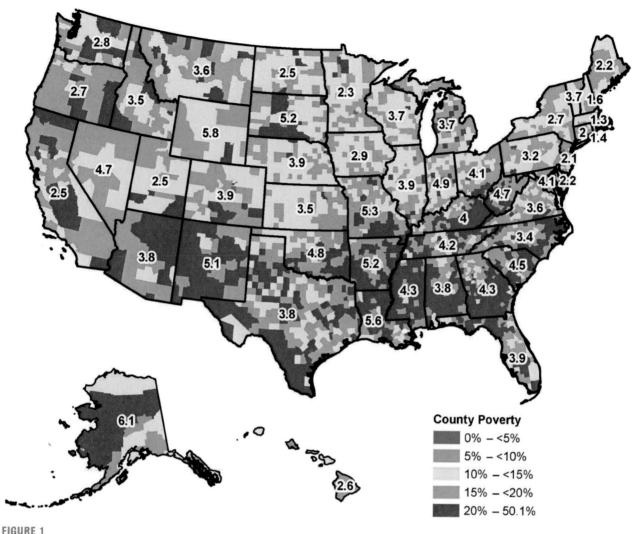

County Poverty
- ■ 0% – <5%
- ■ 5% – <10%
- □ 10% – <15%
- ■ 15% – <20%
- ■ 20% – 50.1%

FIGURE 1

US county poverty concentration (2010) and statewide child abuse fatality rates (1999 to 2014). County poverty concentration is based on 2010 US Census data.[19] The child abuse fatality rate for each state is the cumulative number of child abuse deaths in the state per 100000 children 0 to 4 years old in the population over the study period, 1999 to 2014.

In this study, we analyzed the association between community poverty and fatal child abuse at the national level and demonstrated a consistent association between community poverty concentration and child abuse fatalities across the study period. These results suggest that the economic atmosphere where a child lives may be associated with their risk of suffering a fatal abusive injury.

Theories to explain the relationship between community poverty and child abuse cite lack of community resources, environmental stressors, differential reporting thresholds, and presence of factors related to economic success.[28,39] The greatest difference in fatality rates was seen when comparing areas of low poverty concentration to areas of >10% poverty concentration. This suggests that, for fatal child abuse, there are implications for child health and safety even in the middle poverty categories, where most children in the United States reside. Ideally, this will allow public health officials to target high-risk areas for prevention and resources, rather than rely on post hoc responses to a particular tragedy.

Our results suggest that even in communities of low poverty concentration, African American children have higher rates of child abuse fatalities than white children who live in communities of high poverty concentration. With this data set, we cannot determine if an individual child victim was living in an impoverished neighborhood within a more affluent county. The specific effects of community poverty concentration by race on abuse fatality risk is worthy of additional exploration. Previous studies have reported increased rates of child abuse in minority children,[2,35,40] and African American children have also had higher reported risks for infant mortality, preterm birth, and low birth weight, suggesting increased risk for several poor health outcomes.[41] Although minority children are more likely to be reported to child protection agencies and to have reports substantiated,[42-45] comparison of child abuse to other negative health measures less subject to reporting bias suggests that the increased rates of poor health outcomes of African American children is not simply due to reporting bias.[41] Thus, despite the potential for bias, the difference in child abuse fatality rates for African American children across each poverty concentration in our study warrants attention from health care providers.

This study contributes new findings to previous research by using a national data source to obtain fatality data. The 2011 Government Accountability Office report on child fatalities from maltreatment stated that there are many challenges to obtaining data on child maltreatment

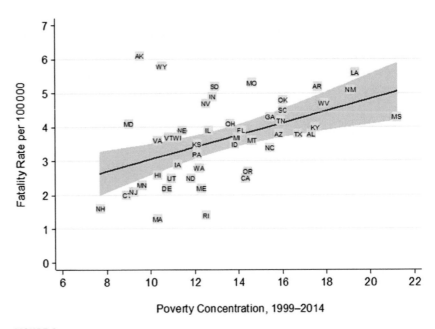

FIGURE 2
Child abuse fatality rates by state and overall state poverty level. Child abuse fatality rate for each state over the study period, 1999 to 2014, graphed over the overall state poverty concentration level (measured as percent living below the federally defined poverty level).

fatalities.[16] To calculate the incidence of child maltreatment, researchers have historically used the National Child Abuse and Neglect Data System (NCANDS) and the National Incidence Study.[32,35,40] Although

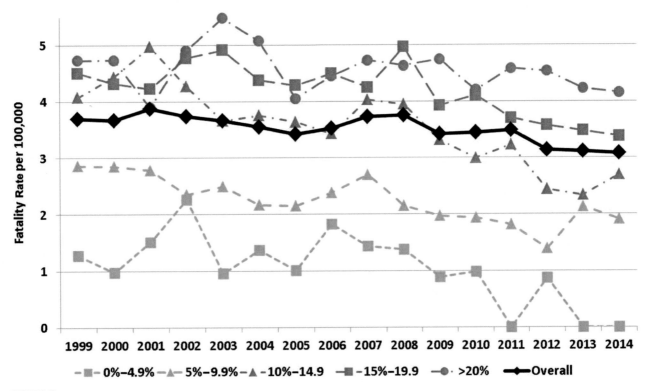

FIGURE 3
Annual child abuse fatality rates by county poverty concentration in the United States, 1999 to 2014. Fatality rates are calculated annually as deaths per 100 000 children 0 to 4 years old. For each subcategory, fatality rates are calculated as deaths per 100 000 children living in that subcategory (ie, 0%–4.9% poverty category).

these are robust data sources, they also carry limitations. NCANDS relies on voluntary reports from child protective services (CPS) in each state and is thus subject to the varying reporting practices of each state's CPS agencies. The National Incidence Study relies on a nationally representative sample of 122 counties. Our study used the CDC CMF, which provides national data from death certificates and, therefore, does not rely on CPS reporting practices or on data extrapolated from representative counties. The 2011 Government Accountability Office report suggests that incorporating data on child maltreatment fatalities from additional sources like death certificates can better inform government agencies. Additionally, our study demonstrates the ability to use ICD-10 cause of death codes to target similar populations previously studied by using ICD-9.[7,32]

These findings should be considered in light of the limitations of the data. The CMF is an administrative database with potential for misclassification, and the data analysis is limited by the included variables. As a result, our study focused only on physical child abuse fatalities, and not on other forms of maltreatment, such as neglect (eg, malnutrition, medical neglect), which are not comprehensively captured with ICD-9 and ICD-10 external cause of injury codes. This may explain differences in the numbers of fatalities reported by other sources, such as NCANDS. Our data are comparable to previous NCANDS results when examining physical abuse fatalities, but not overall fatality rates, which include victims of neglect. Although the Vital Statistics program is a well-maintained reporting system, misclassification of a child's age, sex, race, ethnicity (including Hispanic designation), or cause of death would alter these findings. The use of death certificate data, although a strength of this work, is also a limitation because

it requires the medical examiner to identify the child as a victim of fatal assault. Therefore, the death counts are most likely an underestimate of all child abuse fatalities.

Racial bias has been noted in death certificate review when medical examiners are more likely to record the victim of a homicide as African American than white.[46] It is also possible that the poverty level of the community could influence the medical examiner's determination of cause of death with overreporting of assault in poor counties or underreporting in affluent counties. Researchers have also found census tracts to be more sensitive to economic differences than counties or zip codes.[23,32,38] Counties are larger geographic areas of varying size and heterogeneity in each state, often comprised of smaller communities of varying poverty concentration (ie, a city and its suburbs). As a result, the county poverty concentration is a combination of its communities, which may underestimate the association of community poverty to a health outcome. Additionally, the CMF does not provide information on the individual child victim's economic circumstance. Therefore, any interplay between the socioeconomic status of the individual child and other factors like race and ethnicity cannot be explored with this data set, limiting the analysis for Hispanic children and the interpretation of increased fatality rates seen in African American children in counties of different poverty concentrations. Finally, as an ecological study, we can report an association between community poverty concentration and child abuse fatalities, but we cannot demonstrate causation. Although additional studies are needed to additionally evaluate the complex interplay between poverty and child safety, the findings in this study highlight for pediatricians and community leaders the vulnerabilities faced by children in impoverished communities.

CONCLUSIONS

By analyzing the association of community poverty and child abuse fatality rates from a source of national death data, we found that counties with high poverty concentration were consistently associated with higher child abuse fatality rates across more than a decade of study. As the pediatric and public health communities continue to learn about the undue burden poverty places on children,[47] this work highlights that the poverty found in a child's community is associated with an increased individual risk for fatal child abuse in young children. Community leaders, child advocates, public health officials, and health care professionals must consider community poverty when developing efforts to prevent child abuse deaths.

ACKNOWLEDGMENT

We thank Rebecca Karb, MD, for assistance in acquiring the CDC CMF and the US Census Bureau population data.

ABBREVIATIONS

aIRR: adjusted incidence rate ratio
CDC: Centers for Disease Control and Prevention
CI: confidence interval
CMF: Compressed Mortality Files
CPS: child protective services
ICD-9: *International Classification of Diseases, Ninth Revision*
ICD-10: *International Classification of Diseases, Tenth Revision*
IRR: incidence rate ratio
NCANDS: National Child Abuse and Neglect Data System
NCHS: National Center for Health Statistics

Address correspondence to Caitlin A. Farrell, MD, Division of Emergency Medicine, Boston Children's Hospital, 300 Longwood Ave, Boston, MA 02115. E-mail: caitlin.farrell@childrens.harvard.edu

PEDIATRICS (ISSN Numbers: Print, 0031-4005; Online, 1098-4275).

FINANCIAL DISCLOSURE: The authors have indicated they have no financial relationships relevant to this article to disclose.

FUNDING: No external funding.

POTENTIAL CONFLICT OF INTEREST: Drs Christian and Wilson provide medical legal expert work in child abuse cases; the other authors have indicated they have no potential conflicts of interest to disclose.

COMPANION PAPER: A companion to this article can be found online at www.pediatrics.org/cgi/doi/10.1542/peds.2017-0357.

REFERENCES

1. US Department of Health and Human Services, Administration for Children and Families, Administration for Children and Families, Children's Bureau. Child maltreatment 2014. Available at: www.acf.hhs.gov/cb/resource/child-maltreatment-2014. Accessed October 12, 2016

2. Wildeman C, Emanuel N, Leventhal JM, Putnam-Hornstein E, Waldfogel J, Lee H. The prevalence of confirmed maltreatment among US children, 2004 to 2011. *JAMA Pediatr.* 2014;168(8):706–713

3. Commission to Eliminate Child Abuse and Neglect Fatalities. *Within Our Reach: A National Strategy to Eliminate Child Abuse and Neglect Fatalities.* Washington, DC: Government Printing Office; 2016. Available at: www.acf.hhs.gov/programs/cb/resource/cecanf-final-report. Accessed April 15, 2016

4. Kellogg ND; American Academy of Pediatrics Committee on Child Abuse and Neglect. Evaluation of suspected child physical abuse. *Pediatrics.* 2007;119(6):1232–1241

5. Phaneuf G, Tonmyr L. National incidence study of child abuse and neglect. *CMAJ.* 1998;159(5):446

6. Mersky JP, Berger LM, Reynolds AJ, Gromoske AN. Risk factors for child and adolescent maltreatment: a longitudinal investigation of a cohort of inner-city youth. *Child Maltreat.* 2009;14(1):73–88

7. Leventhal JM, Gaither JR. Incidence of serious injuries due to physical abuse in the United States: 1997 to 2009. *Pediatrics.* 2012;130(5). Available at: www.pediatrics.org/cgi/content/full/130/5/e847

8. O'Campo P, Xue X, Wang MC, Caughy M. Neighborhood risk factors for low birthweight in Baltimore: a multilevel analysis. *Am J Public Health.* 1997;87(7):1113–1118

9. Bhattacharyya N, Shapiro NL. Associations between socioeconomic status and race with complications after tonsillectomy in children. *Otolaryngol Head Neck Surg.* 2014;151(6):1055–1060

10. Lane WG, Dubowitz H, Langenberg P, Dischinger P. Epidemiology of abusive abdominal trauma hospitalizations in United States children. *Child Abuse Negl.* 2012;36(2):142–148

11. Kotch JB, Browne DC, Dufort V, Winsor J. Predicting child maltreatment in the first 4 years of life from characteristics assessed in the neonatal period. *Child Abuse Negl.* 1999;23(4):305–319

12. Gauvain M, Cole M. *Readings on the Development of Children*, 4th ed.. New York, NY: Worth Publishers; 2005

13. American Academy of Pediatrics Council on Community Pediatrics. Poverty and child health in the United States. *Pediatrics.* 2016;137(4):e20160339

14. Eckenrode J, Smith EG, McCarthy ME, Dineen M. Income inequality and child maltreatment in the United States. *Pediatrics.* 2014;133(3):454–461

15. Korbin JE, Coulton CJ, Chard S, Platt-Houston C, Su M. Impoverishment and child maltreatment in African American and European American neighborhoods. *Dev Psychopathol.* 1998;10(2):215–233

16. US Government Accountability Office. Report to the Chairman, Committee on Ways and Means, House of Representatives. Child maltreatment: strengthening national data on child fatalities could aid in prevention. July 2011. Available at: www.gao.gov/new.items/d11599.pdf. Accessed March 27, 2016

17. Cheng TL, Goodman E; Committee on Pediatric Research. Race, ethnicity, and socioeconomic status in research on child health. *Pediatrics.* 2015;135(1). Available at: www.pediatrics.org/cgi/content/full/137/4/e225

18. Hoyert DL, Arias E, Smith BL, Murphy SL, Kochanek KD. Deaths: final data for 1999. *Natl Vital Stat Rep.* 2001;49(8):1–113

19. US Census Bureau. Population estimates, historical data, 1999-2010, 2011-2014. Available at: www.census.gov/popest/data/historical/index.htm. Accessed October 12, 2016

20. Leventhal JM, Martin KD, Gaither JR. Using US data to estimate the incidence of serious physical abuse in children. *Pediatrics.* 2012;129(3):458–464

21. US Department of Health Services. Recommended framework for presenting injury mortality data. *MMWR Recomm Rep.* 1997;46(RR-14):1–30

22. Miniño AM, Anderson RN, Fingerhut LA, Boudreault MA, Warner M. Deaths: injuries, 2002. *Natl Vital Stat Rep.* 2006;54(10):1–124

23. Krieger N, Waterman PD, Chen JT, Soobader M-J, Subramanian SV. Monitoring socioeconomic inequalities in sexually transmitted

infections, tuberculosis, and violence: geocoding and choice of area-based socioeconomic measures—the public health disparities geocoding project (US). *Public Health Rep.* 2003;118(3):240–260

24. Burton DC, Flannery B, Bennett NM, et al; Active Bacterial Core Surveillance/Emerging Infections Program Network. Socioeconomic and racial/ethnic disparities in the incidence of bacteremic pneumonia among US adults. *Am J Public Health.* 2010;100(10):1904–1911

25. Grady SC. Racial disparities in low birthweight and the contribution of residential segregation: a multilevel analysis. *Soc Sci Med.* 2006;63(12):3013–3029

26. Freisthler B, Maguire-Jack K. Understanding the interplay between neighborhood structural factors, social processes, and alcohol outlets on child physical abuse. *Child Maltreat.* 2015;20(4):268–277

27. Garbarino J, Kostelny K. Child maltreatment as a community problem. *Child Abuse Negl.* 1992;16(4):455–464

28. Drake B, Pandey S. Understanding the relationship between neighborhood poverty and specific types of child maltreatment. *Child Abuse Negl.* 1996;20(11):1003–1018

29. Arias E, Schauman WS, Eschbach K, Sorlie PD, Backlund E. The validity of race and Hispanic origin reporting on death certificates in the United States. *Vital Health Stat 2.* 2008;(148): 1–23

30. Rosenberg HM, Maurer JD, Sorlie PD, et al. Quality of death rates by race and Hispanic origin: a summary of current research, 1999. *Vital Heal Stat 2.* 1999;(128):1–13

31. Hair NL, Hanson JL, Wolfe BL, Pollak SD. Association of child poverty, brain development, and academic achievement. *JAMA Pediatr.* 2015;169(9):822–829

32. Krieger N, Chen JT, Waterman PD, Soobader M-J, Subramanian SV, Carson R. Choosing area based socioeconomic measures to monitor social inequalities in low birth weight and childhood lead poisoning: the Public Health Disparities Geocoding Project (US). *J Epidemiol Community Health.* 2003;57(3):186–199

33. Karb RA, Subramanian SV, Fleegler EW. County poverty concentration and disparities in unintentional injury deaths: a fourteen-year analysis of 1.6 million U.S. fatalities. *PLoS One.* 2016;11(5):e0153516

34. Hussey JM, Chang JJ, Kotch JB. Child maltreatment in the United States: prevalence, risk factors, and adolescent health consequences. *Pediatrics.* 2006;118(3):933–942

35. US Department of Health and Human Services, Administration for Children and Families, Office of Planning, Research and Evaluation. Fourth national incidence study of child abuse and neglect (NIS–4): report to congress. Available at: www.acf.hhs. gov/opre/resource/fourth-national-incidence-study-of-child-abuse-and-neglect-nis-4-report-to. Accessed April 7, 2014

36. Huang MI, O'Riordan MA, Fitzenrider E, McDavid L, Cohen AR, Robinson S. Increased incidence of nonaccidental head trauma in infants associated with the economic recession. *J Neurosurg Pediatr.* 2011;8(2):171–176

37. Wood JN, Medina SP, Feudtner C, et al. Local macroeconomic trends and hospital admissions for child abuse, 2000-2009. *Pediatrics.* 2012;130(2). Available at: www.pediatrics.org/cgi/content/full/130/2/e358

38. Weissman AM, Jogerst GJ, Dawson JD. Community characteristics associated with child abuse in Iowa. *Child Abuse Negl.* 2003;27(10):1145–1159

39. Coulton CJ, Crampton DS, Irwin M, Spilsbury JC, Korbin JE. How neighborhoods influence child maltreatment: a review of the literature and alternative pathways. *Child Abuse Negl.* 2007;31(11–12):1117–1142

40. Finkelhor D, Jones L, Shattuck A, Saito K; Crimes Against Children Research Center. Updated trends in child maltreatment, 2012. Available at: https://pdfs.semanticscholar.org/a3cf/5522209a396837089 58514c77d94e3e2468e.pdf.

41. Drake B, Jolley JM, Lanier P, Fluke J, Barth RP, Jonson-Reid M. Racial bias in child protection? A comparison of competing explanations using national data. *Pediatrics.* 2011;127(3):471–478

42. Hampton RL, Newberger EH. Child abuse incidence and reporting by hospitals: significance of severity, class, and race. *Am J Public Health.* 1985;75(1):56–60

43. Font SA, Berger LM, Slack KS. Examining racial disproportionality in child protective services case decisions. *Child Youth Serv Rev.* 2012;34(11):2188–2200

44. Putnam-Hornstein E, Needell B, King B, Johnson-Motoyama M. Racial and ethnic disparities: a population-based examination of risk factors for involvement with child protective services. *Child Abuse Negl.* 2013;37(1):33–46

45. Lane WG, Rubin DM, Monteith R, Christian CW. Racial differences in the evaluation of pediatric fractures for physical abuse. *JAMA.* 2002;288(13):1603–1609

46. Noymer A, Penner AM, Saperstein A. Cause of death affects racial classification on death certificates. *PLoS One.* 2011;6(1):e15812

47. Flores G, Lesley B. Children and U.S. federal policy on health and health care: seen but not heard. *JAMA Pediatr.* 2014;168(12):1155–1163

Injury and Mortality Among Children Identified as at High Risk of Maltreatment

Rhema Vaithianathan, PhD,[a,b] Bénédicte Rouland, PhD,[a,c] Emily Putnam-Hornstein, PhD[d,e]

OBJECTIVES: To determine if children identified by a predictive risk model as at "high risk" of maltreatment are also at elevated risk of injury and mortality in early childhood.

METHODS: We built a model that predicted a child's risk of a substantiated finding of maltreatment by child protective services for children born in New Zealand in 2010. We assigned risk scores to the 2011 birth cohort, and flagged children as "very high risk" if they were in the top 10% of the score distribution for maltreatment. We also set a less conservative threshold for defining "high risk" and examined children in the top 20%. We then compared the incidence of injury and mortality rates between very high-risk and high-risk children and the remainder of the birth cohort.

RESULTS: Children flagged at both 10% and 20% risk thresholds had much higher postneonatal mortality rates than other children (4.8 times and 4.2 times greater, respectively), as well as a greater relative risk of hospitalization (2 times higher and 1.8 times higher, respectively).

CONCLUSIONS: Models that predict risk of maltreatment as defined by child protective services substantiation also identify children who are at heightened risk of injury and mortality outcomes. If deployed at birth, these models could help medical providers identify children in families who would benefit from more intensive supports.

[a]Centre for Social Data Analytics, Auckland University of Technology, Auckland, New Zealand; [b]School of Economics, Singapore Management University, Singapore, Singapore; [c]TrygFonden's Centre for Child Research, Aarhus University, Aarhus, Denmark; [d]Children's Data Network, Suzanne Dworak-Peck School of Social Work, University of Southern California, Los Angeles, California; and [e]California Child Welfare Indicators Project, School of Social Welfare, University of California, Berkeley, Berkeley, California

Prof Vaithianathan acquired the data and participated in its analysis, conceptualized and designed the study, drafted the article, and reviewed and revised the manuscript; Dr Rouland contributed to the design of the study, conducted the data analyses, drafted the initial article, and reviewed and revised the manuscript; and Prof Putnam-Hornstein conceptualized and designed the study, and critically reviewed and revised the manuscript, and all authors approved the final manuscript as submitted.

The results in this article are not official statistics; they have been created for research purposes from the Integrated Data Infrastructure (IDI), managed by Statistics New Zealand (NZ). The opinions, findings, recommendations, and conclusions expressed in this article are those of the authors, not Statistics NZ. Access to the anonymized data used in this study was provided by Statistics NZ in accordance with security and confidentiality provisions of the Statistics Act 1975. Only people authorized by the Statistics Act 1975 are allowed to see data about a particular person, household, business, or organization, and the results in this article have been confidentialized to protect these groups from identification. Careful consideration has been given to the privacy, security, and confidentiality issues associated with using administrative and survey data in the IDI. Further detail can be found in the Privacy impact assessment for the IDI available from www.stats.govt.nz.

WHAT'S KNOWN ON THIS SUBJECT: Administrative information available at birth can be used to effectively risk stratify large populations of children based on the likelihood of future maltreatment. It is unknown whether these children are also at risk for other adverse health and safety outcomes.

WHAT THIS STUDY ADDS: Although a relatively small number of children experience injury hospitalizations and death during the first 3 years of life, these children are concentrated among the highest risk decile of a model built using birth records and predicting child protection involvement.

To cite: Vaithianathan R, Rouland B, Putnam-Hornstein E. Injury and Mortality Among Children Identified as at High Risk of Maltreatment. *Pediatrics.* 2018;141(2):e20172882

The prevalence of child maltreatment in the US population is considerable; by 18 years of age, more than 1 in 3 children have been investigated by child protective services (CPS) (37.4%),[1] and 12.5% of all children have been substantiated as victims of maltreatment.[2] In their research, authors have indicated that beyond any immediate harm caused, child maltreatment is also associated with a range of poor health outcomes, including behavioral risk factors[3] and preventable death.[4,5] Given high disparities in the prevalence of abuse and neglect by socioeconomic status,[1,6] maltreatment may be an important indirect and direct contributor to health disparities over the life course. Support services that engage women early in their pregnancy and successfully prevent conditions that contribute to child abuse and neglect may therefore provide a vehicle for improved health and well-being.

The early identification of children at risk for maltreatment using linked administrative data and predictive risk models (PRMs) has been shown to be both theoretically possible and practically feasible.[7–9] The richness of administrative data coupled with advances in technology mean that computerized PRMs can be deployed to cost-effectively screen entire populations of newborns. In previous research, authors have demonstrated that these models have good predictive accuracy in identifying children at heightened risk of experiencing abuse and neglect.[7,8] Although ethical and practical use cases for PRM are still being developed, newborn screening could be used to improve targeted primary prevention by prioritizing those families with the greatest need of interventions and support.[10,11]

An important question, however, is whether children identified as at risk for maltreatment as defined by CPS involvement, are also at risk for other adverse health and safety outcomes. In particular, if CPS is a proxy for

"surveillance," then it might be that risk of CPS involvement is unrelated or even negatively related to more objective, adverse health outcomes. This has implications for preventive services. If children identified by a PRM for maltreatment are at risk for negative health outcomes beyond simply child protection involvement, these families should be prioritized for a broader swath of higher intensity preventive services, such as home visiting programs. By contrast, if children flagged by a maltreatment model are at no greater risk of other adverse health outcomes, then the justification for offering a broader range of preventive services is reduced.[12,13]

The objective of the current study is to test whether children in an overall birth cohort who are classified as at very high risk (top 10%) or high risk (top 20%) of substantiated maltreatment by CPS, also have a heightened risk of adverse health outcomes. By using a PRM similar to that developed by Wilson et al,[7] we risk-scored all infants born in New Zealand in 2011. We then administratively followed those children until age 3 to determine the prevalence of injury and mortality outcomes for these children relative to other children in the birth cohort.

METHODS

Data

Our study relied on the Integrated Child Dataset, which is a census of all live births in New Zealand between mid-2004 through the end of 2011, and linked to health, welfare benefits, CPS, and criminal justice registers (among others).[14] This extensive data set was developed in 2014 by the Ministry of Social Development (MSD). Birth and death registrations came from the Department of Internal Affairs. The Ministry of Health provided health data from the following: (1) the National Minimum Dataset (NMDS) for hospitalization

records, (2) the Program for the Integration of Mental Health Data, (3) the pharmaceuticals collection for mental health records, (4) the maternity collection for details on the birth weight and maternal age at the time of child's birth, and (5) the mortality collection. Note that because inpatient care for children is universally provided and fully subsidized by the country's public health system, the hospitalizations register offers almost complete coverage of injury-related hospitalizations. MSD incorporated CPS data from the Child, Youth and Family (CYF) register, along with welfare benefits records. Finally, the Department of Corrections provided criminal justice sentencing data. Supplemental Tables 3 and 5 in the Supplemental Information give details on the precise use of these registers in our study.

The 2011 birth cohort was defined as all children identified within 91 days of birth through either: (1) an official registration of that birth on the national register of births, or (2) inclusion in a main public benefit recorded in national welfare data. This methodology was estimated to cover 94% of all live-born children and resulted in linked records for ~60 000 children in each annual birth cohort.[14] Linkages were developed using probabilistic matching methodologies that incorporated identifying information including names and dates of birth of both children and parents. More details on the data linkages (and on the registers) can be found in the MSD's report.[14]

We used the 2 latest birth cohorts available from MSD to define the study population. From all live births in 2010 and 2011, we then excluded children who were involved in Family Start, a home visiting program first introduced in 1998 in New Zealand, as such a program is likely to have effects on mortality outcomes.[15,16] Among children born in 2010 and

2011, 2865 and 2475 children took part in the home visiting program, respectively. After excluding these children, the 2010 and 2011 cohorts consisted of 61 476 and 60 006 children, respectively.

Starting with children born in 2010 (referred to as "the 2010 birth cohort"), we first estimated each child's probability of being substantiated as a victim of maltreatment by age 2. This probability depended on the child's characteristics and family background (referred to as "predictors"). This first step allowed us to generate weights associated with each set of values for the predictors (referred to as "risk scores"). Second, applying the weights generated in the first step, we estimated for each child born in 2011 (referred to as "the 2011 birth cohort") his or her probability of substantiated maltreatment by age 2. We then ranked children according to their maltreatment probability. Lastly, we estimated for children with the highest probability of substantiated maltreatment their mortality and injury rates by age 3.

Maltreatment Risk Score

The first step in our analysis consisted of predicting the probability that a child would have a substantiated allegation of maltreatment by age 2. Our definition of maltreatment included physical and emotional abuse, and neglect. Children who had only sexual abuse as a substantiated finding were excluded from the MSD data because they were too few to report because of Statistics New Zealand confidentiality rules. We estimated a single PRM for the 2010 birth cohort by using logistic regression and including factors at birth, which were earlier shown to be predictive of maltreatment.[7,9,17,18] We included preterm birth (before 37 weeks' gestation), infant's sex (girl), and an indicator for high

parenting demand, ie, more than 3 children in the family (or multiple birth children, or multiple children aged <2). We also included several maternal characteristics measured at the time of the child's birth, such as age (younger than 25 or older than 35), marital status (single), receipt of public income support, history of a mental health or substance abuse, and criminal records in the last 5 years. Additionally, we included maternal and sibling history of childhood maltreatment allegations to CPS. Supplemental Table 3 in the Supplemental Information gives details on the definition of the predictor variables. All predictor variables were entered into the PRM as categorical variables. Supplemental Table 4 in the Supplemental Information lists the coefficients from the PRM of maltreatment at birth, which achieved an area under the receiver operating characteristic curve of 88% (95% confidence interval [CI]: 0.87 to 0.89).

From this logistic model regression that predicted the probability of substantiated maltreatment by age 2, we then assigned a risk score to each child in the 2011 birth cohort. We stratified births to identify those defined as very high risk 10% (also referred to as top 10%) and high risk 20% (also referred to as top 20%). The top 10% comprised 6009 children, whereas the top 20% included 12 096 children.

Outcome Variables

We examined adverse outcomes for children born in 2011 by using information available from MSD. We focused on measures of cause-specific infant mortality and injury hospitalizations using the *International Statistical Classification of Diseases and Related Health Problems, 10th Revision, Australian Modification* (ICD-10-AM). Infant mortality was defined as overall mortality, with stratifications by

inflicted injury deaths, unintentional injury deaths, and sudden unexpected infant death (SUID). We explored both postneonatal mortality (ie, death of an infant aged 29–365 days), and overall infant mortality (ie, death of a live-born infant before 365 days of life).

We also examined injury hospitalizations. We coded long bone fracture injuries by age 2 and intracranial injuries by age 1. Both measures are considered markers of inflicted injuries when observed among toddlers.[19] We additionally risk-scored children falling into other hospitalization groups, including those with any injury hospitalization by age 3, as well as children experiencing maltreatment-related injury hospitalization by age 2, and those with an ambulatory sensitive hospitalization by age 3. Supplemental Table 5 in the Supplemental Information provides details on the definition of the outcome variables we examined based on the code set from the ICD-10-AM.

For both the subgroup of very high-risk children (top 10%) and the subgroup of high-risk children (top 20%), we estimated a log-linear model with robust standard errors for each outcome variable. From the exponentiated coefficients, we computed relative risk ratios for each outcome, defined as ratios of the incidence rates among children in the top 10% (and top 20%) over the equivalent rates for all other children in the cohort. We used Stata MP, version 14 (StataCorp, College Station, TX) for the statistical analyses.

RESULTS

In Table 1, we present the prevalence of each predictor variable for children born in 2010 in the top 10% of the distribution of risk scores and for the whole birth cohort. Relative to the birth cohort overall, children

TABLE 1 Distribution of Predictors of Maltreatment at Birth Among Children Born in 2010 in New Zealand

Predictor Variables (Dummies)[a]	Proportion of All Children who Are in the Top 10% Group (%)	Top 10% Children[b], No. (%)	All Children, No. (%)
Preterm birth (before 37 wk gestation)	17.5	780 (12.6)	4455 (7.2)
Female infant	9.8	2946 (47.7)	29 952 (48.5)
Maternal age <18, y	63.2	666 (10.8)	1053 (1.7)
Maternal age 18–19	35.9	981 (15.9)	2733 (4.4)
Maternal age 20–24	18.5	2037 (33.0)	11 022 (17.9)
Maternal age >35	3.6	495 (8.0)	13 617 (22.1)
Single mother	38.3	5451 (88.2)	14 229 (23.0)
Maternal history of welfare (≥3 of last 5 y)	54.7	4710 (76.3)	8604 (13.9)
Maternal history of a mental health or substance abuse (last 5 y)	42.9	2259 (36.6)	5262 (8.5)
Maternal history of childhood allegations to CPS	53.3	3321 (53.8)	6234 (10.1)
Maternal criminal justice sentence (last 5 y)	67.7	1584 (25.6)	2340 (3.8)
High parenting demand[c]	46.8	1899 (30.7)	4059 (6.6)
Siblings referred to CPS (last y)	96.5	1242 (20.1)	1287 (2.1)
Siblings referred to CPS (last 5 y)	81.7	3900 (63.1)	4773 (7.7)
Total No. children	10	6177	61 746

We applied Statistics New Zealand confidentiality rules to counts, which included the random rounding of all counts to base 3. Data come from the Integrated Child Dataset, a one-off integrated record of all live births between mid-2004 and the end of 2011 in New Zealand, with health, welfare benefits, child protection system, and justice registers. The data set was put together by the MSD.

[a] All variables were measured at the time of birth unless otherwise stated.

[b] Children receiving the top 10% of scores generated by the PRM of maltreatment by age 2.

[c] More than 3 children in the family (or multiple birth children, or multiple children aged <2).

identified by the PRM as at very high risk of substantiated maltreatment (ie, top 10%) were more likely to have a single mother (88.2% vs 23.0%), a mother <20 years of age (26.7% vs 6.1%), and to live in a family with high parenting demand (30.7% vs 6.6%).

Compared with the cohort overall, past or current CPS involvement in the family was more prevalent among children classified by the model as very high risk. More than 1 in 2 children had a mother who had been reported to CPS during childhood (53.8% vs 10.1%). Approximately 1 in 5 children at very high risk of substantiated maltreatment had older siblings who were referred to CPS in the year before the child's birth (20.1% vs 2.1%). The prevalence of mothers receiving welfare was much higher among children at elevated risk of substantiated maltreatment (76.3% vs 13.9%). These mothers also had a higher probability of having served a criminal sentence in the 5 years before the child's birth (25.6% vs 3.8%), and they were more likely to have a mental health record (36.6% vs 8.5%).

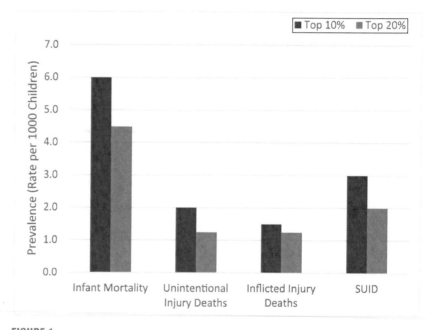

FIGURE 1

Postneonatal (death of an infant aged 29 days to 1 year) mortality outcomes among children born in 2011 in New Zealand and at very high risk (top 10%) and high risk (top 20%) of maltreatment. We applied Statistics New Zealand confidentiality rules to counts, which included the random rounding of all counts to base 3. Data come from the Integrated Child Dataset, a one-off integrated record of all live births between mid-2004 and the end of 2011 in New Zealand, with health, welfare benefits, child protection system, and justice registers. The data set was put together by the MSD in 2014.

Results for children at high risk of substantiated maltreatment (ie, in the top 20% of the distribution of risk scores) are presented in Supplemental Table 6 in the Supplemental Information, and show similar patterns to children in the top 10%.

In Table 2, we summarize the early childhood injury and mortality outcomes for children born in 2011

TABLE 2 Mortality and Injury Outcomes Among Children Born in 2011 in New Zealand and at Very High Risk (Top 10%) of Maltreatment

Outcomes	Incidence No. (Rate per 1000 Children)	Relative Risk Ratio,[a] Coefficient (95% CI)	Proportion of Top 10% Children With the Outcome Among All Children Affected[b] (%)
Mortality			
Postneonatal infant mortality[c]	36 (6.0)	4.8 (3.2 to 7.2)	35.3
Postneonatal inflicted injury deaths[c]	9 (1.5)	9.0 (3.9 to 20.7)	42.9
Postneonatal unintentional injury deaths[c]	12 (2.0)	9.9 (4.2 to 23.3)	57.1
Postneonatal SUID[d]	18 (3.0)	8.5 (4.4 to 16.5)	50.0
Infant mortality[e]	60 (10.0)	2.7 (2.0 to 3.5)	22.2
Inflicted injury deaths[e]	12 (2.0)	7.6 (3.4 to 17.0)	50.0
Unintentional injury deaths[e]	12 (2.0)	8.2 (3.6 to 18.7)	50.0
SUID[f]	18 (3.0)	6.9 (3.7 to 13.1)	46.2
Hospitalizations			
For any injury, by age 3	489 (81.4)	2.0 (1.8 to 2.2)	18.1
For maltreatment-related injury, by age 2	30 (5.0)	9.6 (5.8 to 15.8)	50.0
For intracranial injury, by age 1	Suppressed[g]	Suppressed[g]	Suppressed[g]
For fracture of long bones injury, by age 2	27 (4.5)	2.6 (1.7 to 4.0)	23.1
Ambulatory sensitive hospitalizations, by age 3	921 (153.3)	1.6 (1.5 to 1.7)	15.4
Sample size	—	—	6009

Children receiving the top 10% of scores generated by the PRM of maltreatment by age 2. We applied Statistics New Zealand confidentiality rules to counts, which included the random rounding of all counts to base 3. Data come from the Integrated Child Dataset, a one-off integrated record of all live births between mid-2004 and the end of 2011 in New Zealand, with health, welfare benefits, child protection system, and justice registers. The data set was put together by the MSD in 2014. —, not applicable.

[a] Ratio of the rate (per 1000) of adverse outcomes among top 10% children over the equivalent rate among the rest of children.

[b] Proportion of top 10% children who are affected by the outcome among all children with this outcome.

[c] Death of an infant aged 29 d–1 y.

[d] SUID of an infant aged 29 d–1 y.

[e] Death of a live-born infant before 365 d of life.

[f] SUID of a live-born infant before 365 d of life.

[g] The application of Statistics New Zealand confidentiality rules implies to suppress output if the underlying unrounded count is fewer than 6.

and identified as at very high risk of maltreatment. We first report the number and rates (per 1000) of adverse outcomes for these children, followed by their relative risk ratios. Finally, we calculate the prevalence of children with risk scores in the top 10% who experienced the adverse outcome among all children exposed to that outcome.

All relative mortality risk ratios were higher among children identified by our model at elevated risk of CPS substantiation. Overall, children in the highest 10% were 4.8 times more likely to die in infancy (95% CI: 3.2 to 7.2) compared with other children. The largest relative risk was observed for postneonatal mortality because of unintentional injuries. Children classified by the model as at very

high risk had 9.9 times (95% CI: 4.2 to 23.3) the risk of other children, and accounted for 57.1% of all accidental deaths in the cohort. The relative risk ratio was 9.0 (95% CI: 3.9 to 20.7) for injury deaths overall, and 8.5 (95% CI: 4.4 to 16.5) for SUID. Children in the top 10% of the distribution of risk scores accounted for ~43% and 50% of the deaths in these categories, respectively.

All hospitalization outcomes were also found to be greater among the very high-risk children. Overall, children in the top 10% accounted for 18.1% of all hospitalizations in early childhood for any type of injury, and were 2 times (95% CI: 1.8 to 2.2) more likely to be hospitalized than other children. Not surprisingly, 1 in 2 children hospitalized for a maltreatment-related injury

by age 2 was at very high risk of maltreatment. The corresponding relative risk ratio was 9.6 (95% CI: 5.8 to 15.8) compared with the birth cohort overall. Hospitalization for long bone fractures by age 2 were 2.6 times (95% CI: 1.7 to 4.0) more likely to occur among very high-risk children.

Supplemental Table 7 in the Supplemental Information reports the same results reported in Table 2, but for the larger group of children identified as at high risk of substantiated maltreatment (ie, in the top 20%). Their relative risk ratios of mortality and hospitalization were similar to those of children in the top 10%. Overall, children in the top 20% were 4.2 times (95% CI: 2.9 to 6.2) more likely to die in infancy than other children. They also were 1.8

times more likely to be hospitalized (95% CI: 1.7 to 2.0). Fig 1 compares both groups graphically.

DISCUSSION

Determining the true prevalence of childhood abuse and neglect is inherently difficult because what constitutes maltreatment varies over time and by cultural norms.[20,21] Although administratively recorded substantiations by CPS are a "noisy" and inexact approximation of maltreatment subject to detection bias,[22,23] our findings document that CPS records can be used as the target variable for predictive models designed for use in child maltreatment prevention efforts. A risk model predicting substantiated maltreatment could identify children at heightened risk of a range of significant, adverse health outcomes. In particular, we found strong associations with unintentional and inflicted injury fatalities, as well as a strong association with SUID.[24]

This is not to say that substantiated maltreatment is necessarily the best measure to model in an effort to target children at elevated risk of later adverse health outcomes. Although the authors of a number of recent studies have suggested surveillance bias may be a less powerful dynamic in CPS involvement than previously thought,[12,13,25] the research remains mixed.[23] Rather, with our results, we simply suggest that factors predictive of substantiated maltreatment are highly correlated with factors that predict injury deaths and hospitalization. These factors are less correlated with more general postneonatal mortality or ambulatory sensitive hospitalization. With our findings, we suggest that PRMs trained and built around CPS outcomes appear to target those children at

risk for the most serious forms of maltreatment.

The implications of having an administrative outcome that can be modeled without additional data collection and that is sensitive to the identification of children at highest risk of serious injury and fatality are important. In New Zealand, the home visiting program Family Start is designed and funded to target the 5% highest in-need families.[18] In our cross-match between children enrolled in the home visiting program and those identified by the PRM, we found that only 43% of children who received home visiting fell into the top 10% of risk scores. One possible reason for this is that the home visiting program relied on crude admission criteria (eg, maternal age and poverty status). Another reason could be that the mothers the model identified as at high risk may be less willing to engage with home visiting programs. This is an important area for future research.

Identifying vulnerable children through the use of linked administrative data has considerable advantages, including the ability to look at full population cohorts with the power to detect differences in rare outcomes, such as infant mortality.[26,27] That said, there are a number of limitations that must still be considered. In our study, the data linkages were probabilistic and some errors in matching clients were inevitable. Available data captured only information collected or generated in the process of administering government services, and included few direct measures of children's well-being and parenting behaviors. Furthermore, our analysis was limited to children born in New Zealand and did not account for immigrant children who entered the country. Finally, we examined 1 birth cohort, and looked into outcomes in early childhood. Our findings may not be fully

generalizable to other birth cohorts or to outcomes at older ages.

CONCLUSIONS

The availability of linked administrative records means that it is increasingly possible to use predictive models to stratify large populations and help target services to those children in families where the risk is greatest. The ability to use data to determine the level of services needed would help focus our most intensive and costly intervention efforts toward those families at greatest risk. In the current analysis, we document that although only a small subset of children classified as at high risk of maltreatment experience injury hospitalizations and death, those children who do go on to experience these events are overwhelmingly concentrated among the highest risk deciles. Our findings suggest that by designing effective preventive services and supports for children and families at high risk of substantiated maltreatment, there could be notable reductions in population level rates of injury and mortality.

ABBREVIATIONS

CI: confidence interval
CPS: child protective services
CYF: Child, Youth and Family
ICD-10-AM: *International Statistical Classification of Diseases and Related Health Problems, 10th Revision, Australian Modification*
MSD: Ministry of Social Development
NMDS: National Minimum Dataset
PRM: predictive risk model
SUID: sudden unexpected infant death

DOI: https://doi.org/10.1542/peds.2017-2882

Accepted for publication Nov 15, 2017

Address correspondence to Bénédicte Rouland, PhD, Auckland University of Technology, School of Economics, Private Bag 92006, Auckland 1142, New Zealand. E-mail: benedicte.rouland@aut.ac.nz

PEDIATRICS (ISSN Numbers: Print, 0031-4005; Online, 1098-4275).

Copyright © 2018 by the American Academy of Pediatrics

FINANCIAL DISCLOSURE: The authors have indicated they have no financial relationships relevant to this article to disclose.

FUNDING: No external funding.

POTENTIAL CONFLICT OF INTEREST: The authors have indicated they have no potential conflicts of interest to disclose.

COMPANION PAPER: A companion to this article can be found online at www.pediatrics.org/cgi/doi/10.1542/peds.2017-3469.

REFERENCES

1. Kim H, Wildeman C, Jonson-Reid M, Drake B. Lifetime prevalence of investigating child maltreatment among US children. *Am J Public Health.* 2017;107(2):274–280

2. Wildeman C, Emanuel N, Leventhal JM, Putnam-Hornstein E, Waldfogel J, Lee H. The prevalence of confirmed maltreatment among US children, 2004 to 2011. *JAMA Pediatr.* 2014;168(8):706–713

3. Felitti VJ, Anda RF, Nordenberg D, et al. Relationship of childhood abuse and household dysfunction to many of the leading causes of death in adults. The adverse childhood experiences (ACE) study. *Am J Prev Med.* 1998;14(4):245–258

4. Jonson-Reid M, Chance T, Drake B. Risk of death among children reported for nonfatal maltreatment. *Child Maltreat.* 2007;12(1):86–95

5. Putnam-Hornstein E. Report of maltreatment as a risk factor for injury death: a prospective birth cohort study. *Child Maltreat.* 2011;16(3):163–174

6. Putnam-Hornstein E. Preventable injury deaths: a population-based proxy of child maltreatment risk in California. *Public Health Rep.* 2012;127(2):163–172

7. Wilson ML, Tumen S, Ota R, Simmers AG. Predictive modeling: potential application in prevention services. *Am J Prev Med.* 2015;48(5):509–519

8. Vaithianathan R, Maloney T, Putnam-Hornstein E, Jiang N. Children in the public benefit system at risk of maltreatment: identification via predictive modeling. *Am J Prev Med.* 2013;45(3):354–359

9. Putnam-Hornstein E, Needell B. Predictors of child protective service contact between birth and age five: an examination of California's 2002 birth cohort. *Child Youth Serv Rev.* 2011;33(8):1337–1344

10. De Haan I, Connolly M. Another Pandora's box? Some pros and cons of predictive risk modeling. *Child Youth Serv Rev.* 2014;47:86–91

11. Dare T, Vaithianathan R, De Haan I. Addressing child maltreatment in New Zealand: is poverty reduction enough? *Educ Philos Theory.* 2014;46(9):989–994

12. Chaffin M, Bard D. Impact of intervention surveillance bias on analyses of child welfare report outcomes. *Child Maltreat.* 2006;11(4):301–312

13. Drake B, Jonson-Reid M, Kim H. Surveillance bias in child maltreatment: a tempest in a teapot. *Int J Environ Res Public Health.* 2017;14(9):971–986

14. Ministry of Social Development. *The Feasibility of Using Predictive Risk Modelling to Identify New-Born Children Who Are High Priority for Preventive Services.* Wellington, New Zealand: Ministry of Social Development; 2014

15. Vaithianathan R, Wilson M, Maloney T, Baird S. *The Impact of the Family Start Home Visiting Programme on Outcomes for Mothers and Children: A Quasi-Experimental Study.* Wellington, New Zealand: Ministry of Social Development; 2016

16. Olds DL, Kitzman H, Knudtson MD, Anson E, Smith JA, Cole R. Effect of home visiting by nurses on maternal and child mortality: results of a 2-decade follow-up of a randomized clinical trial. *JAMA Pediatr.* 2014;168(9):800–806

17. Parrish JW, Young MB, Perham-Hester KA, Gessner BD. Identifying risk factors for child maltreatment in Alaska: a population-based approach. *Am J Prev Med.* 2011;40(6):666–673

18. Zhou Y, Hallisey EJ, Freymann GR. Identifying perinatal risk factors for infant maltreatment: an ecological approach. *Int J Health Geogr.* 2006;5:53

19. Schnitzer PG, Slusher PL, Kruse RL, Tarleton MM. Identification of ICD codes suggestive of child maltreatment. *Child Abuse Negl.* 2011;35(1):3–17

20. Munro E, Taylor JS, Bradbury-Jones C. Understanding the causal pathways to child maltreatment: implications for health and social care policy and practice. *Child Abuse Rev.* 2014;23(1):61–74

21. Gilbert R, Fluke J, O'Donnell M, et al. Child maltreatment: variation in trends and policies in six developed countries. *Lancet.* 2012;379(9817):758–772

22. Schlonsky A, Wagner D. The next step: integrating actuarial risk assessment and clinical judgment into an evidence-based practice framework in CPS case management. *Child Youth Serv Rev.* 2005;27(4):409–427

23. Widom CS, Czaja SJ, DuMont KA. Intergenerational transmission of child abuse and neglect: real or detection bias? *Science.* 2015;347(6229):1480–1485

24. Putnam-Hornstein E, Schneiderman JU, Cleves MA, Magruder J, Krous

HF. A prospective study of sudden unexpected infant death after reported maltreatment. *J Pediatr.* 2014;164(1):142–148

25. Olds D, Henderson CR Jr, Kitzman H, Cole R. Effects of prenatal and infancy nurse home visitation on surveillance of child maltreatment. *Pediatrics.* 1995;95(3):365–372

26. Brownell MD, Jutte DP. Administrative data linkage as a tool for child maltreatment research. *Child Abuse Negl.* 2013;37(2–3):120–124

27. Putnam-Hornstein E, Needell B, Rhodes AE. Understanding risk and protective factors for child maltreatment: the value of integrated, population-based data. *Child Abuse Negl.* 2013;37(2–3):116–119